TINY TITAN

A TRUE STORY

BY

ANN YURCEK

Ann Yurcek

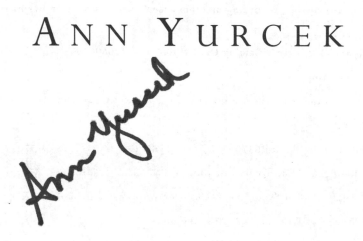

BETTER ENDINGS NEW BEGINNINGS

Better Endings New Beginnings Books

TINY TITAN

Cover & Book Design: Jodee Kulp – Text in Perpetua

Cover Photography (Becca) and Back Cover (Becca/Ann) - Rick Guidotti

Published by:
Better Endings New Beginnings
Minneapolis, MN
763-531-9548 • www.betterendings.org

Library of Congress Catalog Card Number – 2006922946

Yurcek, Ann

A mother's journey to save the lives of two remarkable daughters / Ann Yurcek

ISBN (10-digit): 0-9637072-7-2 ISBN (13-digit): 978-9637072-7-7

1. Rare genetic disorders in children - Noonan's syndrome 2. Adoption
3. Fetal Alcohol Syndrome 4. Children of prenatal alcohol abuse
5. Stories of Triumph – Against the odds

FIRST PRINTING – MAY 2006

06 07 08 09 10 ~ DP/DD ~ 15 14 13 12 11 10 9 8 7 6 5 4 3 2

Printed in United States of America

Dedicated to:

Rebecca Nicole Yurcek

"Adversity is a gift
without it
we would not know
we had been blessed"

— Ann Yurcek

Acknowledgments

For years, I had heard hundreds of time that I had to write our story. People said it was amazing, but the timing was never right. Life, the kids, and crisis always prevented me from beginning. Having to write this book made me return to places I did not want to go. But that was only part of the reason. The real reason was I am 'just' a mom. I was not a professional writer, I was not a doctor, I was not a nurse, nor a psychiatrist, or a therapist, or paraprofessional. I was 'just' a mom who always wanted a large family, and I found one with a crazy and amazing story that needed to be told.

Our story shows that faith, hope, and love, along with a healthy dose of determination allows anything to be possible if God is leading the way and I knew for a long time that *Tiny Titan*, needed to be written. It has taken sixteen years of living and sixteen months to write this. For two years, I struggled with starting and knowing how to write. I almost quit, as I was afraid to tell the story. Then in November 2004, I accepted the Writers' Challenge of 50,000 words for the month of November. That translated to 1,667 words a day. I did a word count on short pieces of earlier writing and decided I could try. A thousand to two thousand words were not really that much. I decided that day; I would finally take a step forward and commit to starting my long procrastinated book. The first day I made my goal, and then I made my second. At times I ran into brick walls where the trauma of a past experience walled me in. But in the process I discovered that writing came easy and the story was cathartic. Our story is real, but the reality is not far from fiction. No one who hears our story can believe it, but it is real and it is waiting to be told so that through our life story others will see the miracles that helped and protected us through the darkest days. Our blessings and adversity changed who we were to who we have become.

This story is far from perfectly written, but to write it differently would remove part of me. I ask the reader to remember that I am 'just' a mom, with a story that needs to be told. I prayed that God would bring me the people to help me along the journey in writing this book. His faithfulness was shown over and over in the many people who made this writing possible. My gratitude goes to the countless people who made this journey possible and it would be impossible to name everyone who helped and touched our family.

▼

A special thank you to my husband Jim, who puts up with all the things that make me, me. To Becca. To all my children for allowing their story to be told in hopes that it helps others understand.

▼

To our parents and extended families for being there, offering support and love when we needed it most.

To the doctors, nurses, therapists, case managers, social workers, teachers, and other professionals our lives have touched.

To the communities we've called home. A special thanks to those people who walked alongside us on our journey.

To Mary, you taught me to believe in myself.

To Pastor Rick and Kim for their support and Spring Lake Park Baptist Church for hundreds and thousands of hours or prayers.

To the Alice's, Zoe, Cheryl, Deb One, Deb Two, Diane, Mary, Maude, Lorraine, and Val for helping our tiny titan be home.

To Colleen, without her I would have given up.

To Manfred, my guardian angel.

To Dr. Prophit, for finding the perfect title for Becca and this book – *Tiny Titan*.

To my friends, thank you for holding me up.

To Jack, who told me I could write this.

To Jodee, for helping me make it happen.

I have no doubt that writing this book is what I have been called to do at this moment. Opportunities for the next step in my life continue to be blocked at the passages.

The book and its writing called me.

I have to do it before I move on.

I am no longer procrastinating.

It's time.

To all who touched our family, thank you.
Your kindness, generosity and support made a difference.

Love,
Ann

Part One

One Small Gift

Part One - One Small Gift

- 1 -
THE BEGINNING

I was 'just' a mom. I was quiet and shy and I most certainly didn't speak to audiences or government officials. I didn't write. I didn't even keep a journal. I didn't have to. I was busy fulfilling my childhood dream of having a large family while being married to a caring husband. I liked being just a mom. With five children ten and under, we were about to have our sixth. Three boys and two girls, and I hoped for another girl to even out the family. I wanted a little girl to spoil and dress up. After five children, I didn't worry about having a healthy baby. Each of the kids was born with some sort of problem, and we learned to cope with them. Little did I know that life as I knew it was about to come crashing down.

The only inkling of the impending struggle was a moment at the grocery store. I was seven months pregnant and waiting at the checkout when I spied a mother with a child about two years of age, both had pale skin. They looked lifeless and like ghosts without a spirit. There was no sense of happiness, and an aura of gloom and doom seemed to hang over their heads. It was obvious the child was very ill. He stared off into oblivion, unaware of what was going on around him. His mother's shoulders sagged and she looked worn. She did not look up as she paid for her groceries with state issued food stamps and she turned as if to conceal the reality of her need for help.

I tried not to look. I felt the embarrassment of her circumstances. A chill ran up my spine, a chill so strong that it left goose bumps on my arms and legs. I wondered how she had lost hope and had given up? I wondered what the future held for the wee boy? As I left the store, the chill remained for a few minutes; I stood stunned by the reaction. I brushed it aside as I hurried home to my children and husband.

▼

I was the oldest of five children in my family and was a quiet and compliant child who felt most comfortable buried in books and learning. I loved reading about large families bonded by love and watching movies of families raising and enjoying children while they survived by mastering the elements. *The Family Nobody Wanted* by Helen Doss in 1954 was my all time childhood favorite. I loved books on history and adversity.

I was different from other kids, I thought of things they knew little about. I befriended the child who had no friends and quietly consoled the child who was bullied. My dolls were always in large families and I loved to plan activities and hold carnivals to raise money for children in need.

It wasn't until the third grade when I found the courage to read aloud for the first time. I had sat silent in the classroom watching the other children.

My mother and father often left me in the care of my grandmother and grandfather. My grandfather rocked me to sleep on his knee, and I remember his warm hugs. He shed happy tears, over the little things. Looking back I am much like him.

During my senior year of high school our family moved to a tiny town in southern Minnesota. My father went to work as a designer and engineer for a company that was founded on his fiberglass designed pick up truck toppers. I started my final year of high school in a class of fifty-six students and I amazingly found a best friend. At a party on New Years Eve I met her older brother and James Yurcek entered my life.

Jim was a freshman at the University of Minnesota and he was everything my parents wouldn't approve of – he had long hair and a knee length coat. I wasn't rebelling, but saw beyond the appearances into a caring person who listened and empowered me. He didn't care what others thought of him; he was confident, bright and caring. The summer he was home from college our friendship blossomed and we spent much of our time together around our jobs as I worked my way through vocational school to be a medical secretary.

Jim and I married in 1977 and at nineteen I went to work to help put him through school. I found a job doing accounting and payroll, and running an office for a mechanical contractor. Jim worked for a fruit wholesaler doing warehouse work. Together we managed to put Jim through school. We had the large family I had always dreamed of. Many thought us crazy to have so many children on a meager salary, but we never went without. The echoes of my stories were now my family.

▾

Our first daughter Kristina was born during Jim's senior year of college and with Kristy in his arms we walked through the college graduation door. Our next son Nathan was born almost two years later. As we rode out the recession of the early 80s, a business degree was almost worthless and a string of long, hard jobs kept us fed. When Ian arrived both of us worked opposite shifts in retail to make sure one of us was always home with our kids. We struggled, and with frugal living we always made do. Our Marissa arrived just as life was getting easier. Jim had finally found himself working in a couple of stable jobs in retail building supplies and we were now homeowners of a two-year-old split-level house in the suburbs. I had begun sewing to supplement our income and Marissa sweetly sat and listened as I worked. Side-by-side we sang and talked. Jim finally worked his way into managing a floor-covering store when Matthew arrived. We had a salary, insurance, and enough money to get by.

Our children were thriving, and our lives were much easier, as easy as it could be with a family of five kids all two years apart. The kids were bright, and with that brightness, it could be a challenge to keep them busy.

▼

One day, our oldest daughter **Kristy** walked in the house and announced that school was for babies. She was playing hooky in kindergarten and had ditched the bus and spent the afternoon reading in the garage. I made a call to the school social worker, and she told me about a lecture on parenting the gifted child that very evening. As I listened to the speaker, I realized Kristy's problem; she was too bright! I thought back to her as a young baby. Her first words came at the same time she cut her first teeth at four months.

At nine months while we were eating Thanksgiving dinner at her grandparent's home, she threw her baby spoon to the floor and demanded "Poons are fo babies. I want a f—k!?"

At age two she was doing addition. One day while taking a bath, Kristy wanted to know about times. I asked her what times. She announced not the clock times, but number times like with the x's. How do you explain multiplication to a two-year-old? I asked her two times two. She announced four. Three time four, and she announced twelve. I quizzed her with the problems up through the fives, and in less than five minutes she had mastered half of the multiplication facts, and she was yet to be three. By three she was dividing numbers and by five Kristy multiplied five digits by five digits in her head. I should have known that this was not normal, but Jim and I both came from families of high intelligence. She challenged my ability to parent, and then Ian followed with his nonstop questions.

▼

Nathan was our quiet one and instead of bugging me he figured everything out in his head. From the time he was a baby he hated going anywhere and from early on, he always got up at thc same time everyday. He woke up at 6:00 A.M., and was ready for the school bus with his backpack and bus button on thirty minutes early. He liked his shirt neatly pressed and he wanted to wear a necktie to kindergarten. He was an organizer and everything had to be just so. As Mr. Neat, he never seemed to have a hair out of place. He kept me close to him and was a Momma's son. He was a truck fanatic and the only childhood trouble he really caused was dumping bags of brown sugar on our shag carpet as sand for his matchbox trucks when he was two. I tried to get the sugar up as it melted in my vacuum cleaner. Carpet cleaners turned it into a harden candy mess. Finally ants enjoying a sugar feast forced us to tear out the carpet a month later. Other than that he was compliant, and thankfully placed between two children with strong wills.

▼

Ian was just the opposite. He was adventurous and made Dennis the Menace look like a saint. He was fast and in perpetual motion. His blond hair was always amuss, reminding us of a little Einstein, and the moment he was dressed his clothes were wrinkled and dirty. We nicknamed him Calvin, (from the cartoon Calvin and Hobbs). He was tiny, scrawny, and I learned to cope with medication and breathing as he struggled with asthma. Nothing stopped Ian from trouble and adventure and his science experiments often called me to the rescue. Ian became known as the 'Little Man of 10 Million Questions' at the ripe old age of four. I spent hours in the reference section library finding answers for his non-stop questions. I learned patience.

▼

Marissa, my little princess invented dances and plays, and made up songs. She is filled with imagination. After two boys, she was all girl. She loved pinks and purples and frills and lace, very much the opposite of her classic older sister Kristy. She was appropriately nicknamed Fluff and was prim and proper. She melted everyone who met her with her little strawberry blond pigtails and round face. She was a patient little girl who could entertain herself with dancing and singing for hours. Her brothers tired of her singing in her car seat, but they couldn't stop the music.

▼

Matthew was an allergic toddler, but was the sturdiest and tallest of my boys. At two was still on formula as he was intolerant to milk, wheat, and corn, but that didn't stop him from growing. We laughed thinking of Matt as he grew up, overtaking the heights of his big brothers. Matt and Marissa were the same size and everyone remarked at our cute twins insulting Marissa who was three years older. Meanwhile Matt loved to find Dad's tools and take apart anything his strong little hands could reach.

▼

Jim had landed a job working with another carpet chain when I had found out that I was pregnant with our sixth child and his new job had more responsibility. He finally had a chance to move up the ladder. We continued paying health insurance premiums to Jim's former employer to cover the costs of this pregnancy. The new job had a pre-existing clause, and the three hundred dollars a month was a struggle. Then the month before the baby's due date we received a letter returning the check for the monthly premium. It informed us that the company was changing plans and they were not continuing our coverage. With the advice of my sister, a nursing home administrator, I made a phone call to the Minnesota State Insurance Commissioner. I found out they had violated the law and should have covered us. With the plan letting us go, we would have to sue the employer with our own money to cover the costs of the new baby and it would take years for us to recoup the costs from the company.

The clerk on the phone told me of another option. We could apply for the State sponsored Medicaid program and for a family of eight, the income ceiling for pregnant women was worth looking into. Jim had just started his new position, and his base salary without commissions was under the Minnesota limit by ten dollars! I felt relieved knowing that our new baby's medical expenses could be covered. With my due date of August 3rd rapidly approaching, I quickly got an appointment at our local social services office.

I was in a foreign world and I realized that these people had so little. I had never been in such a place with struggling families and persons with disabilities. They stared at me, as if I did not belong there. Filling out the twenty-page application was tedious and confusing.

I wondered how these people managed to fill out the form when I struggled with it myself. I was a medical secretary with an emphasis in accounting. I had managed millions of dollars in contracts and payroll for three hundred people, yet I found this paperwork difficult to follow.

The impersonal worker treated me as if I were a number and questioned my being there. I felt unfit and degraded as I walked away, like one of the many still waiting in the hard plastic chairs.

In record time, on August 2nd, my blue Medicaid card arrived. Shortly after midnight, my water broke. We loaded our five children into the car to bring them to my parent's home. Luckily my parents had moved into town a few weeks earlier. They had always lived at least a hundred or more miles away. It was amazing to have them so close just when we needed them most.

Jim was always the one who kept me calm and never seemed to panic about anything. We did not particularly hurry but kept in mind that labor with Nathan was only a little more than five minutes.

Upon arriving at the hospital, labor had just started. In a very short time, less than thirty minutes, the nurses were preparing to deliver our baby. Like with Nathan, my labor progressed quickly. The skilled nurses brought our little one into the world, and she was born in a blur. The doctor hadn't even arrived. Surprisingly, she was still enclosed in the amniotic sac, and the nursing team hurriedly worked to get her out while I tried to get a glimpse of my new baby.

I was not prepared for what I saw. She was not breathing! My baby was blue!

Someone said, "It's a girl!"

She was not like my other five babies, her features looked different. At that moment, I felt the same strange feeling from the day at the grocery store two months earlier when I saw the hopeless woman with the sick little boy. The chill overtook me. Was it a premonition of what was to come?

▼

The nurses turned their backs to me to work on my baby. Then the doctor arrived and grabbed my little one to suction her. I wanted to see her but I couldn't see anything as the atmosphere tensed. I wanted to look at Jim, but I could not draw my eyes away from the professionals fervently working over my newborn. I felt stunned and could barely breathe. It was as if Jim and I weren't even there. We were a silent audience watching a very slow motion movie.

I felt isolated. I began to shake. I still could not see anything. *Oh God, save my baby!*

Then all of a sudden I heard . . .
a tiny . . . very tiny . . . feeble wail.
She was alive!

▼

Seconds later she was rushed from the room.

No one spoke. Jim was now holding my hand; he had barely made it into the delivery room after parking the car.

On August 3, 1989, at 1:57 am,
Rebecca Nicole Yurcek entered the world.

- 2 -

BROKEN HEARTS AND SHATTERED DREAMS

I believe God protects us from things too painful to remember, and when we're ready, he allows some of those memories to surface. I struggle to remember those first days. Much of it is still a blur. Other moments stand out as if they happened yesterday.

After they whisked the baby away, I was exhausted. She had arrived in such a hurry that my adrenaline was pumping and I was covered in goose bumps, freezing and shaking. The trauma of my baby's birth catapulted me into shock. The nurses brought me warm blankets to stop the chill, and a sedative to help me sleep to regain some strength. After I had rested, we made our usual new baby phone calls: one to my parents to let the children know they had a new baby sister and the other to Jim's parents in southern Minnesota to tell them of their newest granddaughter. The rest of our extended family would wait to learn of Rebecca's arrival. It was now well after midnight, and thankfully the hour gave us a reason to not call, besides we had very little to tell about our baby other than her name and her weight. This time the jubilation we experienced announcing the birth of our other five children didn't happen. We held back our fears. We didn't want to worry our parents until we knew more.

Jim kissed me gently and returned home for a few hours of sleep before opening the store. I fell into a medicated slumber and slept late into the morning. When I awoke I asked to see my baby. The doctor told me a nurse would bring the baby to me later. Meanwhile the other mothers held, and smelled, and snuggled their new arrivals. They were busy with bath classes and all those new parent things that happen with new babies. None of it seemed to be happening for me. I stayed in bed staring at the empty rocking chair longing to hold my daughter while time passed slowly. The second hand movement on the clock felt like hours to tick, tock, tick, tock . . .

Finally, the head nurse told me my baby was having problems handling her secretions. The baby was choking and gagging on her own saliva. My Rebecca had arrived in such a hurry that she had inhaled amniotic fluid from the sac that encased her as she passed through the birth canal. She was working on clearing it out of her tiny lungs. As the nurse talked, I remembered she had been stuck in the sack, and they had to open it to get her out. The nurse said they would bring my baby after the doctors made their rounds. The nurse's explanation reassured me and eased my fear and doubt. For me, it's always better to have some information, than none at all.

As promised, shortly before noon a nurse wheeled the baby into my room. My six pound, ten ounce Rebecca was sleeping quietly, and without disturbing her, the nurse gently removed her from her Isolette and handed her to me for the first time.

I examined her from head to toe. Everything seemed intact. But studying her further, I saw she was darker than my other children. Her hair was dark brown while all my other babies were born with very little or blonde hair. Her skin was sallow compared to the skin of my other pink and fair babies. I tried to excuse it by comparing it to my darker coloring. But my instinct in these first brief seconds told me that there was something causing tiny Rebecca, to be strangely different.

Unlike my other children, her ears were low set and she had an unusual thick neck fold. I tried to convince myself that all new babies have some type of misshapen features. I remembered back ten years ago when Kristy was born with a funny cone-shaped head. Today her head was fine. She was also born with a severely misshapen foot and within hours after her birth, she had her foot molded into place and cast in plaster. The doctors told us that Kristy had a clubfoot. In time it would not be a problem. The tiny casts were changed weekly and then replaced by foot braces. By the time she was walking, she only needed her foot braces at night. By age three she was out of her braces and her foot corrected. At ten, the only sign of Kristy's disabled foot was the flipping in of her right foot when she ran and she ran with speed and grace, intuitively compensating her strides to keep from tripping herself.

Tiny Rebecca's cough startled me out of my daydream. The nurse warned me she choked easily, and before she left us alone, she showed me how to use the little blue plastic bulb syringe to clear her airway. She reminded me to use the call button on the side of the bed if I needed anything. Then before my eyes Rebecca progressed rapidly from coughing to struggling to breathe. I held her upright and patted her behind the shoulder blades. As she struggled to move air, I tried to suction the mucous from the back of her throat using the bulb syringe with no success. Rebecca turned blue. *Oh Lord, help Becca. Help my baby.* I prayed for a miracle while I struggled to control my panic and hit the call button at the side of the bed. The nurse came quickly and whisked my baby girl away.

The day continued in slow motion. I didn't venture out of my room. I dozed off in a sedated fog, remembering I hadn't had medication with my other babies. I wondered why they were giving pills to me now. This delivery of my sixth child had been so easy.

My parents arrived for visiting hours and joined Jim and me to see the most recent arrival. We peered in the nursery window to see little Rebecca. She wasn't with the other babies in the row of bassinets near the window. She was now in a covered Isolette along the back wall of the nursery. I knew that the plastic, temperature-controlled enclosures are reserved for very sick or fragile babies. As we watched her, we noticed that she was choking. Becca was turning blue. Jim and I feverishly knocked on the window to alert the nurses that something was drastically wrong with our baby. A nurse grabbed the phone and moved the Isolette behind an alcove, out of sight of the visitors. All around us, parents, grandparents, and visitors smiled and marveled at their new arrivals. Looking into my mother's face, I saw the horrified look of what she had just witnessed. She knew, and I knew that something was very, very wrong with our baby.

After the nursery incident, it took several hours before another nurse came to my room to tell us that Becca was still having trouble breathing, and she was in the covered Isolette to keep her oxygen and temperature constant. They had moved her to where the nurses could monitor her more closely. The nurse's words were encouraging as she explained that it takes time for baby lungs to clear from the aspiration. We busied ourselves with small talk, and making plans for the kids' day ahead. After an hour, Jim and my parents left to be with our other five children. Exhausted, I fell asleep, but dreams caused me to toss and turn through the night.

I awoke at 6:30 A.M. to a young, gentle pediatrician at my bedside that told me what I already knew, something was wrong with my baby. Her features were suggestive of a particular type of syndrome and they were calling in a neurologist to examine her. He told me she had hypotonia, which meant floppiness. I had noticed when I had held her bundled in my arms she seemed floppy. He told me that she had anti-mongoloid shaped eyes. In other words, she had an abnormal eye slant opposite from the slant associated with Down's syndrome. Her ears were very low and tipped back, seemingly out of place. She still had a thickened fold of skin on the back that hid her neck. She was swollen. Each of these things indicated that something was wrong with my baby. They were called anomalies. His most current concern was her inability to swallow and her readiness to stop breathing. He was worried about Becca's condition.

Just as the doctor left, the nurse practitioner from the obstetrics group entered the room. She reviewed everything the doctor said. Even today I can't remember much of what she told me.

I began shaking and sobbing and overcome with obnoxious grief. I had been raised to believe that bad things don't happen to good people. I didn't deserve this. I had been a good person and done good things. I asked her repeatedly why and how this had happened. What did I do that made God so angry with me that he allowed this to happen to my baby?

The nurse was warm and patient as she shared that God was not angry with me, life just happens. She said if I focused on the whys, I'd never get the answers. There weren't any answers and it would cause me to become angry and bitter right at the time when my baby and my family needed me the most. She stressed that there was nothing I did or didn't do to cause my tiny baby to be born with so many challenges. I cried until there were no tears left and for nearly an hour she held me. The hospital chaplain was summoned and he said a prayer for Becca and for my entire family. The prayers calmed my quivering heart.

Looking back, I call the pediatrician, the nurse practitioner, and the chaplain the Doomsday Squad. They had the sad task of offering explanations and comforting parents whose dreams were shattered. I wondered how many times in their jobs they had shared similar life-changing news with new parents. They knew their jobs well, and their thoughtful words and actions helped me continue on the journey that lay ahead. As soon as I could talk without breaking down, I called Jim and asked him to come to the hospital. He needed to get the news about Becca first hand because I could not say the words.

My obstetrician cleared me for discharge and I was given the choice to leave the hospital or stay another day. Becca had been moved to a special nursery for babies needing close observation. I felt scared, and lonely, and sad. There were no flowers for me and no baby to hold, not even my own children could see their new baby sister. Sitting in the hospital in an empty room would be unbearable. I needed to be with Jim and my other children. I needed my family.

I didn't want to watch the mothers strolling the halls to go get their babies. I didn't want to watch their families and close friends arrive with balloons and flowers. I couldn't stand staying for another moment. The phone next to my bed had remained silent. There were no visitors or moments of celebration.

Just time, unending time filled with worry and sadness.

As I packed my suitcase to go home, I found Becca's new sleepers. It was my original plan to bring my baby home from the hospital in one of them. There was blue for a boy and pink for a girl. I would return the blue sleeper. As I picked up the little pink rosebud sleeper with ruffles, my tears stained the soft pastel fabric. Wiping my tears away with the back of my hand, I took the sleeper and blanket, and buried them at the bottom of my suitcase. I hastily finished packing for home, and then when Jim arrived, sat in the wheelchair for the sad exit. I love rocking my new babies and the empty rocking chair in the corner of my hospital room remained unused.

As the chair wheeled over the hospital's highly polished floors, the lump in my throat hurt, my eyes burned with hot tears. I left the hospital with empty arms. I had not even been allowed to say goodbye to Becca because she was down having tests and had been placed in the special care nursery. They didn't make arrangements for me to visit her. They didn't know how to deal with 'just' a mom with a special care infant. They left me alone and I had seen her only five minutes in the whole time I was in the hospital.

Jim and I spoke very little on the trip home and we were both deep in thought. The music on the car radio buffered the silence between us. We both wondered what the future held. He wondered how we'd pay the massive medical bills we'd have for Becca. I wondered what I was going to tell the kids. How do you explain you don't have the baby? How do you answer questions when you have no answers yourself?

I was happy to see my children when we got to Mom's. Grandma had already told Kristy and Nathan that something was wrong with their new baby sister. At ten, Kristy was wise beyond her years and had figured it out. Eight-year-old Nathan knew that sick babies stayed in the hospital. At six and four and two, Ian and Marissa and Matt were still too young to understand.

Once we were settled, Jim returned to work. I filled my day with children and laughter. I needed a respite from the sorrow and worry of the past forty-eight hours. Helping Mom with the kids and my brother's one-year-old daughter Kaitie kept my mind from the thoughts that plagued me. What was wrong with my baby? This question replaced all the whys and what ifs? I spent the night at my parent's home before making my first trip to the hospital to see my baby. A neurologist had been summoned to examine her, and I was to meet him at ten in the morning. Jim and I spoke little of the appointment. Mom didn't bring the subject up. I understood their silence. They didn't know what to say, but the silence was deafening. I was alone with the racing thoughts in my brain.

Since Jim had to work, Mom came with me to the hospital. When we got there, we were escorted to the special care nursery to be with our baby. She looked different than I remembered her. She was less puffy, and her color had changed. Mom and I both noticed the blue veins prominent under the surface of her skin on her head and forehead. I held my daughter and felt her tiny heart pounding under the blankets. She was here. She was real. Becca was alive.

The neurologist took my frail daughter and undressed her to check her from top to bottom. He looked carefully at her little fingers, palms, feet and toes. He turned her over and studied the back of her neck. He was callous and matter of fact. Her little head flopped from side-to-side. He tapped her here and there. He was poking and prodding and tossing her around like a rag doll. He picked her up and dangled her upside down in the air. She flopped and then turned blue. I had noticed her floppiness, so had Dr. Wineinger. As he held her there in front of me, it struck me how much more she flopped than any of my other newborns. Then the doctor laid her on her back and she turned blue again.

Throughout the ordeal Becca remained silent.

When the examination was complete, the doctor sat down with us to share his findings. He used the word hypotonic to explain the baby's floppiness. He told us that her features suggested some sort of syndrome and babies like her often have other problems that would surface later. Only time would tell and we could expect more things to surface.

He seemed to be saying the same things I had heard before.

I was upset over his roughness with my new little one. New babies deserve to be treated with swaddling and tender care. After all, she was a very sick baby. Why had my naked baby remained silent? My other babies liked the security of being clothed and tightly wrapped in their blankets. They protested loudly when they were undressed. Becca's strange bare silence bothered me.

After the exam, a nurse carried in a rocking chair, and for the first time, I got to rock Becca. I buried my head in her soft skin and felt her newness. I smelled the baby scent I longed for. I didn't want anyone to see me crying as I tried to focus on the new person in my arms. The tears were welling up again.

The visit was short and again I had to leave my daughter with a goodbye kiss to return home to care for the kids before Jim left for work. Mom and I talked little on the way home. We did not know what to say.

We quietly made lunch while Kristy begged to see her new sister. I promised her she could go and we tried, but we never arrived. About a mile from the hospital our old car died in the middle of an intersection. Fortunately, on the corner opposite the light was a convenience store.

I quickly put ten-year-old Kristy into the driver's seat. When the light turned in my favor, I started pushing the car through the intersection. I am not that big and had just delivered a baby. I knew I shouldn't be pushing a car, but I had no choice because my car was blocking traffic. Fiery hot tears rolled down my cheeks as I pushed the stupid car. My body trembled. The more I pushed the angrier I became. My car was broken. My baby was not right. My entire life had fallen apart in less than seventy-two hours. Poor Kristy waited patiently and silently through my moment of agony and fury.

Then as I turned to my left, two young men saw my dilemma and jumped out of their car to help me. They told me to jump in and steer as they pushed the car quickly into a parking place. As I reached into my purse to give the Samaritans a reward, they disappeared.

After I had a chance to compose myself, Kristy and I entered the little store to get change for my five-dollar bill to call my dad to rescue me. After calling my dad, Kristy and I grabbed a soda and candy bar to pass the time. Dad was a college industrial arts professor and was well versed in car repairs. He took one quick look and realized that the timing belt had broken. Dropping Kristy and me off at home, my brother Dan volunteered to help fix the car and my son, Nathan, tagged along. The guys managed to get the car running, and thankfully back on the road a couple of hours later.

It had been a very long day, beginning with the disturbing meeting with the neurologist and ending with the car fiasco. Pushing the car left me sore, tired, and exhausted. I wanted my own bed and my family needed time alone. It was time to go home, so Jim and I packed up the five kids. Four kids hugged Grandma and Grandpa while Ian snuck back into the kitchen to load his pockets with Grandma's famous gluten free chocolate chip cookies.

It felt good to tuck my children into their own beds. Then I retreated to my bedroom, taking a few minutes to catch my breath. I rolled on my side only to see Becca's empty crib with the dusty blue ruffled quilt and crib bumper on the other side of my room. Jim and I had planned to keep the baby in our room like we had all of our children when they were tiny. Now the crib was a painful reminder that our daughter was not with us. I took a blanket from our bed and crawled onto the sofa in the living room. I was too tired to deal with facing the pain of an empty crib.

Sunday morning arrived, and we got the kids up and ready for the day. Jim and I wanted to take them to visit our baby at the hospital. They wanted to see their sister. While I was doing Marissa's hair, Matt disappeared. I called to my toddler and he came from our bedroom looking like he had been playing with something he shouldn't have. He had been up to something, but I let his two-year-old mischief go this one time. We needed to get moving if we were to get to the hospital before Jim had to go to work for the afternoon.

While Jim and I were finding the kids shoes and placing them on the correct feet we heard a knock at the door. I was shocked to find a police officer standing there when I opened the door.

He asked if I was Ann Yurcek and my heart sank.

I thought, what's the matter?

He wasted no time delivering his urgent message from the hospital. He was dispatched because the hospital had been trying to call and our phone was off the hook. Now, I knew precisely what Matt had been up to while I was brushing Marissa's hair. He was playing with the phone again. Last week he had read the sticker on the phone and matched the numbers to the buttons to reach the 9ll operator. I thanked the officer and I sprinted upstairs, my feet barely hitting the steps as I ran to grab the disconnected phone.

My hands shook as I fumbled to dial the number the officer had handed me. After three tries to place the call correctly, I was connected to the hospital nursery and identified myself. Hearing the panic in my voice, the first words out of the nurses' mouth were, "She is alive!"

I took a deep breath so I could track the second half of the message. Our baby was being transferred to a children's hospital. She needed to be in the Newborn Intensive Care Unit (NICU) where she could be cared for by a team of neonatal specialists experienced in working with sick babies. Becca was showing signs of heart problems and was getting sicker by the hour. The doctors had discovered a heart murmur. Her heart was unstable and racing. She was increasingly more jaundiced, she was having more trouble breathing and she needed to be transferred immediately. They didn't have time to wait for our permission. They didn't want us to arrive and discover that our baby wasn't there. If it had been a few minutes later, they wouldn't have caught us at home. The nurse gave me a number to call to make a hospital appointment to fill out the paperwork on the coming day.

The officer was gone when I returned to Jim and the kids. They looked up expectantly for whatever news I had.

My news of Becca's tiny troubled heart broke seven other hearts. We spent the rest of the morning trying to be busy. Jim needed to go to work and I didn't want to be alone. So we packed up our tribe and returned to my parents. The kids and I played, and Mom and I visited to fill the long hours of the day, yet whenever I tried to talk about what was going on, the subject was changed, leaving me alone in my head.

Was our baby going to be all right?

Was she going to survive?

How were we going to pay for all this?

Too many questions, maybe Mom was right to not talk about it. I tried to silence my brain and pretend that everything was going to be just fine. I tried desperately to convince myself, but it wouldn't work. My mind was spinning and my heart was breaking.

- 3 -
NICU

On Monday, Becca was now four days old and she was still alive. Both of us needed our mothers. I needed my Mom, as I felt inadequate and alone so Mom joined me on my very first trip to The Children's Hospital. I was nervous trying to navigate my way from the familiarity of the northern suburbs to downtown St. Paul. I knew the network of the freeway systems, but getting off the familiar route to find the hospital scared me. I tried pepping myself up. At least she had been transferred to St. Paul instead of Minneapolis. Jim and I lived there when we were newlyweds. Having Mom with me gave me added courage. We left the kids with my sister, Gretchen, and brother, Tim, who were home from college while we went to the hospital.

Thankfully I had stopped at the bank for money on the way, because the hospital parking cost five dollars a day and they only took cash. The hospital was a huge brick building and it felt ominous and cold to me. As we walked through the front door, Mom and I spied a small pink puppy in the front window of the hospital gift shop. The puppy reminded us of my childhood stuffed toy. My little pink puppy had comforted me through bad dreams and hospitalizations. I had loved all its fur away, and my first puppy was retired at the age of eight. Pink Puppy II was discovered when I was shopping with my Grandmother and Aunt for new shoes for my sister Martha. Mom didn't know, but my little pink puppies still lived in the bottom of my dresser drawer tucked away as a childhood treasure. Without saying a word, Mom purchased the little stuffed puppy for Becca.

The smiling lady at the information desk directed us to the neonatal intensive care unit up on the second floor with a metal door and a tiny doorbell. Little did I know that this was about to become my new home away from home? With the buzzing of the button, we were greeted by a young nurse dressed in regulation blue-grey scrubs. She explained we could come in, but we had to wash and gown to protect the vulnerable babies from infection. It felt strange to scrub with Mom and put on the yellow hospital gown to prepare to see Becca. I was scared and worried.

No one can be ready to see an NICU, much less a mother. Dozens of incubators held teeny tiny babies. IV bags hung from the metal poles connected to little bodies. There were wires and clear plastic tubing everywhere. Bright lights glared and electronic monitors and panels lit up and buzzed and beeped as Mom and I entered. Nurses scurried to help a one pound preemie turning blue, another nurse hastened to help a baby with a misshapen face. Everyone was in such a hurry. There was no welcome package. There was no one to advise us of our role in caring for our sick baby. I stood in this foreign land of tubes and bags and machines wondering how it all worked and what was about to happen next. Where was my Becca?

I was relieved when a nurse guided us to Becca's bedside. Becca looked huge at six pounds, ten ounces compared to the tiny preterm babies that filled the unit.

I noticed a crib in the far corner decorated with toys and a mobile, an infant seat and rocking chair sat nearby. The baby boy seemed many months old, it appeared the nursery had been his home for a very long time. I prayed this wasn't Becca's destiny.

Becca, dressed only in a diaper was lying on a warmer with bright phototherapy lights to help clear the jaundice from her system. The lights were familiar to me, and I took a bit of refuge from them. Matt needed a light system in our living room for a few days to help clear his jaundice when he was a newborn. He was now a big and healthy toddler. Becca was on oxygen to give her a 'little' boost to help her breathe. I hung mentally on to the word 'little.' On her head was a small bathroom paper cup anchored with paper tape to protect the IV port placed in her head to provide her fluids and medicine. I stroked the little pink puppy as the nurse explained Becca's heart problems. My body felt as though my feet had been riveted into the floor. I bit my lower lip, trying to remain calm. I hugged the puppy realizing the heart test results were not in yet.

A young woman with the warmest smile and most sincere eyes I had ever seen stood across from me at Becca's bedside. Her name was Mary. She was a NICU social worker. I had no clue that she would become my hospital best friend who would give me the strength I needed through the months ahead. She offered to answer any of my questions, but I did not know what to ask because this place and my very sick daughter overwhelmed me. I asked if I could give Becca the pink puppy. She said it was fine for her to have a few precious reminders of family and home. She understood that the parents needed to do little special 'somethings' for their babies, especially when they had such little control over anything else. As I placed the puppy with long pink ears next to my baby girl I bent down and gave her a kiss.

Mary helped me fill out the admission paperwork since we had made verbal arrangements for treatment with the hospital until we arrived. After signing the consents for treatment, I said goodbye to my Becca while I tried to fight back the tears.

I was grateful for Mom's company on this first visit to Children's Hospital and I thanked her for buying the pink puppy for Becca. On the way home we talked about my own little pink dog that had accompanied me on my many trips to the hospital when croup kept me struggling to breathe. For the rest of the trip home Mom and I made small talk. I knew that the thirty-mile drive home alone would have been insufferable without her support. Mom kept my thoughts from wandering so I could focus on the road.

I realized today's journey was only the beginning.

The next day greeted me with a phone call from the nurses, saying that they had discovered something wrong with Becca's blood counts. They needed to get a sample of my blood to compare with hers and they ordered me to come down immediately to have my blood drawn. I called Mom feeling that I was imposing again by asking her to care for my kids. I was saddling her with my five and she already had my niece Kaitie. I had no choice; school didn't start until the first week of September.

Hurriedly, I dropped the kids off and raced to the hospital. Once there, I checked in at the front desk asking for directions, but no one knew anything about getting a lab test done for a parent of a sick baby. Nobody knew which hospital or which lab would do the testing. The hospital is a maze of interconnected medical buildings covering two city blocks. There are pedestrian bridges and tunnels that link buildings on opposite sides of the street—a confusion of wards, corridors, and halls. They sent me from here to there to everywhere. I felt like a lab rat in a maze. I was lost, my heart raced and my asthma flared up from my fast-paced, stressed walking and only added to my confusion. I was debilitated from Becca's birth, the strain of trying to care for the kids and worried how to help Becca. I became lost in the labyrinth as the shock and uncertainty of the past four days caught up with me. The long tunnels and stairs and labyrinth wound me up, down, over, and around while skyways and tunnels connected to multi-story car parking garages and offices buildings turned me inside out. I was completely lost. No one could help me and I had still not found the lab. I asked for directions back to the NICU at The Children's Hospital.

I buzzed the door of the NICU anxiously telling them I could not get my labs drawn anywhere.

There stood Mary, the social worker from the day before and I collapsed.

This was all too much. The tears I had valiantly fought back for days were now drowning me in sorrow. The fear of the unknown finally surfaced. I had tried so hard to be tough.

Mary escorted me to a quiet room to sit and help me calm down. "Stay tough."The tapes raced in my head. "It's not okay to fall apart" I heard somewhere deep inside. I was trying so hard to hold it all together, but I couldn't anymore. "Suck it up," my tape shouted. "No blood, no tears" the tape continued. I tried to turn off the tape and stop the tears. It ran round and round. Mary encouraged me to cry and she told me that tears could release the stress hormones to clear my head. She told me I couldn't be tough forever, no one can and I finally found it helpful to cry.

She made arrangements for the lab tech to come to the unit to draw my blood. While they were sticking me she introduced me to the head of the NICU, Dr. Coleman. He explained that Becca did not have enough platelets to clot her blood and her numbers were dangerously low. Her white blood count was five times higher than normal and they needed to test her blood against mine to find the cause.

Mary encouraged me to go to Becca's bedside. She directed me to sit in a soft glider rocker the nurses placed by her Isolette. A nurse carefully laid my sweet baby connected to all kinds of tubes and monitors in my arms. She was bundled in a pink blanket to cover her diapered body. The lead attached to her toe looked like Rudolph's bright red nose was an oximeter and was reading her oxygen levels. The tubing through her head provided her with medicine and fluids. Several bags of medications hung from the IV pole attached to her warmer. They were infusing her with red blood since some of her blood counts were dangerously low.

A nurse explained she had given Becca a transfusion to boost her numbers. The tiny oxygen canula was placed under her nose delivering oxygen. Wire leads attached to a Velcro band around her tiny chest were measuring her heart and breathing rates. Round sticky patches were attached to many different wires. It was overwhelming to see so much medical equipment. Then as I rocked my daughter I was startled by alarms sounding for other babies. The nurse explained that many of the preemies had breathing problems and I shouldn't worry about the alarms. The beepers and alarms helped them keep a close watch over their teeny tiny charges.

The nurses were kind and caring and it was reassuring to hear that in the NICU every two babies had an assigned nurse. I rocked Becca for only a few minutes before she needed to return to being under the lights. I felt torn in two. I wanted to stay and see what was going on, but there was no place to be. At least if I was there I could look at her. I could see she was real, even if we had no privacy and I could not often hold her. I didn't feel like I had had a baby. All the cozy baby moments I was used to had transformed into an NICU nightmare. My heart and body knew I had given birth, but my mind struggled with the reality that I was powerless to care for her. I followed the lead of veteran parents who stood guarding their little one's incubators. I peered at my beautiful baby between the tubes and buttons until I felt in the way of the nurses, then I planted a kiss on my finger and placed it on her soft warm cheek and returned home.

Mary gave me a number to call anytime to see how Becca was doing. Each morning the doctors called to talk to me and other times an urgent phone call summoned me to the hospital to get updates on my baby or sign a consent for more testing. It didn't take long before the thirty-mile hospital trek became routine. I got up in the morning, made breakfast for the kids, dressed the small ones and dropped them all off at Mom's. Then I'd rush to the hospital, pay the five-dollar parking fee, and drive my car round and round the parking ramp looking for a place to park, hoping to beat the doctor's rounds so I could talk face-to-face.

The doctors had discovered that my blood had attacked Becca's. I had some sort of antiplatelet antibody. I have a positive blood type while Becca's is negative and luckily, the blood transfusion had corrected this problem. Still her white blood counts remained too high and they worried that she had some sort of infection. Her white blood counts fluctuated from 35,000 to 80,000 when normal is between five and ten thousand. They placed her on IV antibiotics. But that was not all. They found she was having trouble tolerating any sort of feeding. In addition, the early heart tests showed there were problems with Becca's heart.

One day when I came to my baby's crib I was aghast at her purple mouth. Becca had developed thrush from all the antibiotics and her mouth was all broken out in white patches of yeast. The antifungal paint used to kill the uncontrollable yeast stained her mouth and anything it touched bright purple. With her already dusky blue coloring from her breathing and heart problems, she looked awful. Then she spiked fevers and the blood cultures revealed a major problem. Becca had a systemic staph infection.

More antibiotics and blood tests . . . more ultrasounds and x-rays . . . more tests and medications. I wanted to get a picture of Becca to share with the children and I put the camera down to deal with a new issue. There was always a new problem puzzling the doctors. My wee baby and I were awash in medical terminology and a conglomerate of opinionated specialists. When I went back the camera was gone.

From the start Becca has been an attention getter and she was the Pied Piper of NICU. She puzzled her pediatrician, the neonatal intensive care doctor, and all the residents gaining knowledge from overseeing her care. In addition, she had another pediatric neurologist, a cardiologist, a geneticist, a gastroenterologist, a hematologist, and an immunologist following her progress and setbacks. One day I found a whole team of new University of Minnesota doctors peering into her tiny mouth. They had noticed her mouth had a high arched palate and they had never seen such a palate without having a full cleft palate. Perhaps this was a clue to Becca's syndrome.

Days turned into weeks of up and down phone calls and crises. The nurses placed a child's tape player next to Becca and music comforted her instead of me. It seemed just plain wrong. I wanted to be with my baby. I wanted to be with her every moment, but my other children were not in school and I couldn't go every day. Soon the hospital summoned me more and more often for paperwork and crises and I drove the sixty-mile lonely round trip journey.

By the end of August, Becca was nearly a month old and our children still had not seen their new sister. The NICU rules to protect the welfare of the tiny, frail infants affected visitation for my children. Only children who were immune to chickenpox could visit because exposure to these babies could be lethal. Kristy was our only child we knew was immune. Nathan had the chickenpox at two months of age, but it didn't count as he only had five poxes. Besides, I was told that babies under six months of age who get chicken pox would probably get them again regardless of the severity. My five children wanted to see their sister, but Kristy was the only one allowed to go and she was so excited.

Mom, my sister Martha, Kristy and I made the journey and Kristy looked stunning in her floor length yellow grown trailing behind her as she walked into the nursery. I watched her eyes explore the NICU. She bent up and down, her eyes scanning right and left; I could see the wheels of her extraordinary mind turning in high gear capturing the technology of the NICU. As my gifted child, I knew Kristy was amassing questions to ask. At ten she was already an old soul trying to figure it all out. She was not afraid of this new baby or the unit. I looked lovingly at my oldest daughter with her blond hair and freckled cheeks staring in awe of this tiny little person. She was falling in love with Becca, her new sister.

Because Kristy got to see Becca, the others were now asking, but they would have to wait. The rules were the rules even though the NICU believes in family access. Photographs would be their only connection to the new baby, but my camera had been stolen so that wasn't any longer an option. A nurse rescued me with her instant camera to get my disappointed kids a picture of their new sister.

The picture triggered endless questions. Why did she wear that 'little hat'? Why did they use a paper cup to hide the IV port underneath? We were open and honest answering the questions they asked. They wanted to know when she was coming home. I tried to avoid making promises I could not keep. They asked questions I wanted to ask myself but knew there were no answers. Some of their questions broke my heart, and I choked back the tears trying to answer them. Thankful for the picture of their sister, they went to work producing artwork to post on the wall above her crib like Mary said they could.

We floundered with the day in and day out changing of the

moment. I learned to expect the unexpected and having my parents close by was a welcome relief. I didn't spend much time at home since it gave me too much time to think. Jim and I had lived in the Twin Cities since our marriage in 1977. Now twelve years later, my family was close by and Mom, Dad, and I had lots of catching up to do. It was amazing their new home was less than five minutes from us when I needed them most. Coincidence? Some say so, but in time I began to understand forces bigger than my family or day-to-day circumstances or me controlled our lives. We were being taken care of in ways we didn't understand.

Time continued. I was afraid of being alone. Sleepless, I tossed and turned. Then I got up to scrub, scour and clean to get my mind off the reality until I was exhausted. I did mindless work; I scrubbed stains on the carpet and grout on the tile so I could drop off to sleep.

I couldn't eat; anxiety for my baby took away my appetite.

Jim worked and worked. We lived paycheck-to-paycheck before Becca joined us and now we had even less. I used the little we had to fill the gas tank to get to the hospital and feed the parking ramp. The five dollars a day parking fee was getting harder and harder to find. We were falling farther and farther behind on our bills. The insurance nightmare was becoming even more complicated. We could not hold on if Jim took time off, so I did the hospital solo while Jim worked seven days a week. Having a spouse in the retail management business meant I had often single parented my children and I was used to him working long hard hours. I had become adept at handling the home front alone, and we always made the most of the little time he had for the kids and me. Now I was juggling five children under eleven and a very sick baby in the hospital.

The mailman arrived with a certified letter from our insurance company. Certified letters always scare me, and this one held the tragic news that they were denying coverage from Jim's new company for the baby because of a pre-existing condition clause. Nothing for the new baby would be covered. I sat down on the steps exhausted. I grabbed my head in my hands and wondered…

What were we going to do?

- 4 -
INTENTION

I magically thought the schedule would get easier after Labor Day when school started. Jim was now working more hours than ever, and as the store manager, he opened the store every morning and arrived home long after the kids were already in bed. During the short window between when Jim left and I headed out each morning, he watched the kids while I had a few precious moments to vacuum or take something out of the freezer to thaw for dinner. Jim cherished the little morning time he had to play with Matt and Marissa and he helped me sort and fold the never-ending mountain of clothing. Between juggling giggles and stinky diapers we talked about Becca, our finances, the housework, the groceries and changes in our schedules.

The long summer vacation for Kristy, Nathan, and Ian was now over and they were back to school. It was a neighborhood tradition on the opening morning of school that the moms got together for a breakfast brunch. I decided to take a break from the hospital and do something 'normal.'

With Matt and Marissa in tow I went to the neighborhood party. I sat quietly as the ladies talked about what was going on in their world and I listened as they complained about day-to-day mundane issues. I felt alone with my thoughts. They took the simplest things for granted. The moms didn't know what to say to me and the subject of Becca wasn't brought up. The silence hurt.

Before Becca was born we spent our mornings visiting and letting our kids play. Now, I was in the hospital when other moms visited and socialized and I realized they were afraid of saying something wrong so they didn't say anything. They didn't realize that the silence hurt worse than talking about it. I didn't want to cause discomfort. I felt left behind from the friends in my neighborhood and I distanced myself. It hurt to feel unwelcome. They didn't seem to miss my children or me and they seemed afraid if they spent time with me, 'it' might happen to them.

I thought I was juggling the schedule to meet everyone's needs. Soon, however, I realized my children were having trouble with their upside down life. They began fighting bedtimes, Matt was clingy, and Marissa began hiding in her 'pretend' world. Ian was whiny, Nathan was even more silent than normal, and Kristy was just plain bossy. It became painfully obvious they needed normalcy, including time with Jim and me. I began paying more attention to keeping their schedules as constant as possible while adding new routines to juggle my running to the hospital to see Becca. I already had established a morning routine. I just needed to get the rest of the day under control. Mary had taught me well, explaining that I needed to take care of me first before I could take care of everyone else. I got up in the morning, took a shower and got dressed for the work of going to the hospital. This mom who had never worn makeup even put on some foundation to cover the dark circles under my eyes, then I added lipstick and a little blush for a color. Feeling good about myself and how I looked I was ready for the day. I felt I had some sense of control with a bit of housework done, the older kids off to school, and Matt and Marissa dropped off at Grandma's.

Mom had gotten smart to my not eating breakfast, and she shoved a piece of gluten free toast at me as I walked out the door. I discovered that the thirty- to forty-minute commute to the hospital was shorter if I avoided rush hour traffic, so I left later, to spend a half a day at the hospital, rocking Becca and listening to the doctors explain her newest challenges. Then each day as mid-afternoon approached; I rushed back to Mom's to pick up the little ones and hurry back to beat the school bus. I'd throw in a load of laundry and then corral Kristy, Nathan and Ian at the table with their homework while I started dinner. After dinner I quickly picked up the house and did the dishes. On the rare occasion that Jim was home, we worked together to give the little kids baths, pick out tomorrow's clothes, and read stories or sing songs while getting them tucked snugly into their beds. Nathan helped by packing five backpacks and lunches for the next morning. I would fall into bed sometime between midnight and 2:00 A.M. after finishing the laundry and making sure everything was ready to go. The next day I began my cycle again.

Every day that I kept to this routine I fell further behind and every night I was more and more exhausted. I became afraid to go to sleep and I awoke in the middle of the night startled by a dream I couldn't remember. What was in this dream? It was haunting me in the depths of my sleep. Some nights I woke soaking wet, my heart racing. All I knew was the dream terrified me.

As Becca fought herself into her fourth and fifth weeks of life, her difficulties intensified. Maybe there weren't any more than before, but the doctors were beginning to sort out what was wrong with her. By September, the doctors hoped to start feeding her formula, but she was unable to suck a nipple. She would suck once when the bottle was placed in her mouth, then her instinct to continue vanished. The nurses and I tried unsuccessfully several times a day. Her doctor placed a feeding tube down her throat but knew he needed a more permanent option. He explained that a permanent feeding tube would ensure that Becca received the nutrition necessary for her to grow and thrive. He wanted to place a tiny incision into her stomach for a gastrostomy tube.

The resident showed me another baby who had already had a feeding tube. I watched the nurses feed the tiny baby through the tube with a medical syringe. My thoughts raced and I wanted to run from this place. I wanted to pick up my baby and leave! I wished everything were better.

My heart screamed, "Get us out of here! No more pain for Becca!" My head argued, "You can not escape!"

How would I take care of her? How would I feed her? There were too many things that could go wrong and they would go wrong! This, right here, this hospital was where she needed to be. We had to stay. I could only wish things were different. I had to listen to the doctors despite my wishing otherwise. After the initial panic, I consented to the surgery.

The NICU doctors contacted a pediatric surgeon for a consultation regarding Becca's lack of progress with feeding. He reviewed Becca's records, ordered lab tests and examined Becca carefully. Then he confronted the NICU doctors for not contacting him sooner. Evidently they had known for a couple of weeks that Becca had malrotated intestines, which means that her intestines were clustered together on one side of the body and angled off her stomach in such a way that the stomach was prone to obstruction. The surgeon explained the need for immediate surgery to repair the intestines to prevent Becca from developing a dead gut. If the gut twists it cuts off the blood flow and dies. The consents were signed post-haste and Jim took the day off to sit and wait with me.

I wasn't able to sit still while Becca was in surgery and I tried unsuccessfully to fill my time by watching television and reading. Jim was content with daytime TV while I could not concentrate on anything. When the stress became too much, I followed Mary's advice and went for a walk to settle my anxiety. I tried pacing the corridor as the walls engulfed me. I was scared for Becca. I tried pacing the waiting room and felt as though I was going around in circles. I was so worried. The pressure built as I came to the hospital's five-floor stairway. I ran! I ran up and down, then back to the second floor. I ran up and down, and down, and then up, up to the second floor.

There were many variations. The sweat trickled down my back as the stress seeped out. Suddenly I realized that I was breathing steadily. I was thinking clearly. I was focused. Best of all, I relaxed. I had discovered a new way to help me cope with the many surgeries and uncertainties that followed Becca and me for many days to come.

One step at a time, one minute at a time, one second at a time was how our family would survive.

After Becca's surgery, Jim and I went to the NICU to see her and she looked awful. Her little blue body was grotesquely swollen, and big tears streamed down her tiny face into her little ears. You could see she was in such pain and agony, and we were unable to comfort or touch her. We felt helpless as we watched her silently and waited. Then we were escorted out of the unit.

I didn't want to drive to the hospital alone so the next morning my younger sister, Gretchen, and I visited Becca. I arrived to the news from the nurse that the doctors were changing Becca's pain medication. I saw Becca's tears silently run down her little cheeks. My little trooper was in such incredible pain and the morphine was not working so they ordered a stronger narcotic. Becca hardly ever cried. I was grateful for the doctors and nurses trying to help her. As her mother, it was hard for me to see her in pain, but now even Becca's primary nurse was in tears for her.

The NICU doctor ordered a pain medication and no sooner had the nurse pushed the medication into the I.V. tubing, than an alarm blared and Becca turned a deep purple-grey-blue. Looking at the monitor by Becca's Isolette, I realized her heart was beating slower and slower, and she was not breathing. More alarms sounded. "Code Blue. Code Blue!" rallied over the hospital speakers. People came running.

After months of caring for Becca in the NICU, I knew exactly what Code Blue meant – it means the baby is not breathing and their little heart has stopped. I'd only witnessed it twice before and I knew the drill. Nurses and doctors and machines all running on high alert trying to save a little one. I'd watched the sweat pour off the professionals' faces as they worked with their best skills to save the infant and yet both babies had died. I watched them somberly back away as others turned off monitors and machines no longer needed. And in the end they left the little one in the incubator while they went to call his or her parents with the heartbreaking news. I had said prayers for the parents, and the baby, and my Becca while I stood gazing at my daughter who was still alive as they wheeled the little bed into the small room. The small room I prayed I would never have to enter. I had watched mothers in their grief rock their still child for one last time as father's stood as strong as they could to protect and help the mother. I had seen fathers cry with overwhelming grief while my heart broke watching them and tears of compassion fell down my cheeks. Oh yeah, I knew the drill!

I backed away, grabbing my little sister's hand as the room filled with doctors and nurses, all trying to help my baby. The crash cart was just entering and in my haste to get out of everyone's way, I remembered I had left my purse under Becca's Isolette. I left Gretchen in the hallway and ducked between legs and machines to fetch it. I picked up my head and came face-to-face with my graying precious daughter. I stared in horror; her eyes were open and had rolled to the inside of her head, only the whites remained. I grabbed my purse just as they started to use an Ambu bag. I became light headed as I stood up. The Ambu was a balloon-like thing that had a mouthpiece that fit into Becca's mouth. It reminded me of an old fireplace baffle. In-out, in-out, in-out. The room began to spin.

They were doing CPR and I stood there numb for a moment as if I was frozen in time. In-out, in-out, in-out. One- two- three- four- five, one- two- three- four- five, one- two- three- four- five...

Something inside me snapped.

I wanted out and I ran from the nursery.

Then I bolted, running as fast as I could, leaving my sister standing alone in the hallway. The next twenty minutes are lost to me. I'm told that as I began to run from the NICU, a couple of nurses tried to stop me. I told them that I was running away, and I was never coming back. I punched the elevator buttons until one of the doors finally opened. I didn't pay any attention to what direction it was going, I just wanted out.

Nurses took the staircase to beat me to the lower level. I arrived at the main-floor lobby and ran out the automatic doors as the nurses chased me. They cornered me before I hit the steps leading to the parking ramp. After succeeding in slowing me down, they

silently stood with me, allowing me to breathe and collect myself. Then when I was ready, they gently escorted me back into the hospital and sat me down in a chair in the main lobby.

Eventually they got me to the elevator and back to the NICU. Gretchen gently held my hand. The nurses stayed with us until Mary arrived and took us to a private room. I was now back to reality. We sat in silence as the minutes ticked away. Waiting. It seemed like forever. Time had never moved so slowly. I was beginning to feel my heart rate settling down when one of Becca's doctors came into the room. His facemask hung down around his chin. His gown and cap were drenched in sweat. I could see through the door of the conference room that the doctors and nurses had begun leaving the area of Becca's Isolette.

I had seen this stage before, the unit was now calm and the doctor prepared to speak. I felt my body tensing to run, but his voice was calming, "Becca's pain is under control. Her condition is stable." My tired mind was so completely prepared for the worst that it took me a minute for his words to register.

He said that she was stable. Stable? Becca was alive! I tried my best not to drown him in my tears of elation. He explained the narcotic caused Becca to go into respiratory distress and then she forgot to breathe and then her heart stopped. She was without oxygen for a considerable length of time. The emergency response team had succeeded in bringing her back, but only time would tell the effects the lack of oxygen would have on her brain and struggling body. I could do nothing but sit silently next to my sister, letting my tears flow until I was limp and exhausted.

Then Gretchen called Jim at the store to come pick us up and bring us home.

Becca was different after the drug reaction. She stayed unnaturally still unless she was touched by something or was externally stimulated. The lack of oxygen had caused brain damage, and occupational and physical therapies were ordered to teach her to move her body all over again. They taught me massage and passive exercise techniques. I learned how to move her legs for her, and then her fin-

gers, and her hands, and her arms, and her toes, and her feet. We repeatedly worked with these simple motions and Becca eventually could do them by herself.

When I asked the doctors whether she would have permanent damage the answer was unyieldingly, "only time will tell."

▼

October arrived and the kids still hadn't met their three-month-old sister. After the close call with the pain medication, I knew that every day she was alive was a gift from God. I didn't want her siblings to miss out on knowing Becca and I worried that they would have no memories of their baby sister. Their only connection was the Polaroid pictures that the nurses snapped and sent home. I shared my concerns with Mary and expressed my desire to have all of my children together at least once. As more problems were surfacing, we didn't know how long Becca would be with us. We had almost lost her and this was important! I demanded the kids needed to see their baby sister. Finally the NICU team made arrangements for them to visit Becca in the doctors' conference room.

Like all the babies in the NICU, Becca was very weak and vulnerable to disease and if the kids were going to visit her at the hospital, they had to be healthy. Since Becca's birth, Jim and I were extra careful at home to keep them well for the special day when Becca could come home, but even to visit they had to prepare.

All five kids donned their cartoon-print gowns and facemasks in the gowning area. The masks were necessary as germ barriers to prevent any bugs from reaching Becca. Once they were next to their sister, they weren't allowed to touch her in case they had unknowingly been exposed to chickenpox. We were together for a moment, and if something should happen to Becca, at least the kids had met their sister. It was real and we were a family. The nurse used her Polaroid camera for our first family photo. Ian proudly carried our new family portrait as we left the hospital for home.

The NICU was no longer a foreign world to me. The new routine at home worked for our children and holding my family together took precedence, but I was wearing thin. When I'm physically or

emotionally stressed I am not hungry, so with the new schedule eating wasn't a priority. Some people overeat when bored or anxious; instead I cannot eat because I no longer feel hunger and I have to remember to force myself. I wasn't the only one skipping meals. Jim did everything he could to make sure the kids ate their fill, even if it meant he went hungry too. Our children always had food, we didn't.

Jim had finally reached a reasonable salary but it was not enough to cover the costs for the baby's prohibitive medical expenses. To keep the Medicaid card for Becca our income had to remain around $900 a month for our whole family. He asked his boss to limit his paycheck so we could help our daughter. We had no other known options and it all seemed so backwards to me. Our budget was in shambles. The mortgage was almost $800 and the gasoline and hospital parking ate up what was left for groceries. We were now well below poverty level for a family of eight.

Each month I had to choose whether to pay the house payment or the utility bills because I could not do both. When the natural gas was turned off, bathing nights became a family affair. I was thankful we still had electricity. I covered all four burners of my electric stove with my turkey roaster, canning kettle and Dutch oven filled to the brim with cold water. Once the water was boiling I scurried all five children into the living room and obediently they stayed there while I dashed between the kitchen and the cold porcelain covered cast iron bathtub.

My first effort yielded only a little over an inch of lukewarm water. My second and third batches raised my water level to almost three inches and I could add a bit of cold water to make it hit the three-inch mark. I chose Marissa and Matt as the first bathers since they were the littlest and used the least water. I continued to boil water for separate baths for Nathan and Kristy, who had grown accustomed to rinsing her freshly washed hair with cold water. Last but not least was Ian. He got the final bath with the most, but dirtiest water. He was my bathboy and played in the cooling water while soaking off his accumulated grime. Jim and I struggled with quick cold showers and sponge baths.

The kids huddled together in their beds under several comforters to keep warm and in the morning I opened the oven door to take the chill off the kitchen while the kids ate their breakfast.

There was no money left to pay for family health insurance and I had no choice but to stop paying for it. The Yurceks played Russian roulette with our health, hoping none of us would fall ill. We fell further and further behind as we tried to help Becca.

▼

At three months Becca had not even gained a pound since she was born and she still did not tolerate her feedings. Becca was losing ground by the day. Kind nurses fed her so slowly it took over an hour for two ounces via her feeding tube. Then once it was in, Becca threw it all up dousing her bedding, tiny sleeper and the nurse's yellow hospital gowns. The nurses patiently changed everything and soon repeated the process again. This was not the ordinary spitting up all babies do, but a volcanic eruption of formula that we all had worked so hard to get in.

The doctors ordered barium studies that determined Becca had severe reflux. They wanted another surgery, this time to wrap her esophagus with her stomach to prevent everything from coming back out. This surgery (Nissen) would change her anatomy, and it is only done as a last resort. The doctors warned us that the surgery could cause other problems, but we had no choice for Becca.

▼

Jim's employer faced the next Becca dilemma. Now that our new baby was brought into our family, his health insurance pre-existing clause was running out and he would be forced to add our expensive infant to his company's health care plan. This small company already had faced increases due to two others families recent needs for critical care and adding Becca would tip the scales. Looking at the big picture, he felt he had no alternative and began to force Jim out in order to keep health care for the rest of his employees.

▼

Jim could not take any more time off because his boss was giving him problems if he wasn't at the store for all the hours it was

open. He was afraid of getting fired or being let go and he knew that they seemed to be looking for any opportunity to get rid of him before they had to put Becca on their insurance after the six month waiting period for the pre-existing clause was over. I had to go to Becca's surgery alone and Mary cleared part of her morning to sit with me after rounds. I ran the staircase when I got anxious, and after exercising I could sit and wait patiently.

Hours later, the doctor came to tell me that Becca came through surgery and I hoped it would be her last.

Becca's immune status was now a grave concern. After surgery she spiked a fever from another staph infection requiring more IV antibiotics, more tests, and another 'new' doctor, this time an infectious disease specialist. The high white blood counts, the resistant thrush, and the recurrent staph infections signaled something was drastically wrong with Becca's immune system. He told us that she might have a syndrome called DiGeorge syndrome or she may have Severe Combined Immune Deficiency syndrome (SCID), the same disease of the little boy who lived his life in a plastic bubble.

Devastated, we signed consents for blood studies. And then we waited while each day felt like a lifetime. A week later they called us to come hear the test results. I faced the news alone because Jim couldn't risk losing his job.

With Mary at my side, Dr. Gilmore explained Becca did not have DiGeorge or SCID, but she had some sort of other unusual immune problem. She was developing some immunity, but on many levels she was compromised. The news was better than the doomsday prediction first discussed. She would not have to live in a plastic bubble; she was compromised, but she had some immunity! Some is better than none. Thank you God.

It took three different medications to keep the yeast in her systems in check, and IVs were necessary as she was on constant antibiotics to get rid of the systemic staph in her bloodstream or to keep her from getting something new. She bounced in and out of isolation. Isolation provided Becca and me a refuge from the beeping and alarms and it was the first time Becca and I had undisturbed time alone. We had our own little world away from all the chaos of the NICU. The little isolation room was calm and quiet, I could dim the lights that had been on her entire life and Becca seemed to sleep more peacefully away from the busy twenty-four hour day NICU.

After nearly three months of hospitalization I was a veteran unit parent. Once the staph cleared, Becca returned to the other side of the unit. She was no longer on the critical care side. She had graduated to the side for little human beings waiting to grow stronger to finally go home and she had a private corner sheltered away from twenty-four hour daylight and the commotion of the hospital.

The unit always had a couple of full-term babies or boarder babies to rock and play. The boarder babies were babies who had severe disabilities and were too sick to go home. Families who could not care for them abandoned some. These babies may have lost a family but they found family love in the doctors and nurses who showered them with nurturing and attention. The older babies in the unit got a lot of attention and Becca was developing quite a personality. Everyone in NICU loved my struggling little person.

The primary nurse handpicked a select core of nurturing nurses to attend to my daughter and she ordered the team remain the same. Above her head a sign stated "do not touch her without warning." as Becca was showing signs of giving up on the world, and the occupational therapist was getting worried about her lack of interest in what was going on around her.

I tried to get her to look at me. I jiggled toys to get her attention. I talked high. I talked low. I whispered in her tiny ear. I stroked and massaged her little arms and legs and face. I told her I loved her and blew her little baby kisses through my mask. I created dances for her little pink puppy. At nearly three months Becca still didn't track or respond to faces, she turned away from people. Over time our persistence paid off. Becca learned to grab at our fingers and she looked sad when I had to leave.

One day we noticed that she was watching all of our movements by tracking what was going on in the room using the toy mirror in her bed. She was watching everything through the mirror! I saw her eyes following me in her mirror as I walked to the door and waved to my daughter.

For hours, I rocked my little baby listening to the music tapes that had become so important to her. The music calmed and relaxed her and I savored my moments of peace away from our stressful world. Becca's music collection grew in a bittersweet way. Families who lost their children in NICU gave us their no longer needed tapes. The tapes reminded me of the fragileness of life.

I never knew when I departed for home whether a crib filled with a challenged baby would be empty when I returned. Even babies that seemed to be doing well one day, could be gone tomorrow. Being in the NICU was not an easy place to be and some of the babies died. I no longer liked the color purple. I didn't like watching grieving parents say goodbye. I didn't like seeing the hopeful worry on their faces one day be replaced with sadness and loss as they held their silent and still infant. Each day I left, I worried that one day's goodbye to Becca may be my last. Everyday I prayed for an angel's protection over my tiny titan with my goodbye kiss.

▼

The angels must have heard my prayer because by Halloween the doctors were talking of discharging Becca the following week. I found costumes for the kids in our costume box. I pulled out my dusty sewing machine to sew something for my new daughter. With a piece of pink fuzzy fleece, I designed a costume to match Becca with her pink puppy. Her pink puppy had become like the pink puppy of my childhood, our always-present best friend. Whenever Becca had another poke, puppy was there. When Becca went for x-rays or some test, puppy went too. I purchased an orange plastic pumpkin and filled it with chocolate kisses for Becca's bedside. Becca was treating her caregivers. She had a lot of repayment to do for all the tricks she had pulled on them.

As I sat with Becca dressed up as her little pink puppy, I noticed the spark in her eyes was gone. She was not herself. Something was amiss. I pointed it out to her doctors who reassured me that it was 'normal.' I was just afraid of bringing her home because NICU was a safe place and to bring her home would be scary. They had seen other parents react this way. They didn't understand. I was not thinking about the responsibility of bringing her home.

I was worried about Becca.

That weekend I stayed home from the hospital to spend time playing with my older children and catch up on my household chores. The 'to do' list for Becca's homecoming was long. The immune doctor ordered everything must be clean and disinfected so Becca would not get sick. I washed the crib bedding. I bleached her bed and changing stand. I vacuumed, and scrubbed, and scoured, and dusted until my hands were raw and red and bleeding, but my heart was filled with hope. Exhausted from getting my house spotless, I returned Monday morning to the hospital.

Becca's primary nurse approached me stating she had noticed that something was not right with Becca. The residents at rounds relayed that Becca had a really rough weekend. She was not tolerating her feedings again and was back on IVs to hydrate her. A new neonatologist, Dr. Gato joined her treatment team and she wanted to hear from the nurse and me what we had observed. We explained Becca's lack of spark, her lethargy and change in color. I told Dr. Gato I thought she was sick, something was terribly wrong and I was not taking her home. They had to find out why we were losing her. Asking questions was like a double edge sword. Each time we discovered why, we exposed more things wrong.

I began to despise my intuition since it always signaled another crisis for Becca. It took me a long time to understand that my intuition was my compass to find Becca the help she needed to survive.

- 5 -

LETTING GO

Poor Becca . . . the testing . . . and checking . . . and poking . . . and prodding seemed endless. Every few days the IV port site blew, which meant Becca's teeny tiny vein collapsed and we needed to find another place to start the IV. They held her down while she fought the nurses with every ounce of energy she had left. The only time Becca cried was when they were poking and prodding her.

Dr. Gato, ordered additional tests and more specialists to take a look at her. The cardiologist returned to examine her and ordered even more tests. This time the EKG revealed something had changed with her heart and an ultrasound was ordered to take a closer look. It exposed the source of Becca's ever increasing stress. Her heart was worsening.

Because of my veteran parent status and knowledge of the inner workings of NICU, I knew that when the doctors call you to a conference room to talk the news is not good. If the news was good they approached your child's bedside and announced it to the world. Anything behind closed doors sent shivers up my spine. I already knew Becca's heart was not working, as it should.

The echocardiogram revealed Pulmonary Stenosis which meant the valve between the right ventricle to the pulmonary outflow tract was obstructing the blood flow to her lungs. That was why her little chest shook so hard. It was overworked. In addition, she had a huge hole (Atrial Septal Defect, ASD) between the right and left atriums of her heart, the walls of her heart were thick and not functioning normally and her left and right ventricles were thickened. She had biventricular cardiomyopathy of the heart, and babies with this condition usually don't do very well or even survive and a heart transplant may be her only option. The doctors added more medication. Becca was showing signs of heart failure and the IV pump administered a diuretic through her tiny veins.

My 'mother intuition' was right. I was not afraid of bringing her home, even though I longed for that day. I wanted to bring her home when the time was right. I was not a panicky mother worried about having a sick baby at home as the staff claimed. I knew something was wrong and I wasn't going to let her go until she was ready. The little pink puppy lay next to my very sick little girl. I kissed her gently goodbye and whispered mommy sweet nothings. And then heartbroken and worried, I left once again.

The parking lot was full on the morning when I arrived, so I had parked on the roof. Unlike other days, the doctors had kept me long into the evening and darkness had fallen. The elevator door opened, but to enter felt claustrophobic and I needed to run. I ran with my head down pounding the steps with each foot as I climbed higher and higher. Just as I was calming from my step-by-step climb back into reality I was shocked back into fear by loud noises above me.

"Get the flying elephants! Get the flying elephants!"

I smelled the liquor before I saw the unkempt homeless man waving a liquor bottle at me a half-flight away. "Get the flying elephants!" he roared. I snuck by the smelly crazed man and pushed my way through the third level door. My heart pounded as I ran around the ramp to the rooftop.

Jim had warned me that most of the homeless were mild, but when they were intoxicated, hallucinating or going through withdrawals they could be mean, impulsive and potentially dangerous. Early in our marriage Jim had worked at a produce warehouse to put himself through college and his employer had left the back of his delivery trucks unlocked to provide places for them to sleep. Many mornings Jim had roused the sleeping guests out of their slumber so he could get on with his daily work.

I proceeded with caution, as this was definitely unsafe.

The lights of the city did not console me and my hands were shaking as I opened the door to my car, jumped in, and relocked it quickly. My car would not start and I cranked the ignition over and over until the whining battery gave up the ghost with a click, click, and click. I did what I had to do. Afraid to use the stairs, I walked the half-empty ramp in circles all the way to the bottom. I knew Jim couldn't leave work so I called Mom and Dad to save me. I sat in the waiting room listening to my heart beating, while upstairs my baby's damaged heart was thumping and fighting to keep her alive.

Forty minutes later I saw headlights pull into the entrance. Finally, I could go home. I fell asleep in the car, but once home it was impossible to sleep. Every time I fell asleep, my dreams awakened me. Once again, I got up and scrubbed and cleaned until I drained the little energy I had left.

When I arrived at NICU the next morning, Dr. Gato told me the cardiologist wanted to take Becca's case to the heart specialists at the University of Minnesota. He wanted to discuss her case with the best doctors and researchers the University had to offer. At the university the geneticist and cardiologist concurred. They could identify almost all of Becca's symptom's under one diagnosis. They called it Noonan's syndrome. However Becca had some unusual things that were not known to be associated with the syndrome. Dr. Hesselein said he had once seen a little girl in Canada with the same immune and blood counts as Becca and she was diagnosed with an unusual variant of Noonan syndrome. While Becca had some variants, the doctors agreed that using treatments consistent with Noonan's syndrome would be best for Becca. Finally we had a diagnosis with a name. It did not change anything that was wrong with Becca, but it did provide documented care plans the professionals could refer to. The name Noonan's syndrome was a bright compass pointing us away from a murky path of medical trial to potential error. Armed with a name, my anxiety lessened.

This time I questioned the doctors. I took a deep breath and asked the hard question. "Would she survive?"

They offered me little hope for Becca's future. I had a baby with immune problems, breathing problems, and digestive problems that included failure to thrive and choking on her own secretions. Not to forget, the brain damage from her lack of oxygen when she had coded, and last, but not least, she was now in heart failure.

I slept less and less.

One night the dream that confounded me, awoke me with remembrance. The dream memories were vivid and alive with color and my spirit could no longer run from it by waking. I finally had to confront what I already knew. Becca was dying. I had to accept the dark reality. The little white coffin in my dream shouted at me, "Look, look, you must look." In it was Becca.

I immediately understood why I had been haunted from sleep. I was afraid of my baby dying.

I prayed.

I prayed a prayer of acceptance.

I quit running . . . from the night terrors and bad dreams. I faced them. I determined to love Becca as long as I had her. Falling in love with Becca meant that it would break my heart when one day she would be gone.

I prayed to God to help me through the coming days. I cried. I told Him I couldn't do this alone anymore. He knew better than I what I needed. I asked Him to find a reason for all this pain. I made a promise to Him. I would love Becca for whatever time she had left and I would try to make each moment count. I promised to do what He called me to do, knowing that someday I would have to let her go. I promised that something good would happen out of all this pain. I prayed that Becca's life had a purpose.

In time I would learn how big my promises were, and what His promises would bring. After my prayer, I fell fast asleep, more soundly than I had for months.

The sun woke me with a new sense of calm. I had given over my pain and myself, and most importantly I had returned Becca to her Creator. The November skies were blue and the weather unusually warm. I showered and put on my nicest outfit.

Entering the hospital I stopped at the cafeteria for a glass of soda. Becca's primary nurse ran into me in the hallway and noticed how different I looked that morning. I smiled. I realized that if I took care of myself and made myself look good perhaps I could handle things better as they were thrown at me.

I looked down at my nice outfit.

But she was not talking about my clothes and cleanliness. She told me that she saw a look of peace in my face. She was right. I was at peace. I had accepted the fact that my baby was dying. I had seen the dream that was haunting me for months.

Becca had had a good twenty-four hours and the nurse asked if I wanted to take Becca outside. Her IV had blown again, and before they hooked her up we could go outside to enjoy an Indian summer November day.

I dressed her in the new outfit I had sewn for her homecoming. It was a little pink dress with a ruffled satin skirt I made out of a little pink Onesie. Under the skirt little lacy ruffles rode across the backside. I topped her little head with a matching rose ribbon headband and bundled her in her pink blanket. Then I carried my daughter out of the hospital for the first time.

The warm sun shone on her and her eyes darted everywhere taking in the newness of the outside world. She didn't like wind on her face and she gasped when it blew. I sat on a park bench sheltering her from the wind and enjoying Becca as she watched the birds and clouds go by. The multi-colored leaves danced across the courtyard. I didn't want it to end. My heart wanted to run with her and protect her from the pain and they almost had an AWOL mother with her critically ill baby, but my head knew we must return.

Our Cinderella hour of freedom ended and we walked back through the front glass doors of the hospital. I saw myself for the first time with my baby in the reflection of the glass as I carried Becca. I wished the NICU had mirrors for parents to see themselves with their babies. I was Becca's mother and she was my baby; my reflection proclaimed it. She was my real and forever daughter. All the while my tears dropped on her tiny forehead.

That day I came to a new acceptance of our circumstances. Instead of fighting the reality, I acknowledged the cards delivered to me. I began finding peace in tiny moments when things were calm. And because of those tiny moments I knew I could survive the moments that weren't. The ups and downs would continue. Many days would be hard. Mary suggested I start journaling my thoughts. Sixteen years later, I pulled out the journal I wrote long ago in those earliest of days.

It began . . .

"I settle myself on the roller coaster of Becca's life, with all its ups and downs. This is the way that it has to be to have her in our lives. I know when the ride ends she will be gone."

- 6 -

THANKSGIVING

The diuretic stabilized Becca's heart and she went back on her feedings. Once more we began to hear talk of discharge and the doctors decided she was stable enough to go home for the Thanksgiving holiday. They gave me orders for what I needed to do to prepare to finally bring our daughter home. I carefully checked off each item on my hospital ordered 'To Do' list. Number one was a new item – flu shots for every family member. I discovered the shots were $25.00 each from our clinic, seven times twenty-five equals one hundred seventy five dollars we did not have.

The idea of not being able to make it on our own shamed me so I had kept quiet about our struggles. Finally I confided our dire situation to Mary and she found ways to help me.

The nurses had forgotten to give us the welcome packet with the 'free parking permit' when Becca arrived in the NICU. I should have never had to pay for parking and the State Medicaid program paid mileage for families with children in the program. I turned in my parking slips and the hospital refunded my parking money immediately. I turned in my mileage for all my trips to the hospital and Mary signed the form.

Within two weeks a check arrived just in time for our flu shots and to turn on the gas. Becca could finally come home.

We were grateful. At last, the house was warm. When watching *Little House on the Prairie*, the kids announced that we were just like the pioneers in the olden days because we boiled water, were cold and struggled to have something to eat. I had to agree. Going without heat in November is impossible in Minnesota and the stove and single space heater only warmed one room.

It felt good not to be freezing and have hot water. The kids enjoyed bathing and watching the water run through their fingers. Marissa and Matt put on their bathing suits and had a long November swim in the tub. I loved being able to wash dishes in hot water without having to boil it. It had been two months of rationing and Jim and I had grown used to cold showers. I luxuriated in a hot bath. I had new appreciation for the little things I had taken for granted.

Still, we were barely holding things together. Our cars were giving us trouble and we had purchased an unreliable minivan to replace the dead station wagon. The money for groceries was getting harder to find and I could not pay the upcoming car insurance. The insurance agent would not accept less than three-month premiums. It seemed Jim's paychecks evaporated before they were deposited.

Jim, like me, was too proud to let anyone know what was going on. He believed he was supposed to provide for his family and I tried to explain to him that many families fall into bankruptcy from medical costs too high to handle. No family can make it with catastrophic medical costs without assistance. My words fell on deaf ears. He was raised to believe everyone stood on his or her own two feet and you looked down on people who had to ask for help.

We were excited to have Becca coming home. She had spent four and a half months in NICU and though her holiday time home with us would be limited, we would build Thanksgiving memories as a family. I had a secret plan.

▼

I was happy. I spent the week sewing for her homecoming. I reupholstered Matt's old baby car seat in leftover blue calico with little white hearts. My child was coming home dainty and delicate and beautiful. Finally, I got to put the car seat into the car and pack the diaper bag. I didn't have much to add because Becca's things were mostly at the hospital. I packed two diapers and added the tear stained rosebud sleeper I had stuffed in the bottom of my suitcase when I first came home from the hospital. I hadn't had the heart to bring that sleeper to the hospital with some of the other clothing. Finally, it seemed the appropriate day to include the little sleeper. She would wear her new beautiful dress, but after my surprise I could change her before I brought her home. I took the tags off the diaper bag and added the tiny lacy ruffled pinafore dress.

We loaded the kids in the van to bring home their new sister. I prayed the van could limp along to St. Paul without breaking down.

At home, Becca would be completely in my care. The feedings were still a problem but I knew how to take my time to get the nourishment in. I had learned to weigh her diapers to record her urine output. It was my total responsibility to record her fluid input and output and maintaining it was a delicate balance. I tried not to think about the responsibility of Becca's care, but of the happiness of being a family. I relished watching my older children dote over their new sister. We had good reason to be thankful this Thanksgiving Day. Our family included Becca.

Jim and the children waited outside in the hallway while Kristy and I went to fetch Becca. The nurses packed up her belongings from her corner of the unit. Becca had become one of the 'big kids' who couldn't go home, and at long last the day had finally arrived and someone else could move into her corner. Kristy carried all the ani mals, tapes, toys, and clothing. Staff carried two shopping bags of medical supplies. We reviewed the paperwork.

Then I dressed and primped my wee little daughter in the specially designed pink dress with the white ruffled pinafore. She was a princess in all frills. The staff marveled over the dress I had sewn for this very special occasion. I enjoyed sewing fancy outfits for special occasions for all of my children and while in the hospital, I found comfort designing special sleepers for the tiny preterm newborns in the unit. Some of my tiniest designs were reserved for nurses to give to grieving parents to bury their babies on their final journey home. My creations had provided an added source of money from the hospital gift shop when family members of other children outfitted their wee ones. Sometimes I enjoyed surprising parents with special new outfits for their little people. It was something I could do to help someone else out. While Becca was in the hospital, word spread about the clothes I made for Becca and the other babies and they were featured in a local publication.

We still didn't have a camera so the nurses snapped pictures of Becca in her new dress for her scrapbook. Becca seemed to know that something was up. She was smiling. Her deep dimples were shining. She was at long last going home.

It was hard to say goodbye. I hugged everyone at NICU who had become my second family. They were not just caregivers for Becca; they were friends of my heart who were there when I needed them most. We had been through so much together and Mary had become someone who I counted on and depended on for guidance. How could I say goodbye? She had taught me so much. She held me up when I was falling and provided a listening ear. Even though she was younger than me, she was wise beyond her years. She taught me how to cope.

Someday I promised to be able to return the gift Mary gave me. I would help others on their journey, providing a listening ear or a simple hug when words were not enough.

I bundled Becca in her little pink hand-me-down snowsuit and we walked through the double metal doors of the unit for the last time. We were greeted by my five stair-step children bouncing in their multi-colored snow jackets and boots. They hovered around me and marveled at their new sister coming home in the carseat bucket. The nurse set Becca down in the middle of the floor and the kids surrounded her. Marissa gently stroked her little hand. It was their baby and she was coming home.

Several of the staff followed us out. The nurses and staff were in tears as we buckled her in her car seat. She was so tiny; she weighed only a pound more than when she was born. She looked as though we were bringing home a few day old newborn, not the four-and-a-half-month-old she now was. Soon she fell fast asleep.

Together as a family we left this place of security. I was now responsible for Becca's care and I tucked the emergency instructions and phone numbers into the diaper bag just in case I needed help or support. The nurses in the unit told me to call anytime and they would guide me. It was reassuring that I had people who I could count on and know I was not in this alone.

In the spirit of Thanksgiving we pulled away from the hospital to at long last go home.

- 7 -

HOMECOMING

It was our family Thanksgiving tradition to eat dinner at my cousin's home. The gathering included my aunts, uncles, cousins, and their children. Jim and I surprised everyone by stopping by just in time for dinner. I had cleared the visit with the doctors for Becca to be allowed to see her extended family. They agreed as long as the time was kept short and she was not passed around. It was my secret surprise.

My uncle blessed the food giving special thanks for the gift of Becca being with us. Since the flu and cold season was just beginning, only Grandma was given the gift of holding her. All the other guests had to hold the little guest of honor with their eyes. Becca knew she was special and her little grin melted all who met her. For her, this was a very interesting and exciting day and she stayed awake until we arrived home.

The kids helped carry in her belongings while I changed her into her little rosebud sleeper for her first night in her home. While the kids scurried around her, Becca peacefully nestled in her crib. When everyone, from two-year-old Matt to almost eleven-year-old Kristy, was sure their baby was safe and well taken care of they climbed into bed. Finally the Yurcek team was where we all belonged, at home in our own beds. I snuggled Jim, cocooned in his strength, happy we were once again one unit and thankful for this special day.

▼

We didn't get many happy surprises, and I had fun before Becca's homecoming using Jim's carpet sales incentive points to buy treasures for our children. It wasn't yet Christmas; this was better. The UPS man delivered the secret boxes. One box contained a little red battery powered Corvette to share between Ian, Marissa, and Matt. Another box held a new ten-speed bike to share between Kristy and Nathan. A big box held a fancy stroller for Becca and her support system to allow her to join in the family. I got a treasured vacuum cleaner because I killed the old one getting ready for Becca's homecoming, and we had doctor's orders to keep the dust and dirt under control.

Becca appeared happy to be at home and it seemed like she knew she was where she belonged. She was relaxed, her tiny heart slowed to a steadier beat and she slept well. Caring for Becca was so much more intense than a normal baby. I was getting used to doing the tube feedings, her medication, and tracking her inputs and outputs on schedule.

I rocked and held her while she watched the children play. At least for the moment, everyone was on exceptionally good behavior. Ten child eyes monitored her constantly and no one argued about hand washing before playing with the baby. Ian stood on the bedrail to turn on the musical mobile so Becca was not bored. Marissa tried to get her to look at toys she proudly shared. Matt clung to my leg while I cared for her, he was unsure about being replaced by this new baby. Kristy helped immeasurably, fetching things I needed, and always the neat nick, Nathan scoured and scrubbed and organized without complaint, whatever I asked of him.

▼

This happiness, however, was fleeting. Within three days, Becca had trouble handling feedings, her little body broke out in a sweat after each attempt. She gagged and wretched and was miserable. It hurt me to see her suffer. Even though she was able to keep the nutrients in, she was unable to throw up because of her second surgery.

There was no relief from the dry retching.

On the fourth day out of the hospital we were scheduled for an appointment with our standard family pediatrician. He was an older doctor and I asked questions about her feedings. I could tell he was uncomfortable handling her care and after the appointment, I called NICU and asked what I could do to help Becca. Her primary nurse shared that they had fed her four ounces of formula over an hour's duration. If the nurse took it really slowly, Becca handled eating better via her tube. I was relieved it was something so simple. So over the next few days I fed Becca every other hour around the clock. I took my time, slowly, ever so slowly, helping her eat. In the meantime I made arrangements to transfer Becca's care to the young, gentle pediatrician who first delivered the news of Becca's congenital anomalies. I trusted him and I could tell by his eyes and his presentation of the tragic news that he cared about Becca and about me.

▼

Dr. Wineinger gently held and examined my sweet daughter. Then he looked at me knowing I was desperate for rest. Per my usual super mom self-determination I had tried to juggle caring for five attention-starved children and round-the-clock feedings and I hadn't slept in five days. Without hesitation he ordered a feeding pump to mechanically slowly drip formula and relieve me of doing the same thing. He ordered a home care company to train me in my home. He took care to order an extra feeding tube in case one slipped. He also increased her diuretic dosage to control fluid buildup.

I was thankful to have someone tell me what to do. He wanted me to have in-home health care for Becca. He knew I had five other children and other responsibilities and Becca's heart was worsening. She needed more monitoring than I was capable of doing on my own. I had mixed feelings about having staff in my home because I wanted to care for my baby alone and I questioned my competence. Other parents have sick babies and they don't need help. The tapes of childhood insecurities haunted me telling me I wasn't good enough.

The weekend arrived along with the medical equipment with the new extra feeding tube. I had dozed off by Becca's bedside and awoke to find her feeding tube had been pulled out of the tiny opening in her abdomen. Her bed was full of formula and Becca was covered from head to toe in sticky white foul smelling liquid. She needed a bath. Dr. Wineinger warned me that if the tube fell out, it would need to be replaced as soon as possible or the hole for the tube (stoma) to enter Becca's stomach would close and then she'd need another surgery.

Jim called my mom to come and watch the kids while we ventured to the hospital emergency room where Becca was born. We had been advised to go there for minor incidents and since it was simply a pulled out tube we felt confident this was the right decision.

It was 11:00 P.M., and the emergency room was full of people coughing and feverish with the flu. I explained Becca's immune problems and within ten minutes they accommodated us by moving Becca into the first open bed. The ER was packed and lying next to us, just past the curtain, was a drunken man handcuffed to his bed rails who had come in with the County Sheriff. He alternated between crying and screaming as broken shards of glass were removed from his body. Then the same doctor, without washing his hands quickly replaced Becca's tube. He roughly forced it in and it caused Becca to bleed uncontrollably from the stoma. When the gauze pads stopped the bleeding, we were sent home.

Becca shut down from the pain and the pediatrician on call advised me to get baby Tylenol, but it had to be the right kind and the right dosage. Poor Jim was sent on a three o'clock in the morning scavenger hunt to convenience stores. It took him several stops and many shelf searches before he returned with his treasure. The medicine settled Becca, and I lay on the floor counting sheep waiting for my wee one to fall asleep.

Home health care for Becca meant upheaval of our split-level home. Becca needed her own room upstairs and the girls' pink room across from ours was the only choice to transform into Becca's pediatric care unit. With the help of Kristy and Nathan, Jim moved the girls into the unfinished basement room with the boys. Even though the room was good sized, there was no room for dressers or toys. Two sets of bunks and the toddler bed filled it to the brim. Jim added a damaged carpet remnant and lined up dressers and toys on the other side of the open studded basement.

We moved Becca's bed and dresser from our room to the girls' room. A friend donated a rocking chair. Her stroller sat in the corner. The kids added their most precious stuffed animals as room decorations so Becca had something to look at. It was beginning to look like a nursery and the Yurcek team performed well to prepare for the nurses' arrival.

Becca was quiet. She never cried unless somebody touched or examined her. I read her pain through her facial expressions. Compared to my other noisy children, Becca was too quiet and I asked why. The nurse told me Becca was not strong enough to make noise. It required too much energy for her tiny body.

One night the feeding pump went off and tiny air bubbles occluded the clear plastic tubing. I tried to get them to move like the technician taught me, but I had little patience remembering the recent late night ER escapade. Eventually the pump resumed working and I lay on the floor by her crib to sleep. Staying close to her assured me I could hear if she choked or gagged. I wished I had kept Matt's nursery monitor.

The next day Becca's tiny chest shook so strongly I could count her heart rate by watching and her color sent shivers up my spine. By early evening, her little lips were dark chambray. The dark blue veins across her forehead and temples shone brightly through her skin connected by her tiny capillaries that had also turned midnight blue. She was almost navy. She felt feverish and Becca never had fevers unless she cultured positive for staph. I placed the digital thermometer under her tiny armpit as I rocked her. Her fever was 102.9° so I called her doctor who once again sent us to the local hospital.

The ER was much calmer in the early evening hours, and the on-call pediatrician looked worried as she peered into Becca's last night's chart. She called Dr. Wineinger and confirmed what antibiotics she was taking. With her compromised immune system, they did not want to take any chances. They gave her something to bring down the fever and a treatment to clear her wheezing lungs. Becca stabilized and we were cleared to return home. It wasn't until much later, we realized what was wrong, and understood the malpractice of the attending ER doctor the late night before. He had not used antibiotic prophalixis. He had quickly changed the tube without gloving or using even a bacterial swab to cleanse the site. He put it back in without lubrication and he left her seriously at risk for an infection. The new ER team was aware of the mismanagement of her care the previous night, though it took years before we understood. We were lucky that this new doctor treated at least part of the problem with the antibiotics. Her cardiac doctors had told us at discharge that before any procedure Becca needed antibiotics to keep her heart from becoming infected.

The doctor's nurse called us the next morning to check on Becca and it was reassuring that they were monitoring her so closely. I was comforted that I was not in this alone. I had had no sleep since she came home from the hospital since Becca needed constant care. I struggled to manage the housework, cook and watch my busy two-year-old. As soon as I turned my back he was into something. There was only one of me and three of them not in school. Thankfully Marissa, who was five, was very adept at entertaining herself and she responsibly updated me on Matt's escapades.

For the first thirteen days of home care we had no nursing staff. Becca was hooked up to an IV pole on casters eighteen hours a day to drip the formula slowly into her tummy. I tried to carry Becca and move the pole from room to room because I dared not leave her alone as each pump feeding could cause her to choke and wretch. I was beginning to understand the conversation from Dr. Wineinger telling me I would need help. I finally realized I was not capable of doing this alone. This was my moment of acceptance and his wise words reassured me. He must have done this before for other families. Dr. Wineinger told me that asking for help eased the burden. It was unwise to tackle this mountain alone. He told me to focus on keeping our family together. He told me that families who have children like Becca do not survive intact. I remembered him tossing me a statistic of 90% divorce rate among families with chronically ill children or dying children. Jim and I loved each other. We were forever the Yurcek team. Nothing could separate us. Jim and I were best friends. How could "that be true?"

When the older children returned from school the stress eased. Kristy and Nathan watched out for their younger siblings and entertained Matt while my evening filled with dinner preparation and Becca's care. By the time Jim arrived home from work after 10:00 P.M., the children had already crashed and it was time to start one of my three daily loads of laundry while Jim listened for Becca before he went off to bed. After Jim was in bed, I cuddled alone on Becca's floor in a sleeping bag for another broken night's sleep. Jim was exhausted from overworking out of the home, while I was worn out from overworking in the home with Becca and our family. I was glad the cavalry was arriving. I waved the white flag realizing I needed the nurses.

The day of the Caregivers Nursing Agency case manager appointment at our home finally came. It was uncommon for them to set up care from within the home, but with more and more seriously ill clients from Children's Hospital they were adapting. The nurse and her assistant arrived and were so startled at how tired I looked. They asked me when I had last slept.

I told them I had not had more than an hour of sleep at a time for the last thirteen days. The meeting ended before it began and they sent me to bed. They agreed to watch Matt, Marissa and Becca while I wearily departed for my mattress and pillow. I remember looking back at the nurses reading books and coloring with my kids, and I realized how bone tired I was. I'd hardly realized that I was exhausted. It was the first time in almost two weeks that I had crawled into my own bed.

An hour later a nurse summoned me to Becca's bedside. What was normal for Becca? She was blue, diaphoretic and breathing fast. The nurse called Dr. Wineinger who ordered an oximeter and oxygen. Concerned for Becca's well being and my fatigue, the nursing agency scurried to find coverage for the evening and night shift. As the evening wore on, the equipment arrived along with a relief nurse and I fell groggily back to sleep.

A concerned nurse awakened me again because Becca was "spelling."

"Spelling?" I sat up confused.

"Becca's eyes are rolling and her tongue is protruding." The nurse explained. "It lasts only a minute or two. Her breathing changes when she is not getting enough oxygen."

"My baby!" I jumped up and ran to Becca's bedside, praying as the nurse administered oxygen. Becca did better for a while and several nurses came and went. The phone rang between nurses and doctors and at midnight some new, unknown staff person sent me off to bed with reassurance that if they needed me they would wake me.

I awoke to the doorbell ringing and I rushed up to answer it. The sun was about to rise. It was the next shift nurse arriving, and the night nurse filled her in on the Becca's instability. I overheard the nurses whisper that the doctor will probably want Becca to return to the hospital. I overheard, "I am sure he will be calling soon."

I waited. Return? Return? Return Becca? I waited for the br . . . br . . . bring of the phone. I was prepared in an odd sort of way for the doctor's order. *"The order to bring Becca back to the hospital either by driving her or sending her to The Children's Hospital by ambulance."* I heard, but I didn't want to listen. *"She should not ride alone with the paramedics. Keep the nurses with you until she is admitted to the floor."*

I sent the big kids off on the school bus and the nurses packed a few of Becca's precious belongings while I dropped off Matt and Marissa at Grandma's. We loaded the oxygen, the feeding pump, the oximeter, the recently arrived Ambu bag and finally Becca into my van for the trek to the hospital. After thirteen days at home we were heading back. I knew that this was what had to be. My heart wanted her home with family. Did I fail her? I had been forewarned of the possible ins and outs, but warnings at the moment didn't matter. The reality hurt as Becca, the nurses, and I listened to Becca's music, comforting us on the trip back to the hospital.

The emergency room at The Children's Hospital was much different from our local hospital. Everything was child focused and decorated brightly and cheerily. They welcomed us and said that we were expected. Becca had her own room on the medical floor within the hour. The home care nurse provided an update of the previous night to the admitting resident so I could settle in Becca.

I was thankful for the professionalism of these strangers who had moved into my home.

Then with a kiss on the cheek I left Becca in the care of hospital staff, and again with empty arms I went home to my other five children.

- 8 -

BACK AGAIN

The difference between the medical floor and NICU was startling. I missed the constant care and friendly faces of my old hospital staff friends who I now saw casually passing in the hallway or momentarily in the cafeteria. The floor nurses were busy caring for multiple patients and I was often alone with five-month-old Becca. Mary was a welcome sight from the quietness of Becca's hospital room. She remained in daily contact with the pediatrician, nursing agency and me to keep everything in place.

Becca and I stayed busy watching television and waiting for tests, tests, and more tests. Then we waited for the results to figure out what was wrong with Becca. My sister, Martha, a nursing home administrator, got involved. She wondered why such a sick baby had been sent home with such little preparation. She knew something was not being addressed and a family friend also raised questions on our behalf shaking up hospital quality control. I had not made waves with anyone, I was 'just' a mom and all of a sudden I was being expected to meet with a team of Becca's doctors, the administration of the hospital and a state agency representative at a conference just before Christmas.

My friend Kim asked our pastor to join Jim and me. Each day I felt a twinge of more nervousness while I waited for the approaching conference. I was 'just' a mom. I was doing 'just' mom things.

Pastor Rick joined Jim and me over Becca's crib. Tears streamed down my face and thoughts pulsed in my head as he prayed for my tiny titan's healing. I have always been very shy. I had been happy being 'just' a mom. I didn't ask for this conference! I held on to Jim's hand. I stutter when I speak in public and my eighth grade teacher worked judiciously with me to garner a bit of self-confidence. I felt like I was being thrown into the lion's den. I would soon face a room full of professionals who knew what they were doing, people who knew about the discharge planning that I knew nothing about. The pastor concluded his prayer saying a few words asking God to support me in the upcoming meeting. And then Santa Claus walked in.

Becca looked up at the strange fat fellow. She tracked him with her eyes as he walked across the room. He smiled and laughed like the Santa's I had read of in my childhood. He was the Santa I had envisioned in my dreams, while I waited for the magical drop down the chimney and presents as a youth. His cheeks were rosy red, and his glasses fell off his nose just like in the books and I felt as though I was looking at pictures in a storybook as the jolly fat old fellow reached down to touch my daughter on her tiny head with his gloved hand. He told her in the gentlest of Santa Claus voices how special she was, and then he reached into his bag and pulled out a big brown teddy bear decked out in a hat and scarf for the Christmas holiday.

In the most magical movement of all, he skillfully picked up my wee one connected to medical leads and cuddled her as if he did it everyday. Becca looked deep into his eyes and smiled, and Mary snapped a Polaroid. Then ever so gently, as if he held dying infants in his arms everyday, he returned Becca to her crib. I was mesmerized as he laid his finger on his nose and disappeared from the room. Becca was still smiling!

I heard Mary prodding me to head to the meeting, and I realized that the Santa distraction had removed my anxiety. The miracle of meeting Santa made me forget what was to come. All I could see was my baby girl's joyous smile as we were ushered into a room of a dozen administrators sitting around the conference table with yellow legal pads. I hoped God had listened to my secret feeble prayer.

I recognized a couple of Becca's doctors. The empty four seats at the far end were reserved for Jim, Mary, Pastor Rick, and me. Without meeting Santa it would have been a long distance to pass by the opponents, but we were walking on Becca's smile.

They asked me to tell what happened at discharge and after. They asked what planning occurred ahead of time. Did anyone address the need for assistance? They asked me to relive the thirteen days at home. I'm 'just' a mom. I'm 'just' a mom of a very sick baby and I did what moms do. I told my story. A couple of the administrators shook their heads. They asked how I managed on such little sleep. I told them when you're a mom you do anything you can for your kids. I 'just' did it the best I could. I don't remember planning what to say, I 'just' spoke from my heart.

Mary told me as I left the room I didn't stutter once. I didn't shake and that was a miracle because I always shake. Santa and Becca gave me my bedside wish! How 'bout that? I did it!

As we left the meeting, the infectious disease doctor met us in the hall. He told us they were transferring Becca to the Pediatric Intensive Care Unit (PICU). Some of the results of the blood work and the new heart tests were in, and Becca's heart was failing further. Her white blood count was nearly eighty thousand. The last check of her vitals had revealed that she had spiked another fever. They were not comfortable having her unattended on the floor as she needed constant monitoring.

Becca had already been in the hospital a week and I struggled when it came time to leave her. I wondered why they placed her alone away from the nursing desk? At home she never left my side. I knew how much she gagged and choked and needed to be suctioned with the bulb syringe to help her clear her airway. With Becca in PICU I could go home without being concerned for her safety. I wondered if the meeting and whispers from the administration had something to do with the transfer. God had answered my feeble prayer that I asked Him secretly while Santa stood over Becca if I could be His witness. I asked him to help me stay calm and be truthful. I told God I wanted to be direct when I addressed the men and women in white coats.

Less than six weeks later I ran into one of Becca's nurses from the NICU who whispered that one of their nurses was promoted to be a full time Newborn Intensive Care Discharge Planner, and they were in the process of identifying another. Perhaps the fiasco my sister and friend had initiated along with the conference I participated in had something to do with it. I'll never know for sure, but I did learn that the hospital was written up for improper discharge procedures in Becca's case. Something good came out of my thirteen sleepless nights and Becca's trips to the hospital ER.

My sister Martha's call to the Office of Health Facility Complaints at the Minnesota Department of Health had stirred the pot. She had rattled more cages when she charged the hospital administration personally with inappropriate discharge planning. My sister's outreach of love made a difference not just for Becca, but also for the future safety of other children.

Becca was transported to the intensive care unit with an entourage of new doctors and specialists to oversee the intensive care doctors. With so many professionals there was confusion about who did what, but in time they untangled their respected professional roles and responsibilities. Becca continued to play tricks and each time the doctors felt secure discussing discharge, she plunged back into sickness. Then ten days before Christmas she was diagnosed with pneumonia.

I wasn't looking forward to Christmas, and now I had a baby in the pediatric intensive care unit with pneumonia. On top of that, four of my other children had started sneezing and coughing. Their little noses were red from rubbing and Matt was barking with croup. I was worn out from the past five months and I was incapable of fighting the viruses that plagued my children.

I felt sick and went to bed shivering.

I was highly allergic as a baby. As a small child I was often hospitalized with respiratory symptoms. I remember my Grandfather camping out with me in mist tents because I scared my mother when I turned blue. Finally, as an adult, I was diagnosed with an autoimmune disorder called Celiacs disease, which a couple of my children also inherited from my mother through me. To stay healthy required eating a diet that was nutritious and healthy. It meant cooking everything from scratch, remaining gluten free, and not eating junk food. Keeping a strict gluten-free diet is not cheap. I struggled to maintain groceries of any kind on our dwindling money supply. I had skipped meals to feed the kids and I no longer had the stamina or reserves to fight infection. The virus attacked the outside of my brain and my inner ears. My whole world was spinning. My lungs fought to breathe. The room spun around and around until I threw up and the doctor prescribed medication to keep me sedated. Now I had absolutely no control, even my bed wouldn't stand still!

Fortunately the kids were not too sick; they were shuffled between home and Mom's. Kristy managed simple meals and Nathan assisted. As I lay severely ill in bed, Becca struggled in intensive care with RSV (respiratory syncytial virus) a deadly killer of premature and compromised babies. With the RSV Becca forgot to take breaths and needed oxygen and the doctors gave her aerosol antiviral treatments hoping to stabilize her. Sometimes she needed the ventilator. One moment she seemed better, and then another fever would spike. As if RSV wasn't enough, her recent blood cultures indicated another systemic staph infection.

▼

The Christmas Season lineup of the Yurcek team included Jim, both sets of Grandparents, Kristy and Nathan all pulling more than their share caring for three coughing, sneezing and feverish children. They were busy wiping little noses with soft lotion tissues and tucking feverish bodies into bed. Jim thankfully still had his job and was managing a retail business at peak season, juggling family and holiday shoppers while his sedated wife lay flat on her back and is of no use to anyone. Meanwhile his gravely ill daughter lay in intensive care diagnosed with a compromised immune system, RSV, staph, pneumonia, and heart failure. The doctors were saying they didn't know from one day to the next whether she would live. On top of everything we were penniless.

Jim, my husband, my fearless leader, and my best friend could do nothing to make any of this better. My parent's couldn't and his parent's couldn't. No one and nothing could.

We needed a miracle.

- 9 -
Christmas

I sunk into despair. The holiday was fast approaching and Christmas was the last thing on our minds with Becca critically ill in the PICU and everyone else sick too. There was no money for gifts, and there was no time to buy or make anything. I was sick, tired and depressed over the circumstances we found ourselves in. If the phone rang, I was afraid to answer it because it might carry the news that Becca was worsening or no longer here. The phone was a constant reminder of trouble. It rang with bill collectors waiting for money. It rang when medical personnel had more dreaded news or another crisis for Becca. My emotions rose and fell like tidal waves, up, up, up and down, down, down. I tried not to think; not thinking was how I coped. It was like the stairs I ran at the hospital, up and down, and then I'd stop and sit, empty and mindless. I could not think about my children going without gifts at Christmas, but our lives were impossibly out of control. We had fallen into a dark hole due to no fault of my innocent children. At any moment they were going to lose their new baby sister. They were caught in the tidal wave of catastrophic illness when they needed a Santa most to give them hope. How would I explain to my children that Santa forgot them?

I was used to planning ahead and beginning in July bought two presents each month to cover birthdays and Christmas. Over the years my frugal plan had worked flawlessly. I squirreled away the hottest toys for Christmas gifts with early season purchases. While other families were school shopping I was making wishes come true. It was a challenge to make my kids birthdays and Christmas memorable. I love the holidays and I began to bargain shop for Marissa's September birthday gift. I budgeted a little each month until Christmas, finding sale and clearance treasures, completing my shopping race under budget. In November we celebrated Jim, Nathan and Ian's birthdays followed in December by Matt's birthday, and then Kristy's birthday in early January. The gifts I bought with Jim's carpet points guaranteed the boys November birthday gifts. Matt at age three was easy; all I needed was something big. Big for my little kids were exciting and ten dollars went a long way. Other than that I had nothing. We had already used the house payment money to pay for medicine, throat cultures and doctors visits for the kids and me while we were sick.

I was a rookie in the being broke game. I called Toys for Tots and discovered I was too late. They quit accepting new registrations before Thanksgiving. Luckily I remembered buried in the rafters, hidden from my sneaky children I had one gift I had purchased before things fell apart. Before Becca was born I had purchased the new pirate ship Lego set that had caught Nathan's eye. It was an expensive present, and I could put both boys' names on it. I had already cut out doll clothes and a dance costume for Marissa, but the fabric pieces remained on my closet shelf while I was sick. Now that Marissa was home from kindergarten I would not be able to get the covert sewing done, besides I was still too dizzy to sew my visions for Marissa's holiday present. My eyes were seeing double. We would share dinner with relatives and I hoped I would have a dish to pass, but my cupboards were as bare as Old Mother Hubbard's. My head spun at the thoughts of a hopeless Christmas and the room took another whirl; exhausted I took some Benadryl and fell back to sleep.

While I slept, Kristy took the picture of Becca from the fireplace and sat alone in a quiet place to cry. It was something I never knew she did until years later. People often think children don't know what's happening but they are much more a part of the reality than the adults realize. Kristy never complained and she protected us by caring for the little ones and not adding to our burdens. I worried sometimes about how this would affect her in the future. Today, she tells me it was the substance that made her strong.

The little elves in my family executed a Christmas plan. Kristy found the Christmas tree in the garage, and she and Nathan, my mechanic, assembled it. Ian and Marissa got busy cutting out paper snowflakes and hung them with dental floss from the ceiling and windows. My little red and green sewing pins stuck six stockings to the mantle. When I awoke, they surprised me with their magical transformation. I had not lifted a finger. They had carefully hung each of their hand made wooden, beaded angel and needlework ornaments crafted by Jim's parents. Hundreds of hours of love radiated from the tree centered in a carpet of paper snowflake snippets.

I explained to them that Christmas was about family and being together and sharing memories. What was going to be special about this Christmas was that the Yurceks were a family. Christmas is about the baby in the manger who brings hope to a dying world. Our baby was in the hospital and all we had was hope. After spending seven days in bed, I was regaining my strength.

Why did I feel such shame that Santa might not come this year? I prayed, *"Oh Lord, How can I find gifts for Kristy, Marissa and Matt? It is already December 23. How can I let my children down? How can I face Christmas morning empty handed? The kids' baby sister is dying. They need something good to happen. Please don't let their baby sister die at Christmas."*

My children were ready for Christmas. I was not. I couldn't expect my parents to shower my children with toys; they were struggling with my dad's recent unemployment. My parents blessed my children with attention, but had no financial resources to give.

Becca was transferred to the Pediatric Intensive Care Unit (PICU) just as I had fallen ill. It had been a very long nine days and finally the kids and I were well. I was healthy enough to see Becca and had been given clearance to drive. I was no longer dizzy.

The PICU had a circular desk, and different beds surrounded

it. Off to the side with glass doors were the isolation rooms. One of them housed my Becca, who looked so tiny in the crib in such a big room. She was on oxygen, and they explained to me that she kept forgetting to breathe due to the RSV and pneumonia. The respiratory therapist gave her a treatment to help clear her lungs. She had a blood staph infection, her feedings were on hold, and they were giving her nutrition and fluid by IV. Her heart was in failure. Merry Christmas was far from my thoughts. Bah Humbug! This was not merry, not merry at all. I was dreading Christmas and I was feeling like Ebenezer Scrooge.

Startled out of my doldrums, Mary was standing in front of me saying hello. The nurses had called her to let her know I had arrived. She had something she needed me to sign. That's all I had been doing, signing, and waiting, and hoping, and praying. Bah Humbug!

She took me to her office. I had no idea where her office was as she always brought the paperwork to me. She opened the door and picked up a large shopping bag. Her smile radiated. "Merry Christmas!" she exclaimed. The nurses had shopped for families who would be without for the holidays. They picked out a present for each one of my six kids. They even purchased the batteries for the remote control car for Nathan. They thought of everything. The bag contained a roll of wrapping paper, bows and even the tape. It's nooks and crannies were filled with little treats – a box of candy canes and five chocolate Santa Clauses to peek out of the top of the stockings. Miracles really do happen and my wish had been granted. My kids would have Christmas.

Mary told me that the hospital employees often play Santa for families to make sure they would not face the holidays empty handed. She knew that if I were skipping meals to feed the children, there would be nothing for Christmas.

I returned to Becca's isolation room. She was much too sick to be held. I savored a moment of calm and thankfulness. Slowly I was learning to savor tiny moments of peace and tranquility. I stayed by her side quietly reading before heading home with my miracle sack. I felt so thankful for the graciousness of these kind people. With my ritual kiss goodbye and whispering I love you, I prayed to her angels that she would be here when I returned.

My kids are notoriously nosy and I wanted to surprise them on Christmas morning. I rushed off to pick up Matt and Marissa at Mom's and stashed the Christmas gifts before the older ones had a clue. While I had been sick, Mom had been busy and blessed us with another surprise. She had sewn Kristy and Marissa new Christmas dresses and my aunt had bought sweaters for the three boys. All my five kids would have new matching outfits to wear for Christmas.

Jim closed the store early on Christmas Eve and helped me dress the little kids for the Christmas Eve service. I told Jim my secret miracle and we smiled eye messages across the heads of our stair step sized children sitting between us in the church pew. We sang for the birth of baby Jesus and our hearts cried out for a Christmas miracle for Becca. After the service the kids played in the manger, Marissa and Matt rode the lifelike donkey proclaiming they were on their way to Bethlehem while I stared down at the tiny doll in the manger and said a quiet prayer for my little baby lying so far away, all alone, in a bed in the PICU. We needed hope in the midst of such incredible sorrow.

Mom invited us for cake and ice cream after the service, but I had other plans. Families are supposed to be together and I was not going to allow Becca to be alone on Christmas. We all went to the hospital to visit Becca, but only Kristy and I were able to go to PICU. Jim stayed with the other kids in the lobby while Kristy and I went to say Merry Christmas to Becca. Each child had made Becca a card and the nurse taped the cards to the wall above her bed. I hung Becca's handmade stocking on the foot of her crib, putting on the Christmas music Kristy had recorded. I made a special Christmas wish, asking for a miracle for Becca. I left her again with a kiss on her feverish cheek and wished her a Merry Christmas and a very blessed goodnight. The walk from PICU to the lobby seemed endless, my heart heavy laden with grief, babies should be home with mommies and daddies on Christmas Eve.

Fresh snow had fallen, and instead of hurrying home on the

freeway we meandered past the lighted mansions on Summit Avenue of St. Paul. We passed the Cathedral and the Governor's manor. The children marveled at the beautifully decorated homes. Matt clapped his hands in joy, while the others argued over which house was the favorite. Ian and Kristy engaged in a competitive battle. Marissa's face was lit up from the wonder of the lights and its beauty. The kids were enjoying the ride so much that we wound our way home through parks, and lakes, and residential streets for over an hour. It was peaceful and calming. The kids quieted and Matt fell asleep.

Scattered snowflakes were falling and Jim and I listened to the Christmas music playing from the radio. The radio DJ announced that Santa was spotted circling the globe, and Marissa and Ian excitingly questioned how he managed to get all the work done in one evening?

This explanation I left to Jim, it was his turn to try to satisfy his children's curiosity. His eyes sparkled as he told them Santa was magic and can make anything happen if you only believe. It was a heavenly ride. I reached across the seat setting my hand on Jim's knee. Jim's answer had satisfied the children's curiosity, and Kristy had caught my glare, playing along with the magic of the moment.

It was nearly midnight when we arrived home and the house was pitch black to save on electricity. As we pulled in the driveway, the mini van's lights shone upon dark shadows lying near the door. Jim hopped out of the van to see what was going on. Then he summoned us as if it were nothing.

As I reached in the back seat to get sleeping Matt, the children shrieked, "Santa came! He came! Santa was already here!"

What were they talking about? I grabbed a confused, groggy Matt. There were nearly a dozen or so thirty-gallon black trash bags left sitting by our front door. Jim and the big kids carried in the bags.

The children tore open the plastic bags to discover dozens of wrapped presents with their names on them. It was blessed chaos. There were tons of groceries, toilet paper, and shampoo. Everything we were out of. Kristy, Nathan and Ian were stacking the packages by the tree while Marissa and Matt played mountain climbers scaling the huge mounds of packages. Kristy screamed as she caught the tree from falling. Marissa narrowly escaped a plunge from the top of Gift Mountain. Our children were bouncing off the walls, but we finally convinced them that it wasn't Christmas yet, and Santa required they open presents on Christmas morning like in *The Night Before Christmas.* They didn't argue because we had just read the story.

Marissa wondered why Santa left them outside, instead of bringing them down the chimney. Ian, who always had an answer for everything, announced, "he had so much dummy; if he brought the bags down the chimney, he would get the chimney stopped up." Kristy added "that the house was locked and he could not bring them in the door." Finally they all scampered off to their rooms and soon were snuggled in beds dreaming of Christmas miracles.

Shortly after midnight the phone rang. It was the resident from PICU calling us to let us know Becca had turned the corner and they upgraded her status to stable. She was improving and was breathing easier so they had removed the ventilator; Becca was now breathing on her own and on supplemental oxygen! Becca was getting better! My Christmas prayers had been answered. And someone, some Santa somewhere had fulfilled my wishes. He or she arrived with bags of toys, and goodies, and groceries. My cupboards would no longer be bare. Jim and I had no means to provide for our family, yet someone, somewhere, knew our needs. I thanked the baby in the manger for this Christmas miracle.

Jim and I put away the much-needed groceries. Two turkeys, packages of hamburger and chicken went into the freezer. We put the canned goods on the shelves . . .apples and oranges, carrots and potatoes, and onions . . . bathroom and hygiene products. There were even a couple loaves of expensive rice bread. Whoever brought this Christmas miracle, had not forgotten anything. They had even picked up a double pack of diapers for Matt who was regressing from his potty training in his upside down life.

The real Christmas miracles were hidden in the tiny details. Buried deep in one of the bags I discovered a brand new pair of much needed white Reebok tennis shoes for me. They fit perfectly. We filled the stockings with candy and small gifts from the bags the kids had not seen. With the gifts from the hospital and the one from us for Nathan and Ian, we had more presents than we had ever imagined. Our room looked like a Hollywood movie Christmas morning scene. Where did all this come from?

Jim and I crawled into bed, hoping to get a few hours of sleep before the kids scrambled upon us to open their presents. They were tired from the late night and for the first time ever on Christmas morning; they slept until 8:00 A.M..

Kristy in her sweats and the little ones in their blanketed sleepers tore into the pile of packages. One, two, three, four, five, six, seven, I lost count of the gifts they each received. Nathan screamed pulling out a pair of roller blades, the current hottest trend retailing at $150 a pair. Who had done this? Ian soon discovered he had a pair too! Kristy found a boom box, a jewelry box, curling iron and music to play. Packages marked to the Yurcek family contained a VCR to replace the one that had been stolen when our house had been robbed and ransacked right before Becca's birth. There were movies, games, books, colored markers, and art kits for each child. Even Becca was not forgotten. She got new clothes, a diaper bag, several new pink animals and more music. Marissa found a big package with a dollhouse and furniture. She was surrounded in pink heaven. Matt tunneled and laughed through the wrapping paper and boxes. We corralled him to open his presents, a big floppy eared dog, trucks, cars and a train track. The boys tried to set up their new remote control car racing set in the middle of the wrapping mess.

Jim was not to be forgotten and he discovered new socks, sweats, jeans and a belt. He handed me a tiny box from under the tree that he discovered while we were cleaning up and making sure all the tiny toy pieces were not thrown away with the mountain of boxes and wrapping paper. Inside was a solid sterling silver heart necklace with six tiny stones. The necklace was a reminder of hope, a mother's heart with my six precious children. The six little diamonds sparkled in rainbow colors from our Christmas tree. It was bittersweet to look at as Becca's heart was slowly failing. But I reminded myself that for today Becca was doing better, and this Christmas we had witnessed a true miracle. Some unknown Santa with a caring heart had done all this for us. But who, how, when?

▼

No longer were our cupboards bare. The kids and I made a fresh fruit salad with real whipped cream. Kristy peeled the apples and Nathan chopped them along with slicing frozen strawberries. Marissa cut banana coins with a bread knife and Ian added one handful of marshmallows to his mouth before adding the next handful to the magical miracle bowl of Christmas fruit.

We dressed for Christmas dinner at my cousins. The family celebrated the day together with aunts and uncles, cousins and second cousins. All were there but one, our Becca.

No longer would we be hungry again. We had food for the next month until our food stamp case opened. The kids had new toys to keep them occupied. We had warm clothing and mittens. I later discovered when our bills arrived, that some unknown Santa paid our phone bill, the utility bills, and our car insurance! We will be forever grateful for the gifts of that year, and we will never forget we witnessed a true Christmas miracle. I have from then on remembered to give back to others as you did for us. Thank you! What you did for us that year was unbelievable! You gave us the gift of hope and belief in miracles.

Buried in one of the bags of the hundreds of dollars in gifts we found a card, wishing us a "Merry Christmas and to all, and to all a good night. You are loved! Santa."

Those were the same words whispered in tiny Becca's ear ten days earlier. Was it connected?

Over the next few years, the miracles continued helping us when we needed it most. I tried to find who our anonymous Santa was but we never discovered the giver of the gifts. Whoever it was did not want to be found out. Maybe someday that person or persons will read my writing, and I will finally be able to thank her or him for our Christmas miracle and generosity.

Perhaps, we will never know.

- 10 -

BELIEVE

Becca continued to improve and the doctors turned their attention to discharge planning. This time the home nursing agency was an integral part in helping to get ready for Becca's homecoming. It was obvious procedures of discharging ill children had changed and incredible transformations were happening to make an appropriate transition home.

While I prepared for Becca, the kids ran loose in holiday glee. I had been sick for nearly two weeks before Christmas and the house was cluttered and messy. I spent my days meeting with nurses, training, doing paperwork and caring for Becca. I was overwhelmed with hospital and the nursing agency 'to do' lists. In the evening I tried to keep the kids fed. I no longer had the energy to keep up on my never-ending mountains of laundry and housework.

Becca graduated out of isolation, but she was still too sick to be discharged to the medical unit so she remained in intensive care while the hospital strengthened her to return home. Mary busily coordinated payer systems. She filled out the complex forms to get Becca's homecare covered under a home and community based waiver. She explained that this meant Becca could be at home with the same level of care as a child who needed to be in the hospital.

Because of another mom's fight for her hospitalized daughter, the Katie Beckett Waiver allowed children to qualify for Medicaid and get the supports needed to be at home with family instead of languishing in the hospital. The other Children's Hospital had been successfully getting very sick children home for a year or so. This was very new to Mary, and Mary's first job after completing her Master's Degree was working with the new Children's Discharge coordinator. Minnesota had two hundred slots for people of all ages under this waiver. When one opened up, another person qualified for a slot. Mary applied for Becca to obtain one of those waivers. She applied for the Minnesota equivalent of the Katie Beckett Waiver, called TEFRA (Tax Equity and Fiscal Responsibility Act). Becca would be one of the first children out of our Children's Hospital to come home under the waiver.

TEFRA bases the child's qualifying information for Medicaid on the child's disability and as a family of one. This would allow us to make more money and no longer be forced into poverty to pay for Becca's catastrophic health care costs. We could apply for Social Security Disability (SSI) payments for Becca from the federal government. Mary told us some children were just now qualifying for those funds. It could take months to be approved, but then it would give us over four hundred dollars a month to pay for things that she needed to be at home.

It sounded too good to be true.

We were getting help for Becca.

My training as a medical secretary and working in an office managing accounting and payroll records for two hundred employees rose to the occasion as I waded through the red tape of the welfare system. In filling out the twenty-page application, we learned that the children and I possibly qualified for Medicaid, too. The county opened our case for the food stamps I applied for in December. There was a glimmer of hope. Just as I finished one task another was assigned. I spent the cold dark days of January drowning in paperwork. I signed so many forms my hand cramped. I provided proof: proof of income, proof of mortgage payments, and proof of utility bills. I scrounged for money to get duplicates of birth certificates of my very alive and underfoot children.

I filed for social security cards for Matt, Marissa, Ian, and Becca. I struggled with proof, proof and more proof for the social security cards. How could a person with a disability ever achieve this mass of completed paperwork? I wondered how a struggling parent or undereducated person ever managed. In time I realized many people who deserve services don't get them because they are incapable of jumping through the hoops. They struggled to prove their identities and without a social security card, birth certificate, or picture ID it is impossible. The maze of getting help is so complex; I figured many who needed help the most gave up.

Three new home nurses joined Becca at the hospital for training with her existing ICU hospital team. My friend, Val, who I had come to depend on for help with the kids was a Registered Nurse and was hired by the agency to help coordinate Becca's homecoming.

The doctors ordered an apnea monitor to add to our electronic collection to reassure me Becca was all right when I was out of the room. Anyone who had witnessed Becca's choking and gagging spells would be wary of having her unmonitored. Becca was enrolled in the Apnea program. I didn't realize it, but I had become a trusted advocate for my daughter while I still thought of myself as 'just' a mom.

We fell into a medical training camp; Jim and I were trained in infant and child CPR in the middle of our living room. Not wanting to be left out, Kristy, now eleven insisted on being a team member and she asked such good questions that the instructor gave her hands-on training, practicing on the baby doll mannequin. I received lessons on the apnea monitor at the hospital. I got instructions on using the suction machine to clear secretions from the back of her throat if they began to clog her airways and she began to choke. Becca had floppy muscles in her throat and lungs along with her the inability to swallow and sometimes she needed help to keep her airway open.

Becca's home nursery now looked like a pediatric intensive care center. The oxygen tanks sat next to the side of her bed. The five-foot stainless metal IV pole sat next to the head of the bed attached to the feeding pump. The kid's plastic Little Tykes white toy box with its blue plastic lid held the apnea monitor and suction machine so it could reach the crib. The leads from the monitor had to connect to Becca most times. We found a small folding table to set up for the nurses' paperwork. The huge four-inch binder looked like overkill, but once Becca came home I watched it fill up fast. Jim built shelves above the table for all the medications and supplies to keep them out of reach of mischievous Matt.

A mom from our church gave Jim a changing table for Becca's nursery. I couldn't believe my eyes when he came home with it, it matched the dark wood crib we had bought new when Matt was a baby. The girls white with pink printed wallpaper matched the dusty blue changing table skirt with rosy pink bunnies and softened the medical look of the room. The free blue stroller sat in the last remaining corner. After washing everything, I sewed new white curtains out of an old sheet and Kristy helped me stencil them with blue bunnies and pink hearts. Everything had to be disinfected, so I washed the walls and surfaces of everything. I washed all the clothes from the dresser. The new air cleaner purchased with this month's mortgage money sucked the old air out of the nursery and spit clean air back in. With all the decorating the room did not look like the stark intensive care of the hospital I was used to, but a dainty calm place for Becca to come home.

I told Mary I was tired and running out of energy. My lungs had barely recovered after my bout of influenza. For the first years of my life, I was in and out of the hospital with lung problems and I got winded every time I got sick. I didn't want my asthma to return. Mary talked to Pastor Rick who was involved with helping us get Becca home. He made arrangements with my mom and sister to have the ladies from the church clean my house. It had faced weeks of neglect and my laundry looked impossible to complete. I couldn't do it all; I was getting sick again.

Mom and my sister commented that they were worried about what the ladies in the church would think of my messy house. That was all I needed to hear. I was trying to be the 'good daughter,' it was already Monday, and the helpful ladies were arriving on Wednesday. I couldn't embarrass my extended family in front of the church parishioners so I stayed up all night, running laundry around the clock. I 'Super Mom' cleaned everything, jumping from one area to the next, angrily scrubbing, straightening, and vacuuming. I was angry about how hard and unfair our circumstances were. I scrubbed harder and harder; my anger and frustration surfaced. I straightened more and more. I pushed the vacuum cleaner as hard as I could across the carpeting. I scrubbed the walls, and I bleached the grout in the bathroom with my only toothbrush. Then without sleep I got in my car to drop off Matt and Marissa at Grandma's and proceeded to the hospital to visit Becca.

When I returned home I realized I had made a dent in the disaster but not enough to please Mom and the church ladies. So I scrubbed the floors and scoured the countertops. I washed the walls and changed the sheets. I ran up the stairs and down the stairs putting away clean laundry before crashing at 3:00 A.M.. Mom volunteered to care for the children while the church ladies cleaned my house. My sister, Martha offered to host the event with donuts and coffee. They cleaned my oven and changed the burner pans on my stove. They washed our windows and finished up what little remained. They left after two hours of visiting and chatting over coffee and treats and my house was totally spotless.

Mary noticed I was exceptionally tired when I arrived to visit with Becca. I told her how pressured I felt from my mom and sister about the condition of my home. I trusted Mary and I told her that I had four hours sleep in the last two nights while I tried to get caught up on my housework before the ladies arrived to clean.

Mary shook her head in disbelief. Why on earth had I worked so hard? My baby had been in the hospital for over six months. Our lives were stressed. What on earth was I thinking to expect myself to have a totally clean house?

I told her I didn't want to make trouble and I always did as expected. She smiled a crooked little smile and shook her head again. Then she proceeded to give me a lecture on expectations. She told me that no one could handle all that I had had to deal with without help. From now on she was making the arrangements with Pastor Rick herself and bypassing my family. Obviously if I had to please everyone before I accepted help from others, good intentions would continue to backfire.

The Yurcek's were ready for D-day and Becca's arrival. The state and county paperwork was filed and the doctors cleared our tiny titan as stable enough for discharge. They announced a 'Care Conference' with a couple of Becca's doctors to talk about what to expect regarding her future. The evening before the care conference I felt the same fear and anxiety I experienced before the quality control meeting.

I journaled.

Here I am again. I was so exhausted. I collapsed in sleep last night. I was sure I would get a good night's sleep. Wrong! I woke up and am so wide-awake. My mind is churning so fast. This is getting to be a habit. Usually I wait until at least two in the morning for this. Twelve-thirty is ridiculous. I know what I have to do. Get up, run the bathwater, and find my journal.

I ran the bathwater, nice and hot. I added bubbles and then I slid down to contemplate and write in my journal.

The Mission:

Why I woke up and why I'm stressed.

"Today I get to sit and try to address with the docs what we need to get Becca home and learn the guidelines of what we must do. They will ask questions of me that I have to be able to answer clearly and know what to say. I did it before. I knew my mission from the previous care conference. I knew I couldn't speak clearly and worried

that the words would not be there. I did it even better than I would ever have dreamed possible.

This I need to do again. So OK Lord, this is up to You! Give me the words when I need them. Give me the questions I need to ask. Give me the strength to hear the words that will break my heart when we have to talk about what the future might hold. Make this whole thing go smoothly."

I was so into writing that my bath water turned cold. I added hot water to warm it up so I could relax and continue meditating in preparation for the coming day. I couldn't sleep. I knew this conference should be easier. My entire support network would be there, Val, my friend and now Becca's home nurse, Pastor Rick, our spiritual and emotional guide, and Jim. My poor Jim was struggling so to make financial ends meet. He knew little of Becca's circumstances. At least he was at my side.

I sat in the cooling water thinking that the troops were backing me up, and the reserves were called in. I was learning that when it came to helping Becca I could do anything.

I breathed deeply and took up my pen.

I think ahead sometimes. I hear people telling me that what I am doing and how I am handling things is amazing. I am clouded on this one. I am too hard on Ann. If I quit being so hard on me, perhaps I can see some of what I am hearing. Val says some day I will have to share my experiences with others. She says maybe not now, but later. She has her ideas on how this may work: The women's group at church (Ann does not speak in front of people) I told her. She said, "You do now." Or through this journal, it may have to be shared. (I

> *told her I don't know how to write. She said, "you do now." I guess I am, so I do, don't I) I leave myself open for what lies ahead. If I make no demand on myself and leave everything open, things will come.*

Did Val predict my future or did she plant the seed that tears watered? While writing our story I found my journal of those early moments. My coping by writing opened the door to this book. My public speaking grew as I stood up as a strong voice for Becca. My fear and shyness were laid down as I took up the cross for my daughter to meet her needs.

▼

The meeting grated at the souls of the persons who loved this tiny titan. I asked what to do if Becca's heart stopped. They countered by asking when would we choose not to resuscitate her. When would we stop heroic treatments to prolong our baby's life? I held back the tears that were welling up in my eyes. I asked questions past the lump in my throat that was trying to prevent me from speaking. Do not resuscitate orders would be our decision, how can a mom choose to let her precious baby go?

They talked about her failing heart. Dr. Hesslein, the cardiologist, was afraid that it might stop at anytime. He told us that the stenosis in the pulmonary valve was worsening and the thickened walls in her heart were becoming thicker the harder it worked. He told us some babies with cardiomyopathy (the thickened walls) did well with a heart transplant, but with Becca's unknown immune problems, she would not be eligible for a new heart.

Jim and I expressed our wishes for Becca.

If she was not breathing, and her heart stopped . . . Jim and I agreed . . . we chose to have them try to resuscitate her if she was not breathing just in case it was an airway problem instead of heart failure. Jim squeezed my hand in support.

The doctors forewarned us that she probably would not survive resuscitation. Her heart was too damaged to keep going, but they would try. How could I let her go without a fight? I knew it was far beyond my control and our time with Becca was limited; she was going to die sooner versus later. I understood they expected the time at home to be short and this would be a long road filled with heart-break and uncertainty. We were possibly bringing our baby home to die. Hope was all we had, in the midst of our sorrow.

We would not give up without a fight. As long as Becca wanted to fight, so would we.

I walked away from the meeting in low spirits and was soon accompanied by Dr. Hesselein, Becca's cardiologist. I asked him point blank if there was any hope. He didn't know what the future would hold but he was certain that we could not give up on her. There were good pieces we could hold on to. Her heart had not changed in two months and the diuretic was holding the heart failure in check. He said he was hanging on to hope for now and I had to think of each and every moment we had together as a gift.

It was the first time Jim had to face the reality of his daughter's possible death. I had gotten used to hearing such upsetting news and had chosen to shelter him from the harsh realities. I believed he needed to work while I cared for Becca and our family. He already worried about losing his job and having no money to provide for his family. Jim sat silently and I could tell by his body language he was devastated, yet there was nothing I could say to help him. I hate quiet! The silence between us was deafening. We sat next to each other isolated and alone in our independent thoughts.

From my journal I read,

They all sounded so bleak. They sounded like there was no hope. I have accepted that we may lose Becca at any time. Hearing people saying it was so hard. I lost it afterward. No matter what, I have to learn to deal with all of this. I know I have to allow myself to be sad. Damn it all! It hurts like hell!!! I shouldn't feel disappointed in myself when

I lose it, I am Becca's mother and I love her so.

Sixteen years later new tears fell as I relived these moments to write our story.

The next day, the hospital had a second care conference to merge our wishes and the capabilities of Becca's service teams. Jim's employer had been giving us trouble about adding Becca to our insurance plan. He told Jim that if he went to this conference he was walking away from his job as manager. They could not fire him, but he would be demoted to a carpet sales job and be on straight commission. We talked about the options Jim had been given. How could someone be so cruel as to demote someone on the day of discharging his daughter after her months in the hospital? He proclaimed to be a man of faith and he preached to his employees about church and the road to heaven. He certainly didn't practice what he preached. No one should force anyone to make that kind of decision.

Jim always wanted to do the right thing and he was now in a no win position. He wanted to provide for his family and he wanted to care for his family. The two were opposing forces. Between the stress of the job and the complexities of his family he had been having a hard time getting out of bed each morning to go to work. He bravely took the demotion and decided to begin to look for a new job.

Jim, Val, Pastor Rick, and I entered a room full of new faces. I recognized the social workers, the doctors, and the nursing agency personnel. I heard people names and agency names. There were so many. I tried to catch the agency names and their job roles. It was confusing and my mind was bending as the county public health nurse, the independent school district early intervention coordinator, the school district physical therapist, the school district occupational therapist, the caseworker from the county department of human resources, and a liaison from some sort of non-profit organization for families with children with disabilities introduced themselves. It was a standing room only crowd.

Jim counted twenty-eight persons and noted that thirteen of

Becca's doctors were missing. Was this what it would take to get his little daughter the help she needed?

I remained quietly astounded, remembering Becca's first discharge in November. If this is what it took to get her out of the hospital and to support her care I was grateful that I no longer had to do it alone. It was an awakening to Jim and me of the enormity of the care our Tiny Titan required as each agency discussed what they were prepared to offer.

Mary and the new discharge planner had thought of everything. They had to protect the Yurceks and all the professionals who provided care, but most importantly Becca.

The physical therapist would work to strengthen her floppy body and help her learn to control her muscles after she had lost oxygen when her heart stopped at two-months-old. The occupational therapists would look at fine motor and daily tasks. The speech therapists would work on feeding, eating, and swallowing issues. They would help our silent daughter learn to use her mouth and to make noise. The county agencies would control the hours on her waiver and the services she would receive. The nursing agency explained how they would provide the nurses and coordinate the care plan with the treating professionals. Then there were food stamps for the family and Medicaid for our other children to keep everyone at home healthy.

Plans were discussed about how Becca would return to the hospital when she needed to come back in. Plans were laid for calling the physicians for the updates. The heart and immune doctors explained the severity of Becca's conditions and what to monitor.

The meeting discussion changed from strategy to future outcomes. We discussed the plan if Becca's breathing stopped. Yes, Jim and Ann had been trained to use the Ambu Bag to help her breathe and initiate CPR. They discussed Jim's and my resuscitation wishes and our decision about the DNR order. They discussed the emergency procedures to be activated in case Becca died at home.

Second by second they dissected Becca's mammoth needs. I kept telling myself to think with my head as they stomped on my heart. If Becca died, we would call the pediatrician's office to document the time of death with the nursing agency. This would help us avoid our family having to face the inquest and allegations of the police and the child protective service interviews. I was told that all children who died at home, had to be "investigated and questioned" by the authorities. By doing this we could protect against the removal of our other children to shelters or foster care by child protective services while the investigations were in process. What? Why child protection? We never hurt any of our children. I wanted to scream, but it was no use. We are fighting to help Becca, but because we could not prevent her from dying, we could be blamed and were guilty until proven innocent. It seemed unforgiving to me, when a family is in crisis over losing a child, that we would be forced to worry about losing our surviving children. I kept telling myself to think logically, but everything seemed very upside down and twisted.

Arrangements were made for medication orders. Lines of communications were put in place for updates and orders from the doctors. Everything was documented. It was profound the number of details assembled for one very small and fragile human being. One phone call later, we were approved for a waiver slot. Becca was ready to come home.

I sat astounded at the magnitude of it all. Twenty-eight professionals representing a multitude of agencies were committed not only to help Becca survive, but to help her succeed in hopes of a miracle. We had support; we did not have to face the uncertainty alone.

Jim and I walked to see our daughter. She smiled, her eyes sparkled, her deep dimples made us laugh. She was a Tiny Titan all right and if she believed, then we believed. And if we three believed then perhaps, just perhaps, anything was possible.

- 11 -
HOME SWEET HOME

Since a hospital is the worst place in the winter months for a baby with immune problems we needed to get Becca out of the hospital. We couldn't let wily hospital bugs and germs of influenzas, and viruses and staph kill our baby.

Everything was set to go! At long last Becca was coming home!

The last six months were hard on everyone. Our family needed time with Becca. Matt was clingy and had regressed completely back into diapers. Once we talked openly and honestly about the facts, even little Matt and Marissa felt more at ease. The older kids had always been filled in on the truth. I learned early on that keeping secrets from them was not the right thing to do and they were smarter than I gave them credit for. Kids sense something is going on and they react to the stress. It was important when their whole world was seemingly falling apart they could still trust us. We told them that their baby sister may die, and as sad as it was, at least we had the truth out in the open. In time I found the kids were resilient, they were affected but they survive, if we do.

Just as I explained to the kids I didn't have ten dollars to buy diapers to bring Becca home, Pastor Rick called saying he had a hundred dollar check for our family from the benevolent offering they take on communion Sunday. It was the miracle I had prayed for and it was just in time to buy diapers, paper towels and kid smelling disinfectant liquid soap for the bathroom so the kids could easily wash their hands anytime they wanted to play with Becca.

I was so excited I called my Mom to tell her the great news and she immediately burst my bubble. She and Dad were just getting back on their feet after his time of unemployment and she worried about what people would think of a family that couldn't take care of its own. It saddened me that she felt judged because they also were going through a difficult time. Mom and Dad had helped for so many months when Becca was in the hospital; they fed my children hundreds of meals, watched Matt and Marissa every single day and gave the older children attention when they returned from school when I had to be away. They bailed me out countless times when I became stranded from a broken down car, or provided a ride when Jim couldn't get away from work without losing his job. I couldn't have done it without them and I was grateful to my parents. But my parents were proud people and they didn't want anyone to know we were struggling. It felt like they were ashamed of me.

I tried to return the check to Pastor Rick, but he refused to take it. It was the policy of the church that no one knew the recipients of the offering except for him. According to Pastor Rick, Mom should let go of her worry and let others have the gift of being able to help. Who cares what it looked like to anyone else? Pastor Rick told me he'd keep a secret if I could. I needed to cash the check, go buy diapers and fill my empty gas tank for the trip to bring Becca home at long last.

The mailbox held our next miracle "two months of food stamp coupons!" Nathan screamed as he counted them, "it was over six hundred dollars!"

I had worked diligently to stretch a hundred dollars to feed all seven of the Yurceks for a month. Now we had hit the food lottery! Finally, the kids could eat until they were full and Jim and I could eat again. I frugally filled our pantry, mixing store sales and specials with coupons and food stamps. I didn't want to waste a dime; I was afraid this windfall would disappear. Stocked with groceries and baby supplies we were ready for Becca's arrival.

Jim wanted to come to the hospital to fetch Becca, but he

couldn't. Jim's new demotion agreement was simple; if he didn't sell carpet, he didn't get paid. His boss made it very clear he did not want Jim with the company. Val offered to join me and drive her own car to pick up our tiny baby, along with an excited Matt and Marissa. We were down to one car. With Val's offer, I didn't need to worry about taking Jim to work and picking him up after Becca came home, plus with two adults we could handle both little kids and the baby. Once again we signed the discharge paperwork and loaded up all the gear to bring Becca home. This last month stay in the hospital seemed like an eternity.

At six-months-old, Becca barely weighed ten pounds with much of that weight being fluid build up from her failing heart and impaired lymphatic system. The doctors now were pretty sure she had Noonan syndrome and the syndrome commonly included lymph problems. In rare cases fluid even leaked into the chest cavity, lungs and gastrointestinal tract. We later learned that was just another of Becca's many anomalies associated with her syndrome.

Val got the honor of dressing Becca in another new designer outfit I had sewn for her homecoming. Sewing and designing clothing was the one tiny creative outlet of sanity I had left. I busily made itsy bitsy sleepers with pink roses, blue sleepers with little puppies and teeny, tiny booties. I made others with sweet little ruffles and others with footballs. I dropped off a number of the tiny new outfits along with my invoice to the gift shop on the way out, thankful for their support in keeping our family afloat. I tucked the business and discharge papers into the diaper bag and we said our goodbyes and were on our way home, to a very different home than any of the Yurceks were used to.

Becca's homecoming created the need for a new routine. The nurses came and went seven days a week with the first shift starting at 7:00 A.M. and continuing with the second shift leaving at 11:00 P.M.. Having someone in my home felt reassuring and I looked at our tidy little group like the Brady Bunch with 'eight' Alices. We had 'Alice' Val, my friend and 'Alice,' Diane the Becca spoiler. We had Grandma 'Alice' Zoe who raised six children and now enjoyed her grandchildren, including a little granddaughter with Downs. And we had 'Alice,' Deb One, a pastor's wife and mother of three and 'Alice' Deb Two who was married and childless. We had 'Alice' Cheryl who surprised me when we discovered I had worked for her father while Jim was in college when Kristy was a baby. And last but not least we had 'Alice,' Mary, the Jim surpriser. There are no secrets when you have shifts of nursing in your home day in and day out.

We had nurses to offer stability and help through this unplanned and uncharted journey. I felt relieved and settled in with a new 'normal' for our 'new family.' The 'Yurcek Bunch.' I realized that I had a choice. I could fight the intrusion or turn it around as part of the job description of a family with extra-ordinary needs. I had already tried to care for Becca alone, and I knew it wasn't feasible, even though my heart wanted to be able to do it all. I had accepted my limitations. The nurses would have to stay if Becca stayed.

While I enjoyed and felt secure working with the Alices, Jim had a hard time with the nurses in the house. He was not used to the intrusion of working with in-home professionals. For six months he had worked diligently as he struggled to provide for his family, while I, almost single-handedly, managed Becca's being in the hospital. Jim struggled with the Nurse Vaders who did things like pop into the bathroom without knocking as he climbed out of the shower. Red-faced nurse 'Alice' Mary quickly departed to leave him to dry off alone. Later she shared her embarrassment over the moment and we joked about it. She told me it was just part of having in home care.

With so many people coming and going for Becca and taking over his family, Jim felt pushed out. There were no male nurses to talk to, only nine strong and passionate women caring for a dying tiny human being. He had originally felt abandoned when I developed a close relationship with Mary, the social worker. I shared all my thoughts and details with her believing I was protecting Jim from the trauma of the reality of Becca. Neither he nor I understood the different way that men handle the stress of a critically ill child. At that time no one supported the dads who are too busy at work trying to financially save the family.

The time Jim had left for free time after working eighty or more hours a week he spent with his feet up relaxing in front of the television or sleeping. Or as he appropriately stated, trying to stay out of the way. He felt forgotten in 'no man's land,' dumped out and pushed aside.

Having five kids in the house and nurses coming and going sixteen hours each day made for busy days. The phone rang with news from the agency. The phone rang with information from the therapists. The phone rang with updates from the doctors. The nurses and I shared ideas of care for Becca. While they taught me nursing skills, I filled them in on what was normal for her and taught them how things were done in the hospital. We worked together and learned from each other. From their experiences with the special needs of kids in other homes, they shared tricks that the hospital staff had not thought of to manage Becca's feedings.

The nurses and I used creative ingenuity to help Becca. We needed to vent her tube. Poor little Becca couldn't tolerate feedings directly into her G-tube and her little tummy was puffed and swollen with gas. I ran to my sewing box to get red bias tape. I ran to the toy box to get red and blue and yellow plastic links. The tape would suspend over Becca's crib, a plastic link would securely hold an open sixty cc syringe. The feeding pump tubing dripped a drop at a time into Becca and allowed the air bubbles to escape so she would be less uncomfortable. The pump with its thin tubing carefully measured 50 cc or less than two ounces of formula one drip at a time to help her impaired GI tract have the best chance of absorption. Taped securely this trick eliminated stressing her as she was fed.

The nurses worked with the doctors to find a formula she tolerated better as she was not gaining weight. While we played the music on the tape recorder, Becca played musical formulas and no formula seemed to work. We had soon exhausted nearly a dozen varieties before settling for one that caused the least amount of discomfort, though it was still inadequate. The doctors worked to get the calorie count up with specialized formula, all while limiting Becca's precarious fluid balance. The nursing agency seemed well versed in handling anything that came up.

I learned to document everything. I learned military time as medication was charted, eighteen hundred hours, was 6:00 P.M.. I became skilled remembering to record when I had to give Becca meds or change and weigh her diapers. Ian thought it funny to answer time questions in school in military time and when he got them marked wrong on his test papers, he delighted in proving to the teacher he was right! How do you argue with a seven-year-old who is well versed in military time? I got a crash course in metric conversion, grams and cubic centimeters. Everything is measured, recorded, and documented.

Becca had good and bad days. We enjoyed the good times. When she had bad days, her constant care kept both the nurse and me busy. Bad days signaled trips to the doctor, a call for more medication, or another piece of equipment. Becca's breathing became compromised; the drops in her oxygen saturations brought more care and more interventions. Her x-rays showed her lungs were solid white. White was not good!

The respiratory therapist was sent out to teach us a technique to clear her tiny lungs. We were taught to give her breathing treatments using the Nebulizer at home every four to six hours around the clock. When she really struggled, the treatments were upped to every two hours to keep her lungs clear. In addition, we had to pound on her chest and back with our hands holding a little pink plastic, flexible cup. We drummed on Becca every other hour for ten to fifteen minutes to dislodge the sticky white mucous plugging up her lungs and bronchial tubes. I was one of the first people trained and it felt weird to now be the trainer of the nurses to do BD's (bronchial drainage) on Becca. I was the parent and they were the professionals. The nurses assured me it was okay and that often the moms of these kids knew more about their children and their procedures than the professionals.

Maybe I wasn't 'just' a mom?

The tape recorder Becca loved was left at the hospital, though we had a basket full of tapes. 'Alice' Diane bought Becca a new tape player for her ever-growing collection of inseparable music tapes. Her room filled softly with baby lullabies and bounced to the Beach Boys. The nursery was now a place of laughter and song and every treatment was done with play and music.

We made life fun and loving no matter how dismal it appeared, and I was beginning to understand why children thrive in home care versus institutional care. The nurses welcomed the siblings with open arms. Each morning the children ran from their beds, warm and soft from sleep in their pajamas, to say good morning to their baby sister. The nurses smiled as they reassured the kids that she was still home.

Marissa started the tradition of bringing a book to Becca. From that point on, nurses filled Becca's days with reading, and any number of ten additional little ears shared the stories while hanging along the crib rail or sitting quietly listening on the floor.

I tried to maintain a routine. I was home when the kids arrived from school. With five kids in the house, cleaning was a constant battle and I had to become strict on keeping a routine. I threw in loads of laundry in spare minutes throughout the day and I nagged the kids to pick up and to wash their hands. There were days it felt as though nagging five children was my full time job. But, all in all, it was a welcome relief to be home and away from the stress and juggling when Becca was in the hospital. The days home with Becca were busy and the busyness intensified when they included trips to the doctors or short stints in the hospital.

Wherever Becca went her medical equipment followed. Juggling all the leads and equipment was like putting together a 3D jigsaw puzzle. We placed the suction machine in the basket under Becca's blue stroller and suspended the open syringe with Becca's feeding tube with a toy plastic clip, and then we clamped the feeding pump to the stroller handle. We stationed the apnea monitor on top of the hooded canopy. The nurse carried the huge diaper bag while she pushed the oxygen connected to the oximeter that was hooked up to Becca's toe and placed inside the stroller. I pushed the stroller out of the house.

Then when we got to the minivan we moved all the equipment

inside, secured everything in its place, and bungeed the oxygen so it would not move during the trip. I was forever grateful to Dr. Wineinger for helping us get a handicap sticker for the van, the consolation prize of having a child with disabilities.

Things could change at a moment's notice, and so did our plans for everything when Becca was really sick, and it was always unexpected. She was fine one moment and critically ill the next. Stints in the hospital disrupted our home routine while Becca struggled with fevers and breathing problems. The doctors ran blood cultures, stool samples and adjusted medications. Then magically our Becca returned home and everything was back in place. The agency coordinated and timed everything, including upping our nursing care temporarily to twenty-four hours a day until we had Becca stable again. The intermittent demands of so many hours and nursing shortages on the nursing agency sometimes left them so short staffed I covered many open shifts. When I had to cover those shifts, Kristy was a great help. She watched over Matt and Marissa while Nathan, my nine-year-old veteran chef, prepared simple casseroles and hamburgers or hotdogs without help. When things were really stressed, the kids were happy with an old standby of my childhood called 'Sunday Night's supper' consisting of cereal, fruit and milk. This was our new normal.

We tried to find time to be together by having the nurses bring Becca out of her room to watch Sesame Street with Matt and Marissa while the kids were in school. The nurse sat with the little kids while I quickly washed breakfast dishes. Then the older kids played with Becca. They loved their new sister. Marissa performed dances for her or showed her pictures that she had colored. Matt hung on my legs. Ian, the little man of ten thousand questions, had an audience of professionals who helped him understand the hundreds of questions he had about his tiny baby sister or anything else that he was already wondering about. Ian is now planning on being a doctor. Kristy rocked and watched Becca so I could do something with Matt or change a messy diaper. She was a capable young lady, and her maturity and giftedness were a boon when I faced several open shifts per week. On the flip side it was nice to temporarily be 'only our family', but I struggled to get everything done and I played catch up when the nurses returned.

I was in charge for most of the night shifts, and that caused a chronic state of sleep deprivation. Our home was filled with round-the-clock beeping alarms that went off far more in the nights than during the days. From pseudo sleep I'd jumped up to answer alarms for occluded feeding pump tubing, the oxygen saturation drops signaled by the beeping oximeter, the low or the high heart rates of her gagging or the short apnea spells when Becca forgot to breathe. I'd gently shake and stimulate Becca to rouse her from her sleep, making sure she was awake enough to remember to continue breathing. When her airway was clogged, I used the suction machine to suck out the mucous from the back of her throat. I kept a sleeping bag on the floor of her closet to pull out and crawl into when I was too concerned for her welfare or too tired to go back to my bed.

At first I set the alarm, showered and greeted the nurses when they arrived in the morning. Then as exhaustion set in, I awoke to the front doorbell, and padded down the stairs to let a nurse in. Finally I left the front door unlocked and the nurses walked in at 7:00 A.M. without knocking. Many mornings I was startled as a nurse carefully stepped over me to care for Becca. The nurses smiled and shook their heads in wonder at me. Then once the kids were off to school, the professionals grounded me to my bedroom to a welcome nap while they played with Matt and Marissa and cared for Becca.

- 12 -

MIRACLES OF THE HEART

Except for visits to the hospital and Dr. Wineinger's office, we were homebound for our Minnesota winters to protect Becca. I missed attending church and I wanted to have Becca dedicated to the Lord on dedication Sunday. Surprisingly, her doctor cleared her dedication. Becca could be dedicated at the Baptist church I'd attended since childhood. Pastor Rick continued to be a huge support to our family and he was honored to be able to dedicate Becca to God. My church had felt like a homey sanctuary since my parents, my siblings, my aunt, uncle and cousins were all a part of our congregation. For months my daughter's name was on the church sponsored prayer chain, and the entire congregation invested time to pray for my tiny daughter.

During the service Pastor Rick called Jim and me forward with Becca and his treasured words and their meaning were sealed into my heart. They carried me on angels' wings when I struggled. He told the congregation, "This tiny little one has a purpose. In her short life she has inspired many who have come to love and hear her story. She has a mission. She is here for a reason. Through her challenges she helps us realize that life is short, and we need to make each day matter." Little Becca looked up at her mommy and daddy and Pastor Rick. She smiled. The tender magical moment moved the flock and even the old men wiped their eyes.

After the service an elderly lady really named Alice came to me and gave me a huge hug. Alice had been sending me cards and notes, of encouragement and support, over the past few months. She was encouraging me while fighting Leukemia and her last days were spent helping others cope through cards and prayers. She told me that we were blessed by our adversity. From this experience we will understand that life is precious. Having this type of life trauma this early in our lives was a gift. We would grow up to understand what life is all about while we were young and we would be better for it. Months later she peacefully lost her battle to cancer. She was not afraid to die; she wrote me that she was moving on to a place of perfection. In time I would understand what she meant. That day set the stage for the future. *"We would come to find incredible blessings in the face of adversity, and we would be changed for the better."*

After the service, Pastor Rick presented us with a check. For the first time in the history of the church, they had taken up a collection from Sunday school classes and services to raise the funds to save our home. We were two payments behind; the check was exactly what we owed. It was $1500. Through tears of joy, I hugged Pastor Rick. Once again, God answered my prayer. As always, God knew exactly what we needed.

He provided. I just had to trust and have faith.

Word had spread through our congregation that I had to move the girls from their bedroom into the boys' unfinished room in the basement, and volunteers worked weekends and evenings to finish their new rooms. Jim's dad had owned a hardware store and he plumbed the new bathroom. My uncle and Dad wired the basement. Jim added scraps of gently used cream carpet that he had salvaged from one of his customers. The freshly taped sheetrock made the rooms look nearly complete. We had applied to the waiver program for the basement bathroom fixtures. With eight people and all the nurses one bathroom was not enough. Every time we wanted to use it with Becca we had to disinfect it and most often there was a line waiting to shower or use the toilet.

And Jim was locking the door!

▼

Becca was almost six-months-old and a recent stretch in the hospital had confirmed our suspicions that her heart was failing further. The doctors agreed to try to do a cardiac catheterization, when the cardiac surgeon tries to balloon the obstructed pulmonary valve on her heart to see if they could open up the valve relieving the pressure. The procedure was very risky for such a tiny, fragile person, but we had little choice. We chose to risk her life to save her.

It was almost February, the month of hearts and love. Becca's heart screamed for help. Red and pink hearts shouted from all directions. Hearts covered the windows of retail stores. Hearts hung from the ceilings of grocery stores. Hearts, hearts, hearts and more hearts surrounded and called at me. Hearts were bittersweet, her failing heart was broken and our hearts were filled with love for our tiny baby. My children cut out hearts that now lay all over my kitchen table in paper piles.

As I was sitting at Becca's bedside with Mary, I had a brainstorm. I needed a moment to celebrate Becca's infinitesimal life. She may never see her first birthday, and her sixth month birthday was two days away. We could throw a party for her! Since our camera had been stolen, we had few pictures of our tiny little tike except for the ones taken by the nurses.

Mary suggested I borrow a camcorder from someone, but no one in my family or circle of friends had one. We continued to banter around ideas, and Mary decided we should call Make-A-Wish and tell them about my wish for Becca. Surprisingly when I called, I reached the Executive Director, who listened to my wish for a camera to use for a few hours to remember Becca. She told me that Make-A-Wish grants children their wishes, but Becca was only a baby and she was too little to have a wish of her own. I thanked her and hung up the phone, it had been worth a try. Reaching out to ask was not as hard as I thought it would be. I was saddened; it was unfair that my baby could die before she ever got a wish of her own.

I shared my party idea with my friend, Val. We could invite family and friends. It could be after dinner, a potluck dessert party and I was psyched. I barricaded myself in my room after the kids were in bed and turned two pieces of fabric into a beautiful party dress for my little Cinderella. Becca had been rehospitalized and was coming home on a two-day pass preceding her risky heart procedure. Those two days gave us time to party and Val spread the word to friends and Becca's support team while I called family.

While the nurses cared for Becca, I cleaned the house. Val's four girls and my kids made posters and decorated the dining room. We hung red and white heart streamers from the ceiling, looping and twisting them in fine party fashion. As word spread offers of paper cups and plates poured in. Red Valentine napkins arrived. Everything was coming together in record time as I put the finishing touches on the secret little dress. While we were busy festively transforming our home, the phone rang. Kristy shouted it was Make-A-Wish and they made an exception for Becca. The simple act of wanting to have a memory as a family to cherish moved them and they made a way for us to borrow a camcorder, and use it for a few precious weeks.

The camcorder arrived via messenger, and Val happily volunteered to document the event. I presented the new dress to Cheryl to put on Becca for her party. Val and the camera followed the arrival of the guests bearing Valentine's Day presents. The nursing agency sent a huge bouquet of helium heart balloons. Valentine gift bags, red heart wrapping paper, balloons and more balloons arrived. Flowers, gifts, heart shaped cookies, heart shaped cakes, and heart candies magically appeared and filled the dining room table. Soon the top of Jim's grandfather's antique buffet was mounded with scrumptious goodies of all sorts. Our heart-themed home was lovely and ready to welcome guests.

As we were getting ready for the party, we were surprised by a knock on the front door. It was a photographer and camera crew sent by Make-A-Wish to professionally document the party for the creation of a special video of Becca and our family before the guests arrived. The camera crew captured my mom and dad, brothers and sisters, aunts and uncle, and cousins as they shouted 'Happy Half Birthday Becca!'

The camera crew captured the over a hundred people who stopped in to share Becca's special half birthday, friends from church, old family friends, and neighbors joined us to celebrate our little girl. When the camera crew and the guests gathered together, the nurse brought Becca out in her new heart dress.

The dress was my gift to my daughter, a one-of-a-kind creation. The delightful little pinafore dress was white with red hearts, decked with tiers of ruffles capped by dainty white lace. The front neckline was a ruffle of red with white hearts, which matched the dress underneath, peeking out from the dress were darling teeny tiny fancy bloomers to match with a heart appliqué on the backside of her diaper. Her little head was crowned with a matching lace headband made with ribbons and a red heart. I had been sewing for a crafting friend, and she surprised me with a new, unique creation, a hand painted heart dress for me to wear that evening.

Pastor Rick was right, Becca inspired hope in others. Her tiny presence was a vehicle of healing wounded hearts. I was moved when Marissa's little friend, Amy; held Becca. Amy had heart surgery as a baby. My aunt held Becca; she had given up her daughter Cindy with Down's syndrome back in the 1950's to foster care before I was born. Cindy ended up in an institution and died at age thirteen from heart problems. It was a family secret until Becca's birth. She looked at Becca with tears in her eyes; Becca's presence opened the path for her and me to safely discuss the differences that time had made for children with disabilities in the future.

Kristy took out her cello and offered a recital of her new repertoire of songs for the guests. The kids and their friends ran through the house with smiles and laughter. It was a miracle we could send them all downstairs to play as the basement now had partitions and newly hung sheetrock for two new bedrooms, a bathroom, a laundry room and a large family room.

Kids ran up and down the stairs to get food. Marissa packed her round little cheeks like a squirrel with peanuts and candy and scurried off to her friends. The boys dumped out all their Lego's. Ian was chased and taunted by the girls who thought he was cute. Val's daughter was in love with him and caught him to plant a kiss on his cheek.

Val called all the kids upstairs, and everyone gathered to sing Happy Birthday to Becca. My mother held her sweet little granddaughter as Kristy opened the huge pile of presents. Kristy appropriately took her time, reading each card aloud for the watching guests and passed them around for guests to admire. The gifts were caring and thoughtful; picture frames and photo albums, musical animals and furry little stuffed critters, outfits and sleepers. Someone filled a box with diapers, lotions and baby bath products.

On the spur of the moment people drove for hours. Jim's mom and dad drove 180 miles to celebrate with us, and Aunt Mitzi joined them. Another aunt surprised us when she arrived in from Wisconsin. She always lived with my grandmother who had passed away the month before and we had been unable to travel out of town for the funeral.

Big sister, Kristy handed me her special present for her little sister. She had used all her savings from neighborhood babysitting to buy Becca a little two-piece pink and mint green bunny outfit. She was so proud of doing it all herself. That evening the house was alive with laughter . . . the laughter all of us needed in that time of stress and uncertainty. We found hope. We were surrounded by love and so blessed by those individuals who reached out to us as a family.

As I was eating my ice cream, I took a little bit on my spoon to give Becca a birthday dessert sample on her lips. Since the first early days when she quit accepting a nipple, she had never had any food item touch her little lips. Tonight she seemed to understand that this was her party, and she was going to try something. She squished up her nose from the cold and then licked her lips not quite knowing what to do with it. With everyone in the room laughing she smiled in the excitement.

As the evening wound down, we had a house full of company, and three-year old Matt had slept through all the noise and commotion. He woke up in time to go back to bed as the last of the guests left. Matt stared with half sleeping eyes at the overflowing table of goodies, and he grabbed a handful of gluten-free heart cookies. Then he snuggled in his father's arms, quite unsure of what had transpired while he slept.

Cheryl readied Becca for sleep while Val and I cleaned up the party mess. Tomorrow, bright and early, we would depart for the hospital, this time to try and help Becca's teeny tiny heart.

▼

Heart surgery morning came too quickly, and we loaded Becca and her boatload of equipment into the stroller . . . and then into the van, and then out of the van . . . and into the stroller . . .into the lobby and up the elevator . . . back to the intensive care unit. After six months I knew the drill. Labs, labs and more labs . . . wait, wait and more waiting. This time I didn't run.

I sat. I waited.

I prayed for everything to be all right.

I looked up at the approaching doctor.

"Becca was out of surgery. The passing of the balloon through the valve was not successful. The valve was too misshapen to be helped. He had taken biopsies of the thickened wall of the ventricles of her heart to see if it would shed light on what kind of cardiomyopathy Becca had. As he was slowly pulling out the catheter during the procedure Becca gave him quite a scare. Her heart went into ventricular tachycardia and raced out of control. Fortunately with administration of medication he got it to resume a normal rhythm. We could not go through any procedures without Becca scaring her family and physicians with some heart-stopping prank. She kept us all on our toes, and when the moment passed those gargantuan episodes strangely eased the huge fear and uncertainty of the moment.

She remained under close observation in intensive care for the next couple of days. With every surgery Becca seemed to require IV antibiotics and she always spiked a high fever. The blood cultures revealed deadly systemic staph infection, even though they had given her IV antibiotics. The medical staff worked to get her temperature down and her feedings back on track so she could go home to her private pediatric intensive care nursery.

▼

The home-nurses were set to greet us when we arrived, offering welcome home smiles and support unraveling and navigating Becca and the stroller back to where she belonged.

The news of Becca's heart was not good, but for today she thankfully was still alive and home.

▼

I knew in my heart of hearts we were on borrowed time. She was destined to the fate of many critically ill babies. Becca was as sick as it gets and I didn't know any other Noonan syndrome babies with as many complications as Becca who were still alive.

Sometimes I wondered if making her stay was wrong. I wondered about her quality of life. She was in such pain and it was so hard to see her suffer. Were we right to allow it to continue?

I chose to honor my promise to God.

I would love Becca no matter where it would take us.

- 1 3 -
QUARANTINE

After Becca's failed cardiac catheterization, the doctors presented Becca's case to the University of Minnesota cardiac surgeons. They came to a consensus that Becca's heart was waning. A renowned pediatric cardiac surgeon, Dr. Foker thought it might be worth trying to fix the parts of her heart that could be repaired to give her a little more time. They could not repair the thickened walls, but they could remove her blocked valve, and repair the huge hole. They explained to me that children can survive without a pulmonary valve, and they could patch the hole between the two chambers. However, changing the anatomy of her heart could backfire and make it fail faster. We had little choice; risk surgery or she will die anyway.

Dr. Hesselein, our cardiologist felt the surgery was risky. She had already scared him during the last heart procedure and could develop life-threatening problems post-operatively even if she survived the surgery due to her weakened immune system and 'newly discovered' leaky lymph system.

He explained, "after heart surgery, some of the kids with Noonan syndrome develop lymph fluid in the chest walls and lungs that can be life threatening." We knew with previous surgeries Becca developed systemic staph infections and the odds were not good for our little one. Since this was our only hope for any sort of future we gave them permission to schedule Becca for surgery in early March. She will die without surgery; she may die if we try. We decided to try and pray for a miracle. Her home nursing staff was commissioned to build her strength to help her survive the upcoming open heart surgery.

As Becca was getting sicker the doctors ordered Becca's nursing care to cover additional shifts. The 24-hour a day nursing care was welcome security. The nurses adjusted her formula to double the strength while keeping the fluid level down. We added special oils to increase calories without adding extra volume or stress. The diuretic was adjusted to keep her stable until the surgery. But Becca seemed to need increasing oxygen and her doctors did not understand why.

Jim finally had had enough with his job, his boss was making it impossible for him at work and was finding fault with every little thing he did or didn't do. He gave Jim's customer orders away to other salesmen when the customers returned to place their orders. Then he had the gall to ask Jim why he was not selling enough. When Jim confronted the owner with his concerns, he fired Jim immediately. The carpet company held his final paycheck an extra week and they fought Jim's application for unemployment. A month later we won an unemployment appeal, but the two hundred dollar a week unemployment check was not enough for us to be able to make the house payment.

While awaiting surgery Becca became too sick to stay at home, and she landed back in the hospital on the medical unit. Becca had a virus that was causing her heart to work too hard; her lungs were struggling to breathe. The residents on the unit call kids like Becca 'frequent flyers.' The chief resident asked if I would help give a know-it-all resident a lesson in humbleness. I was all for the challenge and he filled me in on his plan. The chief told the intern that he needed to get a complete history on Becca. It was all I could do to hold back my smile. I needed a welcome break from the worry of waiting and watching my hurting Becca sleep fretfully. The intern grabbed 'one piece' of paper and assured the chief that the history would be done before lunch. The chief laughed and told him he should get more paper and grab a quick snack, as this may take a while.

I began as 'just' a mom answering his questions, and I went on, and on, and on, with the important dates and medical details for over an hour and a half. The rattled intern left the room with Becca's chart, but the chief still had unanswered questions. The humbled intern returned to get more answers to the questions he'd missed. The doctors and the chief commended me with smiles on a job well done. We had tamed the intern who learned that parents are the experts of their children, they have much-needed knowledge, and are valuable partners in their children's medical care.

Becca's homecare nurses warned me that kids like Becca should not be left alone on the floor of the hospital. Too many mistakes get made and the nurses are so busy they cannot adequately monitor children like Becca. That was all I needed to hear, Mom managed the kids and I moved in with Becca. They provided a cot for me and I helped provide much of Becca's care. The nurses were astonished when I fixed the alarms on the equipment like a seasoned pro. One of the doctors recommended I return to school and become a nurse and told me that I would be able to test out of much of the coursework. I am already a nurse for my daughter and the thought of doing it forever was something I hoped I would never have to face.

By the time Becca was stabilized enough to return home, we only had a week before her open-heart surgery. Then on the day before surgery, Ian awoke covered with red spots. He must have picked up the dreaded chickenpox. The nurse placed a panicked phone call to the pediatrician, who alerted the infectious disease doctor, and we were given twenty-four hours to administer a shot to provide Becca chickenpox immunities. The doctors ordered quarantine and the kids could not be at home with her. Now, we had to postpone the surgery for three more weeks until we knew that Becca was not infected. We could not risk her getting chickenpox before, during or after surgery and she could not be in the hospital exposing others. What was it with chickenpox? First, the childhood illness stopped her siblings from seeing Becca for months, now the dastardly chickenpox was stopping Becca from having her urgent life saving surgery.

Kristy, the only child with some immunity stayed home while we moved the other four kids to Mom and Dad's house for Becca's safety. Poor Mom and Dad's little townhouse was quarantined with four additional permanent children. I packed suitcases for the duration, trying to calculate enough clothes for two rounds of chickenpox outbreaks. Since Ian already had them, it would be up to three weeks before round two started. Hopefully all the children would get them at the same time and our epidemic would be over.

I struggled running between my house and Mom's to help her with my itchy crabby children and managing Becca's home care. I could not contaminate Becca so I had to shed my clothes in my freezing cold garage. I shivered standing in my bare feet on the concrete garage floor. Minnesota winters are downright cold and I put on a clean oversized T-shirt to cover myself on the way to the bathroom where I had to shower every time I returned home. Afterwards I scoured the bathroom with bleach to disinfect it to make sure we did not give Becca chickenpox. My hands were red, and raw, and cracked from all the washing and scrubbing. I ran back and forth between our house and Mom's some days more than once . . . shivering. . . .showering . . .checking in to make sure the nurse was there to staff the next shift and then head back to help Mom with the kids. There was one ray of hope to this dark time; Kristy had time alone with her mom and dad.

▼

Meanwhile Becca was worsening. At the end of three weeks we worried she could pass away before the surgery. She started having spells causing loss of oxygen to her brain. The nurses and I watched the numbers on the oximeter fall. We upped the oxygen and prayed.

▼

Marissa came down with the second round of chickenpox the date we admitted Becca to the hospital for her heart surgery. Mom and Dad's townhouse was filled to the brim with four grandchildren in the isolation, Kristy, my two-year-old niece Katie, my brother Tim, and sister Gretchen, who came home for college spring break.

Then Matt and Katie, still in diapers, broke out in round three and Marissa developed a secondary infection and now was a very sick little girl. Poor Mom soaked little sore bodies in baking soda baths and covered them in calamine lotion. Grandma rocked the irritable toddlers while caring for a feverish nauseated Marissa. The toddlers' were barely scabbed over when Gretchen and Tim called from college needing to come back home, as they had just become round four.

When it was time for round five, we waited for Nathan to finally get the chickenpox. It was too late for us when the federal food and drug administration announced the release of the chickenpox vaccine. Mom's quarantine term lasted from early March through the end of May when Nathan was finally allowed back home. The two chickenpox Nathan had as an infant had spared him from a full-blown onslaught from this pandemic. Pour Nathan had spent over two months living away from home and never got sick. That spring Saint Grandma earned her angel wings.

Jim and I became distanced from each other after the nurses arrived. I didn't need him to help me care for Becca; I had the Alice's. Jim on the other hand had been nurse-invaded, he sat off by himself, overworked, underpaid and felt responsible to fix an impossible situation. His glasses were gray with depression and I was sick of him looking lost and moping around feeling sorry for himself. It was though he had become frozen since he had no job and he was not helping at home. One night a nurse called in sick and I blew up. I confronted his depression when we had no audience. I had handled much of the load alone and I gave him an ultimatum. If he wouldn't start helping and supporting me, he might as well just leave!! I would do it without him since I already was doing it alone.

Cross words flew in both directions and Jim walked out the door. The frustration and anger had been building for a long time. Was this the final straw? Were we going to join the 90% of families who fall apart because of the stresses put on them by having critically ill children?

▼

Three hours later he returned home and he had thought about his depression and our circumstances. How could he feel sorry for himself, when his daughter was smiling through all her pain?

▼

The day of open-heart surgery arrived and Jim was right beside me. The nurses sent me through the now familiar maze of medical corridors to go and get Becca's medical records. The medical records clerk asked if I needed help with the charts as she handed me the three volumes of binders each at least four inches thick. I tried to carry them and finally resorted to wheeling them in an unoccupied wheelchair.

Jim and I stayed with our daughter in the pediatric intensive care unit until they were ready to take her down for surgery. Mom had her hands full with our kids who were still quarantined, plus now we had added Kristy. Pastor Rick arranged a twenty-four-hour prayer vigil for Becca's healing. The day was broken up into fifteen-minute segments and church members and family took turns praying. Amazingly there was not one open break through the entire day.

Once again I sat and waited, but this time I was not alone. Jim was with me. My new tennis shoes were broken in as I ran off my anxiety on my five-story treadmill. Jim and I laughed with Mary to pass the time. Homecare nurses and church members stopped by to support us. For six hours we waited, but we were not alone.

▼

A tall cardiac surgeon with huge hands came to the waiting room to discuss the surgery with us. How could those hands and that big man perform surgeries on the tiniest of hearts? He had patched the hole and repaired the pulmonary outflow tract after removing the damaged valve. He found Becca's valve was one of the most severely thickened and misshapen he had ever seen. He asked for our permission to file the damaged valve on a registry for further research. In addition, Becca's atrial septal defect was one of the largest he had come across. Becca had weathered the surgery, but because of the changes to her heart, her heart may not be able to function and only time would tell.

Jim and I visited our little Becca in intensive care. It hurt to look at her. Her little body had filled with fluid and she was unrecognizable through the swelling. A ventilator helped her breath and many bags of drugs hung from the IV pole administered by at least seven different medication pumps. Three or four tubes protruded from her chest connected to more bags. That evening she was too unstable for us to leave the hospital so the social workers arranged a room for us inside of the hospital in case they needed us. As we went to bed we wondered if our tiny titan would be alive in the morning. But this night, I was not alone on a cot while Becca hovered between life and death, Jim held me and I held him.

▼

Becca was still in critical condition in the morning spiking a fever that signaled the need for more blood cultures. Her kidneys began to shut down as the doctors scurried to stabilize her. Becca had developed a plural effusion and her chest was full of leaking lymph. She was barely hanging on and they used experimental protocols to try to save her.

After the surgery Becca had no immune system and even lab values that used to be normal were no longer normal. Every lab result showed us her entire body was out of whack; there wasn't one normal value in two pages of lab work. The church continued praying around-the-clock, each fifteen minutes handing off pray responsibilities to the next prayer warrior. Pastor Rick called every couple of hours to update the prayer chain.

Jim and I sat next to each other talking; trying not to think about what was going on. The next night we went home to be with our family, in our own home with no nurses. The hospital promised to keep us posted and call if they needed us. We hoped and prayed that the phone would remain silent and it did.

The following morning we returned early to wait. We spent hours talking and reminiscing about the pranks and escapades of our children. Jim's smile radiated when he talked about Ian and all his silly Calvin and Hobbs shenanigans. He lit up when he described Marissa's theatrics and the boys complaining about her constant singing. Jim described to Mary his deep intellectual discussions of world politics, statistics and world events that he had with his very brilliant, growing up daughter, Kristy. I could feel how dear her sunshine was to his heart.

Jim described how much Nathan was like me and how close Nathan and I always were. He asked for suggestions of how he could reach out to his son, and by doing so he reached out to me.

We were both worried about our little Matt. How would all this affect him? We needed to make a conscious effort to find time for him, or he would become lost in this chaos. Kristy and Nathan were seemingly more parents to him than we were. Matt had spent so much time with his grandparents; I was worried my legacy would become his. For the first four years of my life my mom had been working, ill, or busy as we moved from here to there. My grandparents spent so much time with me that I had become confused regarding the roles of my parents versus my grandparents. I didn't want that struggle for Matt. I wanted to be 'Mom' and I didn't want to give my mom control of my children even though I appreciated all her help. I could not have done it without her. I told Jim I wanted to be there for our children. I needed to be there for our children. I knew how it felt to be Matt. It had hurt so much to let go and trust my mom so I could help Becca.

The more we talked, the more our relationship healed remembering the past and our children. Each of our children were unique and special and remembering their antics and the happy times brought us back together. We tried not to talk about Becca. We couldn't go there, it was too uncertain. Yet the more we tried not to talk about her, the more our minds stirred us back to our little one lying in intensive care.

Jim intuitively knew what troubled me and he used quick humor as a distraction while we waited.

And waited.

And waited.

▼

Five days later our little fighter began to turn the corner.

I watched as the doctors prepared to take her off the ventilator, but Becca, like Marissa, didn't do anything without theatrics. Shortly after removing the ventilator the alarms sounded. Becca had stopped breathing and they ordered me to shake her!

Shake my baby with all these tubes and dressings on her?

They yell again, "Mrs. Yurcek shake Becca! Now!"

I grabbed her tiny chest with the three plastic tubes connected to bloody bags draining out of her chest cavity. She had another bag with a catheter. They tell you not to shake babies. Were they nuts? I began to shake all the while the heart monitor showed her heart rate was dropping further and further. They ran for the crash cart and the medical team took over. As I turned my back to my dying baby the monitor showed me that her heart was down to ten beats per minute.

A father of another 'frequent flyer' joined me and we walked out of the unit to wait and pray in the visitors lounge. This caring dad held my hand and prayed with me as they worked on Becca. It seemed like forever while we talked about watching, and waiting, and shared our feelings about how little control we had in our children's lives. I had shared with other preemie parents before, but this time was different. He and I had kids who would not get better, or bigger, or stronger. Our kids had challenges and conditions that before long would kill them. We talked about our fears of our children dying; about how hard it was to watch them hurt so. For the first time, I had the chance to connect with another parent of a child with special needs. My pain and feelings were not unusual. There were others.

Then Becca began breathing. Once again the narcotics had put her into respiratory depression. That night as I slept at the hospital, I remembered back to when Becca coded when she was a two-month-old, and I hoped that this downtime was shorter; I didn't want her to have more brain damage. I cried myself to sleep and my mind finally quit blocking out the trauma of nearly losing Becca the first time. I remembered my running from the hospital and yelling at the nurses that I was leaving. This time I had faced Becca's near-death, all the while knowing that all I could do was wait.

And pray.

I knew I had changed.

▼

It was ten days before Becca was allowed to return home with sixteen-hour-a-day nursing care. My 'little actress' needed more attention and she was not improving. The doctors upped her to round the clock care and she taxed the nurses with her constant care.

▼

Meanwhile, it was time for the unspotted Yurcek children to return home and Kristy's time alone with Mom and Dad ended when pox-free Ian was sprung from quarantine. Matt and Marissa stayed another week and left Nathan at Grandma's for another month because of his exposure to his aunt and uncle's chickenpox outbreak. After almost three months, every Yurcek was under one roof.

- 14 -
NURSE VADER

The months after Becca's heart surgery were full of constant care and she remained on oxygen much longer than the doctors had predicted. Newborn-size, nine-month-old Becca was very fragile and it took all her energy when I gave her a bath in her infant bathtub. She turned dusky blue, while I juggled the oxygen tubing and soaked her slippery body. If we tried to do anything for longer than a couple of minutes, she became exhausted and fell asleep for a long nap.

As if the chickenpox were not enough, Becca was exposed to measles in the hospital after her open-heart surgery. Her doctors ordered gamma globulin treatments to boost her wavering immune system. The infusions every three to four weeks helped her gain strength, improved the constant thrush in her mouth, and seemed to stop the recurrent staph infections. Every four hours we used anti-fungals on a sponge tip swab to scrub out the white patches that plagued her little mouth. Becca hated the procedure.

She learned she had control of one thing — her pacifier became her protection. As long it was in her mouth, we weren't. She hung onto it by sucking as if her life depended on it and her suck became stronger and stronger. The 'Nukie' was her constant companion, and the nurses looped a receiving blanket through the little handle to keep the pacifier from popping out. The pacifier had to be changed when we used the antifungal so our schedule now included sterilizing pacifiers so we had a fresh supply. Early on, Becca learned to suck on the pacifier to calm herself to sleep. The pacifier encouraged her to swallow, and as she used it we did not have to use the suction machine as often. Finally the suction machine was only needed for times when Becca had a virus or a cold.

After surgery we realized that Becca had trouble regulating her body temperature and was sensitive to dust and other allergens. Summer was coming, and we were concerned about how we could stabilize her temperature once it got warm outside. Our split-level home had trees so small that they couldn't block the hot sun. We would need air-conditioning if Becca were to remain out of the hospital for the summer. On hot days in early spring we moved Becca and her entourage of nurses and gear to my parents climate controlled townhouse where she remained on oxygen for the entire day.

We didn't even have the money to buy a small window air conditioner for Becca's room, so I called the public health nurse to ask for assistance. She put in a request for a window unit from the county. A window unit was better than nothing but it wasn't good enough. It meant Becca would be confined to her room and I wondered how I could care for Becca and still keep an eye on my active three-year-old, not to mention the others.

I sent letters to every agency and community group on the North Side of Minneapolis. One day we received a phone call from someone from the Blaine Lions Club; they wanted to meet Becca and our family. With letter in hand, they presented us with a certificate for central air conditioning for our home.

Within a week Becca's environment was a constant 72°. Becca had access to the entire house and our family, and I began to wrestle with higher electricity bills. I had to trust my process of creative juggling or hope that some unexpected windfall of money arrived just in time to save us. Somehow miracles always kept my family fed and the utilities turned on.

Becca was not the only family member to be helped by the air-conditioning. For the first time in my life, my asthma didn't flare out and Marissa and Ian's asthma and allergies greatly improved. The kids happily wrote thank you letters to the Lions Club and the people at Blaine heating and air-conditioning for their amazing gift. The list of incredible people who joined us on our journey to help us make it through was growing.

Jim's previous employer offered him a management position with a small salary and insurance for the family excluding Becca due to her pre-existing conditions. We were grateful for a job and a paycheck. Jim was happier working for his old carpet company and he felt relieved to be out from the pressure of his former boss. With Becca's discharge from the hospital, we were no longer limited to the $900 a month to qualify her for Medicaid. We had freedom to make more money.

I found an ad for a Minneapolis Star Tribune newspaper carrier position. A paper route could help us pay for the utilities on time. We got the job, and Jim and I took turns getting up in the morning to deliver nearly two hundred daily papers. The eight hours a week investment kept the power on.

We spent the summer playing with the kids and helping the nurses. We were now accustomed to having people in our home, and Becca was gaining strength. She was still very silent, yet in her sweet way she communicated clearly. She smiled at the kids who were now her best buddies. Marissa taught her to show us her tongue and now whenever she accomplished something she gave us a toothless grin with a tiny tongue sticking out proudly. Becca's audience of clapping siblings and nurses encouraged her to try new things while the surgery provided her with the stamina to be able to do things most babies do easily. Every milestone was celebrated; the smallest progress was monumental.

In July, Becca at almost one-year-old began to sit up for the first time; she showed us her toothless grin as her eyes sparkled. She was so proud, she did it all by herself! Becca had proved the occupational therapist wrong when she blew their goals away. The therapists thought this mom was nuts when I set a goal of sitting up for thirty seconds by her first birthday. Becca showed them. She sat up a month ahead of schedule. Then one day Becca took a bite of a rice cracker. I asked Deb the nurse if it was in her walker or in her lap? Deb explained she had witnessed Little Miss Becca putting it in her mouth and actually swallowing it! From that moment on I learned to never say never with Rebecca, because she would prove us wrong.

▼

Finally the Yurcek children had a life that was much easier and resembled normal. At home they had their toys, friends, and routine. They were accustomed to the nurses coming and going and they no longer acted up or tested to see what they could get by with when the nurses were watching. Mom and Dad were no longer afraid to discipline because the nurses were in the house. Many of the nurses were parents themselves and they helped me understand the need for setting limits for my budding adolescent, Kristy. Kristy with her giftedness had always done everything early, so why shouldn't I expect that she began to act like a teen? My kids knew they were up against the wall when Mom and a nurse confronted them in unison.

Our house had always been the neighborhood Kool-Aid house as children ran in and out from early morning until dusk. Sadly, the neighborhood children could no longer play inside our home because Becca was under isolation. Happily for Becca, their friends played in our backyard and she watched the kids play from the window with her nurses. Little Miss Becca did not want to miss out on a single thing as she stood with the nurse holding her on the back of the couch. The children waved and shouted while they performed somersaults and stunts for their tiny tongue-protruding audience.

The majority of the nurses were wonderful and only a few did not succeed in our home. Sometimes our family values differed, and other times we had different expectations of care. I was growing accustomed to managing a family plus a team of nurses with differing personalities.

One of our nurses spoiled Becca with extravagant toys and gifts. This began interfering with Becca's relationships with her siblings and my relationship with my daughter. Somehow this kind woman's heart got in the way, and I felt left out. She loved Becca and she laughed and made life lighter. Becca loved her and unfortunately she got so close I began to feel replaced. When I confronted her with my feelings, she got mad and quit. Even though she had been good for Becca, we still needed to be a family. In retrospect, part of this was my fault. I let my jealously get in the way.

Another nurse I disliked from the moment I met her. My gut wrenched each time I saw her. I usually give everyone a chance, but this time I felt different. Something was wrong. She spent one shift with Val and had been oriented to Becca's care and schedule, but I still felt uneasy. Staff told me to give her a chance to see if it would work, but when I saw how many shifts she was assigned to my home, I became more agitated. This woman was driving me crazy and she hadn't done anything. The more I thought about it, the more worked up I became. She supposedly had spent the last 20 years working in pediatric health care. I figured it must be a personality clash, but something in my intuition told me otherwise.

One day she was at the house with Val for another shift, when the supervisor called to check to see if everything was all right. This was unusual as normally a nurse works alone during the second shift, but the agency sensed my insecurity with the new caretaker. The case manager could tell from my voice something was wrong and I shared my feelings and my frustrations. She asked for examples, yet the only two things I could pinpoint was that once she shoved Marissa out of the room saying she needed to stay away when the nurse was doing the baby's care and she had told me she had other ways to handle things from how we were doing them.

Halfway through the shift, Val got an emergency phone call telling her that her daughter had broken her arm at school. As Val was leaving, I walked down the hallway to Becca's room and witnessed the nurse about to administer an orange medication in a plastic medicine cup in Becca's wide-open suspended syringe attached to her feeding tube. I was so shocked I couldn't find my voice to yell stop!

I bolted toward her and knocked the medication cup out of her hand. The orange medicine splattered all over the crib, Becca, and the pink and white wallpaper. I was horrified. The only orange medication that Becca had was her diuretic and a dosage that high would have killed my daughter immediately. She screamed at me that I was crazy and Val ran back to see what caused the commotion. I told her what I had witnessed and Val asked the nurse to check the medication sheet. She was giving five CCs or a teaspoon to Becca. The dose ordered by the doctor was .5cc. It was ten times the dose ordered by the physicians. Val confronted the nurse. Then Val left to take her daughter to the emergency room.

I could not stand to see this nurse's face and I wanted her out of my house now! I called the agency just as Jim walked through the door. Jim had no idea what was going on when I asked him to call the new nurse to the phone to talk to the agency director. The incompetent nurse refused to leave my home and wanted to know whether she should restart the feeding pump. It was as though nothing was wrong. The director told her again she needed to leave, and she would only leave if they guaranteed her remaining days wages. We threatened to file charges against her to finally get her out our door.

I had been drawn to the hallway just in time, five seconds later we would have lost Becca and believed her heart stopped from congestive heart failure. I wondered if this was an accident or had I caught her in the act of mercy killing my baby? The nurse was fired immediately and a complaint was lodged with the state on her license. The nursing agency immediately instituted a new policy for all nurses that included specialized training and testing in administering pediatric medications before being allowed with children and they beefed up their background checks. Yet, there still remain many unanswered questions concerning the nurse who was in our home that day and I am incredibly thankful that I felt summoned to the hallway to stop the life threatening disaster.

Once again my Becca's life was spared.

- 15 -

ONE

The doctors had given us little hope that Becca would live to see her first birthday, but it was gloriously now August. Becca's first year of life had been filled with tragedy and triumphs. I had watched my daughter nearly die many times, but my tiny titan had never given up despite the life-threatening problems she faced.

Personally, I had unfinished business as I prepared for her first birthday. The memories of the past year spun through my head as I tried to sleep, and I tossed and turned every night during the week before she turned a year old. As Mary suggested, I had begun writing as a coping mechanism to organize my thoughts while I struggled to care for my critically ill baby.

Finally, at three in the morning I sprang urgently from my bed. I needed to write. I needed to never forget all we had been through. I sat with my pen through the wee hours of the morning. I turned back the pages to read what I had written so long ago when I was so incredibly stressed and Becca was close to dying. I realized I had come so far since that time. Becca had defied the odds. We all had.

I cried as I relived those early days and read from my first entry eight months ago.

Ann's Life (January 1990)

I am writing this in hopes that I might make some sense and order out of what is currently bothering me. Mary keeps telling me I am not going crazy. Circumstances around me are causing the pressure. Sometimes the pressure is so great I can't breathe. Maybe by writing them down I can find an organized way to look at them so it is easier to deal with them and gather some conclusions.

What I need to handle and feel.

I have been thrown a curve. It is not fair and there are no easy answers. This is heartbreaking but rewarding. Running away is not an option for me. Many people can't do it and quit, but they have a price to pay for it. So I am making the choice to face it head on with all my energy and love. Becca is my full time job.

I have another full time job. Five of the most precious kids who throw another curve at me. They need me, and I need them, but time is precious and there is so little of it these days.

Jim, we are each shutting each other out. There's no time to talk, and if there is our minds and energy are in different places. I know the statistics of marriages in our situation. They are BLEAK. If something doesn't change, we're headed that way. I cannot raise five well children and a chronically ill child by myself. It hurts me to see him in such agony and this too becomes another pressure for me.

Pressures of handling day-to-day with Becca:

l. It is a job that requires stamina, a strong heart and a lot of time.

2. When she is in the hospital life has no normalcy. There are too many demands, too little time. If I stay away Becca becomes angry and pushes me away. If I go the other children resent it. When I stay away many things at the hospital go astray. I lose touch with doctors and what is happening with Becca.

The uncertainties of now and in the future: I CANNOT dwell on this, or I will definitely lose it. I keep trying to enjoy today and find some good that is coming from all of this. (Ann taking care of Ann).

Dealing with the doctors and caregivers of Becca: Sometimes I have to fight or play the advocate to ensure she's getting what she needs. I feel as though I am the only one who cares that anything is done. I know I shouldn't feel that way, and they care, but still it's there. They need to listen, and when they don't Becca pays a price. Too many mistakes.

The new realization that Ann cannot take care of Becca alone. The staff asks what I need, but I don't know where to begin. I want to do it, but all the pressures prevent me. Then I wonder what do they think? Am I a complete incompetent? Ann being too tough on Ann. I don't know what is expected of me.

The five months we have been on this roller coaster is not going to get better. If it does it probably means one of two things: Becca has gotten better; we can always hope for a miracle. Or Becca is gone and we have to learn to go on without her. So we settle for the roller coaster and not think of anything different. I reach out to find someone or a group of people who know what it is like. This I am working on.

The demands of watching and caring for this special daughter of mine whom I love with all my heart is emotionally exhausting, physically taxing, and watching her hurt is heartbreaking. This is my toughest job.

The always having to be on guard and watch for signs coming from Becca signal another ride is on its way. Up and down the coaster again. Waiting until the doctors see it. I wish my intuition would be wrong. It's frustrating having to tell them all the time and not knowing if I am right or over-reacting.

Jim and all that go with it

I. His job leaves no room for him to help me with anything. Thus I resent him.

2. Jim is trying to protect me from the knowledge of our finances, and we need to talk and work together. He is quiet, and I don't know how to get him to work with me instead of each of us doing our own thing. Two people = twice as much power.

3. It bothers and hurts to see him isolate himself. I know he has to want to move forward and that is up to him. But it's an added frustration.

Five other important reasons

Watching my well children be thrown into a situation and having to deal with it is hard. Each one hurts in a unique way. I work to help the best I can, but there is only one of me.

*Time and quality time are hard to come by because of all the other pressures. *All the kids want is everything to be normal again and that is impossible. We'll never be back to simple again.*

The kids' cares require time...homework, baths, mess picking up, laundry, cooking, cleaning, and hugging. There's not enough time for everything.

I worry about how all this will affect them in the long haul. Will they be all right?

Outside stress from other people:

I. Family questioning every move I make and always telling me I am wrong.

2. Other people not understanding and running, being afraid of Becca and us. They do not understand, they do not know what to say.

Finances, the other major stress

1. We're falling further behind all the time. Jim is concentrating on this, and I know it is killing him.

2. The bills, forget them, that's all we can do if we want a house and a car.

Conclusion:

It's not fair. There are no answers. What do I do? Put all this together, and no wonder why I am overwhelmed. Maybe I can start to gather up my reserve and go on with the battle and face the frontline again, instead of trying to retreat.

I began to write, and write, and write on fresh sheets of paper. For a couple of hours I filled these pages with the joys and sorrows of our journey with our tiny daughter to the final words . . .

Becca has changed our lives. Jim and I have been beaten and worn down, we've been tested and downtrodden, we faced fear and sorrow, but somehow we survived. We are now stronger than our family has ever been. We have a new appreciation for the small things and see the blessings we used to take for granted. Becca's first year is over. She made it! I wouldn't change anything, because I have my daughter. The time we spent with Becca and learning to deal with the harsh realities of life has been tough. I can't explain it, for there are no words that cover it. The year has been physically and emotionally exhausting, but I am a better person. I'm stronger because of all I've been through and my priorities have changed. No person can go through this and not be affected by the adversity. I remember the moment I accepted our circumstances and vowed to fight for Becca.

Becca gave me new strength to carry on. It is a battle, but it is a battle worth fighting for . . . the bat-

tle for the survival of my tiny daughter.

I had a choice, I could let the circumstances cause us to give up and to lose hope, or I could choose to live for the day and love well. My Becca may not have a tomorrow, but today she is here, and that is all that matters. I cannot imagine not having Becca and everything that she brings with it. Someday I know that I will have to let her go. I will continue to cherish this precious one who has changed our lives for the better and I am honored to be Becca's mom.

For now, I will give Becca all the love that I can, as long as she is with us. We settle ourselves on the roller coaster of life, for being on the coaster means that Becca is still with us. Someday I know our ride will end, and Becca will be gone, but for today we have hope, and with faith and each other we will survive.

Becca has a purpose, as Pastor Rick foretold. Becca's purpose has become clear to me. Becca is here to teach the lesson of living one day as though it is your last by loving, caring, and giving to each other. Life is too short to spend our time waiting for tomorrow. We need to cherish today, because we are not guaranteed tomorrows. We do not know what the future holds. I must not let the pressure on me get too great or I lose touch with living one day at a time. I have to keep living this way because thinking to the future is presently more than I can handle. I cannot think too far ahead because life is too uncertain.

While writing this story I realize how truthful those words have become. My early journal scribbles led me to being published and then to writing this book so many years later. The reflections of the eve of Becca's first birthday were published in the *Minnesota Parent Magazine* entitled "How a Family Copes with A Chronically Ill Child." The article and pictures of our family with Becca opened the door to sharing our lives to help others. My friend Kim entered it for publishing and I was surprised when there was little editing. I realized then that my best writing came from the depth of my heart when I need to journal. The Ann's Life entry turned into another article for parents coping with trauma. My daughter's pain led me toward a new passion, my writing.

▼

Becca's first birthday was celebrated on a sunny day in August. The nurses, our family and friends partied at a lakeside park. The potluck picnic was a day away from the isolation of the nursery and the day was beautiful, the lake warm and peaceful. At a year old Becca was barely twelve pounds. The kids ran in their swimsuits as they played with Becca and made friends with other children at the beach. The men and boys threw footballs and baseballs, while the nurses took turns trying to keep up with the kids on the swing sets with their baby sister. Becca swang with Marissa and she slid down the slide with nurse Mary. She smiled with her little protruding tongue while she bounced on the park fiberglass ponies. We took a cherished family picture while all 'six' Yurcek children played choo-choo-train on the slide from oldest to youngest. Becca joined her siblings in play and loved every moment. The short time at the beach was a welcome celebration from the realities of her early months and her pediatric home nursery.

Life with Becca had changed everything, she survived her first year. I thought back to the day of the care conference when I asked Dr. Hesselin if there was any hope and he told me we couldn't give up, so our family didn't give up and neither did Becca. Only time would tell what the future held, but for today Becca was here and that was all that mattered.

▼

August 3, 1989

It's Becca's birthday. She seems to know it's her day. Marissa and Matt woke her up by singing "Happy Birthday" at the side of her crib. Becca read her birthday cards. Matt helped her open her presents. She got a My Little Pony Baby, and Marissa, our pony enthusiast, was thrilled. They can play together.

Then Becca gave us a present. She rolled from her back to her stomach and then proceeded to long roll four feet to come to Mom. She knew what she was doing and she was all wrapped up in the tubing of her feeding pump. She smiled at me proudly with her little tongue sticking out between her teeth. Unbelievable!!! She hates being on her tummy and for months we tried to get her to roll over. But today, her birthday, she rolled to come to me. Thank you, Becca.

Mary from the hospital called to wish Becca a happy birthday. She cared enough to think about both of us. I remember how small and sick Becca was. Look where Becca is now.

She's alive. It's a miracle.
Becca, I love you.

Mom

- 16 -
A NEW NORMAL

Becca's first birthday was a milestone, and each day life became easier, relatively speaking. Her heart surgery was a success. Becca was growing stronger daily and we had tools to help her. We were accustomed to the various people who came and went from our home.

The diagnosis of Noonan's syndrome provided us with a knowledge base and from that base we were guided to help Becca. At first, we found a few short articles regarding the syndrome because little was written about this rare disorder with its many complications. Then, over the years, as research papers were published with new findings, we often discovered Becca had many aspects of the syndrome. If anyone had told me all the things that were wrong with Becca at once, I would have been too overwhelmed. Thankfully we found the puzzle pieces of Becca's Noonan syndrome a bit at a time.

Ups and downs became our new normal, and we lived life day by day. Becca made the most of time she was healthy and had energy to play, she would not stop until she was exhausted. She enjoyed playing with the kids and the nurses, learning new skills, and entertaining everyone who met her. On the days she was sick, we survived moment by moment, while Becca shut down to cope with her pain. Becca would wake up and have a good morning and yet by evening we could be back in survival mode. The nurses were a blessing as it took two of us to maintain the enormous care she required on the bad days because each minute was filled with special care for her.

Vacations away from home became going for follow-up appointments to Becca's thirteen specialists. We needed to see the hematologist, the ophthalmogist, the cardiologist, the infectious disease doctor, the pediatrician, the gastroenterologist, the endocrinologist or whatever -ologist they wanted her to see next. I tried to spread those out to one to two appointments a week. Three times a week the early intervention program of our public school sent out their specialists. Becca had physical therapy, occupational therapy and speech therapy in our home. The county caseworker stopped by once a month to document Becca's progress and assess her needs, and the nursing agency supervisor came out to check on the care Becca was receiving. Home care was just as busy, we just lost the long distance commute. Becca's care was intensive, and our home had been turned into a PICU, with one major difference, Becca's whole family surrounded her with frolic and love.

Our days were regimented to keep everything even for Becca. Every hour was filled with something that had to be done. The different medication types and doses were overwhelming. Medications were charted on multiple pages and the nursing charts kept everything organized and timely. Breathing treatments happened every four hours on good days and every two hours on bad days.

▼

From my journal:
It is three days past Becca's birthday:

Becca has right lower lobe pneumonia, and we don't know if it is viral or bacterial. She is not feeling well. Her eyes look sick and she is limp. Her little body seems to whisper "I want to sleep. Leave me alone."

Becca really does not like her BD's. Her temperature is 102°. She is requiring oxygen all the time. Her little heart is shaking her tiny chest. Three days ago we forgot how sick she was. Today we are reminded of her fragility. We are calling the doctor once again, and the doctors are worried.

▼

The doctors prescribed another medication to liquefy the thickened mucous plugs clogging Becca's lungs and treatments were added to help break up the congestion. She hated BDs! After every treatment we pounded her little chest and back to help open her lungs, and she fought us until she seemed to realize that it was helping her breathe, despite not wanting to be touched and prodded.

There was so much to keep my little baby viable. She had meds to keep the gas down in her tummy and medication for helping speed up her touchy tummy. She had antibiotics to keep down the chronic infections and medication for thrush and yeast. Becca was still on gamma globulin treatments every three or four weeks to help boost her fragile immune system. On those days we spent the entire day at the hospital while the four to six-hour infusions were administered.

Becca hated the gamma globulin treatments; the doctor had to poke her repeatedly trying to get the IV's started. The nurses held her down, and I worked to calm my little girl as they hurt her time and time again. . . in multiple places . . . six or seven tries . . . to get the catheter in a good vein. Watching as the doctor and nurses hurt my daughter I wondered what the long-term repercussions for trauma would be. Did they have no regard for her pain?

The immunologist added another antifungal because the thrush was not responding to the first antifungal, and the second antifungal didn't help the systemic yeast so they added another antifungal. We put meds in her mouth and scrubbed out yeast patches and Becca fought us and turned away. I tasted the bitter medications thinking she had good reason to fight us. They were awful and left a terrible taste in your mouth.

Because we were always putting something into her mouth feeding Becca was another challenge and she developed a severe oral aversion. Who could blame her? Every time she choked, we used the suction catheter to clear the mucous from the back of her throat to keep her airway open. Now multiple times a day we used nasty-tasting medications to try to stop the yeast from growing. Becca pushed us away, and nothing got near her mouth without a battle except her pacifier. The therapists believed this behavior was learned, and we had to figure out how to help her get over it. The nurses and I both felt there was more to it. It seemed as if Becca was protecting herself from something and once again we were right.

The nurses and I stayed busy with the pages of doctors orders that were assigned daily, and the therapists required care plan of exercises and activities. We squeezed in the exercises the therapists taught us between the medical cares. Becca bounced on a ball to learn balance and strengthen the control of her body. We encouraged her to reach for toys and we tried to get her to maintain eye contact. Between cares, therapies, and medications, we played, and read, and rocked Becca or relaxed and hung out with the kids.

Becca was in and out of the hospital a few times, but with the in-home help, we managed sickness and crises with outpatient therapy and lab draws, keeping her away from being exposed to more pathogens while recuperating from another. The communication between the hospital, the doctors, and the nursing agency was smooth and provided early intervention, thus saving trips to the hospital. It was healthier for Becca to be at home and more cost effective for the health care system.

The Medicaid program now covered most of Becca's bills and she was approved for benefits from Social Security. The four hundred plus dollars a month helped pay to keep Becca at home. It provided funding for our temperature controlled home. It paid for the extra water, soaps, paper towels, disinfectants and travel to the doctors and hospital. We were finally able to buy things that the professionals said Becca needed.

Since we were down to one car, I drove Jim to work and picked him up after the store closed. I was thankful the nurses were there to watch Becca with all her medical paraphernalia and I could let little Matt sleep in. We had kept the kids in a different school district near my mom's so when Becca was in the hospital, they could walk to school from Grandma's. I drove them back and forth to school and home, and the time alone with the kids on the school jaunts were important times for all of us. The five minute alone time I had returning to the house was 'my time' to regroup and regain strength. I claimed this as 'heaven sent' and I lingered over each moment of freedom from the responsibilities I had when I walked back through my doors. People often wonder how I did it. I did it by savoring the miniscule seconds and moments as if they were weeks and weeks of vacation. My one-minute vacations still get me through.

One morning, a calm male voice said, "Stop." I began to slow down to stop at the streetlight that was glowing green.

I looked in the back, it was empty. I looked to the left and right, no one was coming.

Then the voice continued, "Someone is going to run the light."

I stopped at the green light.

Just as I was at a full stop, a blue midsize car speeded through the intersection going at least sixty in a 30 mph zone. I pulled into the parking lot shaking. Once again we'd been protected. This time I turned fully around to see if someone was hiding. No one was there.

I had heard such whispers as a child and I was scared of them. Today, the calm direct voice comforted me and I was glad I listened.

▼

It took us twenty minutes to juggle Becca and her gear, so going anywhere needed careful planning. Things got much easier when one of the nurses saw a new feeding pump being used at one of her others kid's home, the portable Flexiflo Companion Pump fit in a con venient backpack. The battery lasted eight hours, and Becca didn't have to be tied to the IV pole in her room. Becca and the pump went everywhere providing us new freedom. She played out of her room with her siblings. We went for walks in her stroller during nice weather. We used the pump for doctors, hospital and therapy visits.

The nurses did not just pay attention to Becca; they included the other kids, and the kids and I became comfortable around them. The kids intuitively seemed to understand when they might be in the way and then found other things to do.

The nurses and therapists were now all part of our life.

Jim on the other hand felt like it was a health provider intrusion. He was not as comfortable with having so many professionals in and out of our home, even though he understood this was the way it had to be for Becca.

I learned to be assertive with the caregivers when boundaries were crossed or expectations were not working. I realized I couldn't disinfect the kids or sterilize the house, or live in a 'perfect' world. Eventually I relaxed as I got used to differing opinions and styles of parenting and housekeeping. At first it was hard to speak up, I tried to please them all, but as time wore on, I realized I was the home-front manager. It was my home and my baby.

-17-

YURCEK'S OF OZ AND TOTO TOO

Loving a critically ill child definitely had its bumps and potholes, but even now those surprises were part of our day-to-day life, and we were settled in. Except for medical visits, picking up kids from school or sharing a gluten-free snack with my mom I was homebound. All the outpouring of caring that we had when Becca was first born was now gone. We were forgotten, struggling on our own, and no one called just to say hello or ask how things were going.

Homebound adds to the isolation of families who are already taking care of sick family members and I began to want the "normal" family things we had before Becca arrived. The children were showing signs of jealousy. The tiny baby took too much time. The kid's felt there were too many strangers going in and out of our home. Kristy did not like the opinions of two adults when she voiced arguments for freedom. At twelve she was wise for her years, and the psychologist warned us that her milestones of independence would be early.

Another school year was fast approaching, and costs for school supplies were staggering. The nursing agency enrolled my children at our local mall's Back-to-School program sponsored by a non-profit agency. People adopted anonymous children to get them ready for school and each of my children had a new backpack filled with school supplies and something new to wear on the first day of school. Because of the Back-to-School program my children did not have to face school empty handed and their school supply lists were filled by generous strangers.

▼

While strangers blessed our family, Jim struggled with depression from not being able to provide. It is quite a common outcome for fathers with critically ill children. Men are expected to provide and protect their families, but no one can afford the costs of a child with special needs like Becca without assistance.

Jim didn't talk about his overwhelming struggle and his parents are three hours away and didn't know the reality. When they knew that we were struggling, they somehow knew when to 'pop in' with bags of groceries in just the nick of time to say hello and lend a helping hand. Jim's dad is an excellent cook and got right to work fixing a feast and Granny helped him.

At this time pride was still in the way and if Jim had shared with them, they would have been right there beside us.

▼

I had the support of social workers, doctors, and nurses who helped me understand how to cope; Jim had no one but me, and much of the time I was too tired to listen to his needs. I was too busy trying to meet the impossible demands of an impossible situation.

Jim's thousand dollars a month salary was supplemented by Becca's four hundred dollar SSI payment. That meant the house payment was covered. We could pay for utilities and car insurance, but little was left over, especially when the car kept breaking down. Compared to earlier in Becca's care, life was better. And the children, except for Becca, were off Medicaid with the insurance Jim's employer provided. Now we had co-payments to meet and the added costs of paying for the monthly share of our medical premiums. We still qualified for Medicaid, but Jim wanted us to do it ourselves, even if we had less money in our budget because of it. He needed to pay his own way. He was ashamed of our needing assistance especially with the holidays again approaching.

▼

Last year I had turned Becca into her little pink puppy for Halloween. This year I had another idea. I needed to create something and my sanity needed a return to the past when the kids were little. I had always created holiday costumes for my children and my kids needed to have a 'normal' holiday again. I loved sewing for my family and for others; and I missed my designer doll and children's clothing I had sold at exclusive shops and craft fairs before Becca was born. All I needed to create was a piece of newspaper, a tape measure, and an idea.

The trip to the fabric store was like a vacation back in time. I happily dug through pattern books for ideas. There it was, the Wizard of Oz, and it only cost 99 cents! I was on a mission as I visited two wholesale fabric houses. All I had to do is come across the right remnants. I was having fun again, thinking about what child I would transform into which Oz character and how I could do it.

It was four days before Ian's most favorite holiday, and I sewed night and day to meet the Halloween deadline. Ian's personality and straw blonde hair matched the identity of the Scarecrow. A patched forest green shirt and brown broadcloth pants were transformed from scraps in the 88-cent bargain bin fabrics. I found an old felt hat and added yellow yarn for straw. He was the most perfect Scarecrow imaginable.

I used my silver ironing board replacement fabric for Nathan's Tin Man suit. I scrounged through buttons in my old button box and spray painted some old rubber boots shiny silver.

Mom offered to help me by sewing Kristy's Dorothy dress. I sprayed her almost outgrown Sunday shoes with red spray paint and used spray adhesive to glue on red glitter. I lined a cast-off wicker basket with red gingham and it became a perfect basket for Dorothy's tiny dog Toto.

Little Matt became the Cowardly Lion and a big piece of fur quickly turned him cute and cuddly, while pink lace and satin took shape as Marissa's dream dress for Glinda the good witch. Marissa as a little princess pranced and twirled with her dollar store crowned jewels and magic fairy wand.

I could not forget Becca, she was cast as the smallest of the Oz characters. The dark furred piece of fabric was expensive, but she only needed a yard since she was so little. She would be bundled up as Toto, Dorothy's tiny dog with a big red ribbon to top off her head.

Everyone was excited!

▼

They marched in their new costumes in the community parade, and they won a small prize for the group costume contest. Everyone could see they were a family and little Toto was the most magical part of all with her tubing and medical equipment.

Fall was ending and this would be one of our last opportunities to sneak Becca out before the winter set in with cold and flu season and we were completely closed in. Costumed and attached to her equipment Becca joined her siblings with tag along Nurse Deb at the church Halloween party for the evening. My aunt captured the moment with pictures.

I wondered as I placed the photos into our family album who needed this holiday fun more, the kids or me? In the midst of our chaos, we had an evening of normalcy and laughter.

- 18 -

HOME ALONE

With Halloween over, November ushered in the official Yurcek birthday season. Nathan starts it on the second, Jim on the sixth, Ian's on Thanksgiving this year, Matt on the seventh of December, with Kristy right after Christmas on January sixth. The kids had grown used to our being broke, and I knew anything that I was able to get, would be appreciated. A small toy and much needed clothing would have to do. The boys were growing fast, and their pants were flooding high above their ankles.

Becca was back in the hospital when the Toys for Tots program adopted our family for Christmas. We hoped she would be home to celebrate with us. I had found a 'Baby's First Christmas' embroidered sleeper in my hand-me-down bucket of clothing given to me for Becca. She was still so tiny, that the little sleeper fit just right. This was her second Christmas, but her first at home. Her hospital visits had been short and not nearly as often and her doctors wanted her out as soon as possible to avoid the sickness in the hospital so they limited her stays to two to three days. Yet every time she was in, she caught something. Becca had been exposed to measles and chicken pox twice each while in the hospital or following up with the specialists and hospital staph made Becca sicker than the virus she was admitted for in the first place. Becca was far safer at home. The gamma globulin infusion visits were exhausting and Becca's tiny veins continued to collapse as the nurses struggled to insert the IV needles. I cringed as I held my tiny screaming daughter who was fighting with every ounce of energy she could muster. Becca struggled so hard, that she had bruises on her tiny arms and legs from the nurses hands. Down the back of her spine, she had a line of little round bruises from the pressure of the vertebrae from holding her down. I prayed for an uncollapsed vein to be found as attempt three . . . and four . . . and finally five made an entry into her little body. Watching Becca struggle was something I never got used to. I hated watching her hurt. It broke my heart. It's a mom's job to protect her child and provide comfort and help make everything better and in this case the better felt much worse.

It was the beginning of the long Minnesota winter of infection control. Flu shots were mandatory for everyone. Marissa screamed at the thought and continued to scream uncontrollably through the inoculation, and then she burst into uncontrollable laughter when the anxiety of the inoculation was over. Ian and Nathan argued about whom was the bravest, and Matt hid behind me from the needle. I thought of little Becca and all the pokes she had tolerated. My little soldiers certainly could do this for their bravest of all little sister.

▼

Kristy was now a budding teenager, and having her share a room with three brothers was no longer working. The kids needed the added rooms, we needed the bathroom, and people were helping us. Jim's parents and church friends volunteered to help. We skimped to buy the two by fours for the walls and church friends bought the sheetrock. Jim and his dad hung the wallboards while my uncle and my Dad put in the wiring. My little brother and cousin helped spray the ceiling.

The county had gotten approval for the plumbing fixtures and flooring for the downstairs bathroom and sent the voucher to Menards. All we had to do was pick up the new bathtub, vanity, sink and faucets. Jim's dad plumbed in the fixtures when they came to town for the weekend to help.

My asthma flared up when they taped the sheetrock and I ended up gasping for breath, but I said nothing to anyone. Thankfully by Christmas we were ready to paint.

The newspaper route manager asked us to take on a Saturday and Sunday newspaper motor route. We felt as though our prayers had been answered. Now that Becca was on a waiver, we could increase our income without losing her Medicaid benefits. She was a family of one, and she qualified on her own, so to help our finances we added the new route. Jim and I took turns doing the papers during the week and we shared the job on weekends getting up at three in the morning because the big Saturday and Sunday routes needed to be done by seven thirty. We spent Saturday afternoons preassembling the three sections of the newspapers with the ads so in the middle of the night, we would be ready to only add the news, stuff them in plastic bags and load them into the van. We were on our way with papers delivered to the customers before the sun rose.

One Saturday the day nurse called in sick, so Jim and I took Becca with us to assemble the Sunday newspapers at the depot four blocks from our home. Kristy, at nearly thirteen, volunteered to watch Marissa and Matt with Ian. Nathan joined Jim and me to preassemble the three sections of the Sunday morning paper. Becca sat on the workbench in her carseat hooked up to her medical equipment. She watched us as we made quick work of the papers. We were nearly done when we heard sirens coming from the corner fire station. Jim, Nathan and the depot manager informed us that the fire trucks squealed out of the station heading south out of sight into our neighborhood, while my chest tightened and stomach started turning upside down. I hoped it was not my house.

At home Kristy was running the washer and dryer trying to lessen the mountain of dirty clothing. She had gone upstairs to play with Matt and Marissa when all of a sudden the house filled with smoke and the smoke detectors began wailing. She grabbed Matt and yelled for Marissa and Ian to get out of the house. Ian the curious ran to the source of the smoke and told Kristy it was the dryer. The house was quickly filling with putrid black billowing smoke. Kristy and Marissa grabbed Ian at the bottom of the stairs and dragged him safely outside. Kristy and Ian's asthma inhalers were forgotten inside and the kids were coughing and wheezing.

The next-door neighbor had heard the commotion and saw the children run out the front door trailed by black smoke. He had been a volunteer fireman and he ran for his fire extinguisher while his wife called 9ll. Duane bolted into the downstairs to discover the laundry room blackening. He pulled the plug on the dryer and blasted the leaping flames. Needing oxygen, he sprinted back up the stairs and was handed a fresh extinguisher by another neighbor who came to assist. He held his breath as he ran to try to put out the ever-growing flames. By the time the fire department arrived, the flames were shooting as high as the ceiling. They had moved up the walls to the upstairs kitchen.

The neighbors sent someone to the depot to alert us of the crisis at home. We arrived as the firemen were finishing up their work and packing away their hoses. Huge fans were posted at each door pumping out the black smoke that had filled our home.

Our neighbor saved our home from destruction. If he had not blasted down the flames after the dryer had caught our clothes on fire, it may have been the whole house instead of just clothes and my laundry room walls. Everywhere a thick black coating of smoke and dust lingered.Thankfully, the fire department was only four blocks from home, and our house was saved from being engulfed in flames.

Luckily our homeowners' insurance was paid with our mortgage and it had not lapsed as our finances deteriorated. We were banned from the house until the fire inspector did his inspection, and then we were told that the smoke damage was too great for us to return home, especially with a medically fragile baby and three asthmatics. A service company had to clean the entire house and reseal and clean all the ductwork. Every piece of clothing had to be sent out for cleaning and smoke treatments. Every toy had to be washed. Every stuffed animal had to be decontaminated. The insidious smoke had curled and snaked into everything, even into the corners of our closed dresser drawers and cupboards.

We had managed financially to hang onto our home and now we were homeless anyway. Our homeowners' policy did not cover temporary accommodations. As if the chicken pox fiasco wasn't enough, the snaking smoke damage forced our family of eight and two shifts of nursing care to stay with my parents in their two bedroom townhouse. Mom and Dad were already used to living with my children through quarantine, but now with the fire they had the nurses and 'all' of us. Jim and I thanking heaven that my parents had moved to town the month before Becca had been born. My parents were probably thinking, "what on earth got them to move so near." Their poor house was bursting at the seams. Twice a day Mom answered the door to let in the nurses. In, out, in, out. Up and down went the patter of many little and big feet.

Jim grabbed a few clothes from the house. He got all Becca's medical equipment out and picked up the special cleaners. The cleaning service provided directions on how to scrub them down and get the smoke smell out. A crisis phone call to the home care supply company brought new medical supplies and the pharmacy provided emergency medications. The nursing agency transformed the second bedroom into a pediatric intensive care nursery. A portable crib functioned as Becca's bed. We added wood blocks to give it the same fifty-degree incline, as she had at home, to keep her lungs and breathing clear. We filled the dresser with medical equipment. At night, Kristy and Marissa snuggled in the twin bed next to Becca and somehow slept through the sounds of the apnea and feeding alarms. Becca now slept through her night breathing treatments, and I set my alarm to administer them every two-hours.

We made do. My parents thankfully had a downstairs family room for the kids to hang out during the upcoming school holiday, and having their aunt and uncle home kept them from being bored. We helped Mom and Dad with groceries and our food stamps fed our army of hungry kids.

Mom babysat the children while I stood in line at the Armory to choose two gifts for each child. Mom sewed beautiful Christmas dresses for my two older daughters and the boys each received a new sweater while we waited for the arrival of our emergency cleaned clothing. The few clothes Jim had captured from our home took four washings before the smell was finally removed, but at least each child had two outfits. They wore Grandpa's t-shirts for pajamas and we made do.

All their toys remained in our home awaiting cleaning, and their stufffed animals had been shipped off to be renewed. Our family had been adopted for Christmas, and kind strangers delivered the boxes of Christmas fixing to the garage to await Christmas morning.

Christmas was a distraction from the worries and chaos of the fire. All my siblings came to my parents for Christmas and the house was filled with people, and tradition. During the middle of the night we placed the presents 'from Santa' under the tree. I was not into Christmas this year, I was going through the motions for the kids.

In the morning they awoke at the break of dawn and tore into their presents. Santa delivered some good presents, but he also delivered a broken toy and a smelly stinky missing one ear stuffed animal that left my small receivers in tears. It was unbelievable that Santa would do such a thing. From that Christmas forward I opened the presents to make sure my children would not be hurt by the charity they received. I wanted to make sure the gifts were giveable.

One day when I had stopped at our smoke damaged house, I found a card in the door from social services. We were facing child protection investigation and possible neglect charges for leaving our children alone. The fire department and the police had notified them about our home alone kids. The basement was in the process of being remodeled, the kids had been squished in the one room, the laundry room floor was filled with a mountain of wash and toys were strewn all over the floor. My house before the fire had been a temporary mess due to Becca's immediate cares and after the fire it was now a disaster. I shook for two days as I waited for the meeting with the caseworker.

I did the dishes and faced the worker with an imperfect house. There was nothing else in the cleaning department I could do as the smoke residue triggered my asthma. Kristy had passed the Red Cross babysitting class, and I gave them her certificate. She had handled herself with skill and expertise to keep her siblings safe. We had the backup of respect and understanding from the nursing agency, and Becca was with us packaging papers. The meeting was business like, but from that moment on, I had a healthy fear of social services, and I panicked if everything were not perfect for a very long while.

Gretchen and Tim went back to school after the holidays, and we were looking forward to the return of the older kids to school after the New Year. Then the school district announced the teachers voted to strike! Never in the history of our school district had the teachers gone on strike. Now, when we needed school time the most our kids were granted another week and a half of vacation while the teachers argued for increased wages.

The tiny townhouse was a busy place with someone always walking on or bumping into someone else. We ate dinners in shifts. We fed the kids first and then the adults sat down to dinner and a moment of peace while the kids watched TV or played a game. We made the most of our time at my parents; we had the necessities, and most of all we had each other.

Mom enjoyed the nurses' company, and Becca enjoyed watching her two-year-old cousin Kaitie play. Becca's eyes followed Kaitie's every move studying what being a toddler was all about. I noticed her trying to imitate Kaitie's actions as she tried to play with the older toddler learning toys.

- 19 -

BLESSINGS IN DISGUISE

I never expected the fire would become a blessing in disguise. The fire inspector discovered our dryer's tumbling barrel had dropped down due to faulty clips and when the clothes quit tumbling they heated up until they caught on fire. A year later the manufacturer recalled our dryer's model as other families had lost their homes to fires. The insurance settlement paid for replacing the clothing that had burned in the laundry room, all the carpets in the house, all the cleaning and fresh painting. The check covered the extra costs incurred, and those monies were enough to keep us on our feet. The carpet allowance with Jim's discount at work was enough to carpet the upstairs, plus the bedroom and family room in the basement. Once again God provided for us out of adversity.

As the year wore on, Becca's needs kept all of us busy. When Becca felt well, she astounded us with her progress. Our kids thrived with the consistent structure demanded to have Becca at home and the nurses' quick responses with early intervention kept our very sick kiddo out of the hospital. Our days were filled with treatments, therapy, and play to convince her to put something other than her pacifier in her mouth. Her thrush and mouth sores were still troublesome and her medication regime to keep it under control did not help.

The therapists said it was learned behavior and I wondered why we should blame Becca who was becoming a fun little gal. Four times a day we swabbed out her mouth a with yellow 'anti'fungal and twice a day we used some other 'anti'fungal mixture the pharmacist specially mixed up for patients with weakened immune systems after chemotherapy. Then one or two times a week we painted her mouth with a purple 'anti'fungal.

Becca sealed her mouth in self-protection.

I felt it was something more, but no one listened to me.

I was 'just' a mom.

Matt was now a very quiet four-year-old and had become a shadow in Becca's wake. When Matt was home he had learned to be busy entertaining himself and staying out from under foot. Luckily, he had the stability and structure of his grandparents. He had my dad as an amazing grandfather. He let Matt sit in his lap as he read his airplane and car magazines and watch the history channel. One day, Matt disappeared. We quizzed the kids, but no one could figure out who last saw him. We scoured the house, we searched everywhere, but he was nowhere to be found.

We formed a search party consisting of our kids and Jim's parents. Jim looked in the grasslands to the east near the highway and they looked across the street. We panicked that he may have ventured into the rain soaked swamp, or wandered off into woods near the trailer court on the highway. We had looked everywhere when we finally called 9ll to report him missing. We were frightened someone grabbed him as a couple of sexual predators were known to live in the trailer park outside of our neighborhood and parents now kept close tabs on their children.

While the police were making search and rescue plans, a sleepy little boy plodded into the living room rubbing his eyes. He had come from Becca's room and was curious about what was going on. He had curled himself into a tiny ball between her wall and the dresser and was covered by a hanging chain holding Becca's stuffed animal collection. When we asked him what he was thinking, he simply said he needed a quiet place to hibernate for a nap. The police and the neighborhood laughed at Matt's escapade. I wasn't sure whether to laugh or cry. We were relieved he was all right.

During the first two years with Becca our budget evaporated, and it was one crisis after another as we struggled to keep ahead of the shut off notices and foreclosure on the mortgage. Now life was getting better. Jim's company paid our health insurance and we were off of food stamps! The added income from the paper route allowed us to stand on our own. We still needed help for Becca's care, but we had our home, food, and clothing.

Just when things seemed to even out, Jim got word rumors were circulating that management feared the state was going to make us put Becca on their health insurance plan when open enrollment came around. There was no way this small company could afford to take on that increase, as they had a couple of employees with catastrophic illnesses in their families. The thousand dollars a month was little compensation for the nine-to-nine shift he worked Monday through Saturday, and the six extra hours he worked on Sunday. By the time he finished his paperwork, he was making less than three dollars an hour on an eighty-hour week.

Once again his job was in jeopardy and Jim fell exhausted into a depression. He was discouraged he could not provide for his family again and he worked too many hours for family time or providing help at home. In addition, he wasn't even making a living wage. Nurse Cheryl excitedly shared that her husband had returned to school.

Umm, we had the paper routes and we could get Medicaid for five dollars a month per child. Maybe at long last Jim too, could return to school. Our life was so out of whack it seemed like the perfect idea. We had nothing to lose.

I approached Jim, "Since we are already broke; why not improve your education and change careers?" Jim's business degree in finance had been useless in the recession of the eighties. For twelve years he had been a bystander watching his children grow up. Most of the week I parented solo. Our children had to visit Jim at work to see him and their earliest memories were playing in the store on massive rolls of carpet they turned into an obstacle course. Our kids jumped from roll to roll, performing somersaults, and flips on the cushioned carpet mats. They gleefully remember the teen employees chasing them around the carpet after closing pretending to be carpet monsters.

A few days later Jim announced he had an appointment at the University of Minnesota admissions and was considering going into health care. What better way to insure his daughter than enter the business! Jim's best friends both had gone back to school when we were first married and become pharmacists. They still loved their jobs. Jim was interested in physical therapy or perhaps pharmacy. His mood brightened at the thought of bettering his career. We talked about how we could make this happen.

Jim's father assured him, he believed in him and that if Jim wanted to go back to school, he should do it. It would be hard, but he had the intelligence to make it.

Jim was not a person of much faith, but even he had noticed that when things were tough magical things happened. I felt we were being taken care of. It was a miracle we were alerted to the plan from the carpet company. Jim could not handle more failure and I encouraged him to move forward with his appointment. Our credit had been destroyed by the late mortgage payments, and we had been running from bill collectors. Since he already had a business degree, grants were not available. With hope and faith I pushed Jim reluctantly forward. If it was meant to be, I believed God would provide.

Jim met with the admissions counselor who gave him pamphlets on Pharmacy, Physical Therapy, and Occupational Therapy Programs. The counselor handed him brochures on the Medical and Dentistry School. Was there a remote possibility to get into Medical School? His two failing math grades and his mediocre grade point average from his first time at the university concerned him.

The counselor offered hope that we could borrow the cost of the tuition and the books. He needed two years of hard-core sciences. He filled out the paperwork and applied for financial aid. Jim took a leap of faith the day the loan paperwork arrived; he turned in his notice to resign to the chief executive officer at the carpet company. He took a chance. We took a chance. We knew we needed to jump to better our futures. Jim needed something to hope for if our family was to thrive. With hope, faith and a student loan Jim returned to school. We hoped that someday, maybe, he could provide for our family and for Becca's extraordinary needs.

School gave Jim a new confidence and mission. He had graduated the first time without opening a book and had played and partied without a vested interest. This time he had a dream and a family. He had Becca's medical needs. This time he took his education seriously. In his first quarter he took physics, chemistry, biology, medical terminology and his labs. He passed them all with straight A's. His second quarter he took higher-level science classes, anatomy and labs and again aced them all. He announced he was going to get into Medical School.

Our children watched Dad study and they studied as he studied. The kids began to take their academics very seriously. Their dad was setting a good example, as school became his fulltime job. Jim was happy, and so were the children. They had their dad! We ate dinner each night as a family. Dad surprised them by picking them up at school. We had family time and for the first time in thirteen years I had help raising the children.

- 20 -

HANDS UP

The question people ask when they hear our story is how did we make it on so little? Jim and I had never had financial stability. Living paycheck to paycheck in the years before Becca was born taught me to be frugal. We struggled, and that struggle provided me with the skills to make the most of what little we did have. I was used to bargain shopping, hitting garage sales and feeding a growing family on very little.

Before I knew about food stamps or assistance programs, Jim and I went days without eating. We learned that after a day or so, you no longer feel hunger. We drank water to fill our stomachs when our stomachs grumbled or ached from lack of food. Jim and I fed the kids and told them we were too busy to eat. Then we ate what was left on their plates after they had eaten their fill. We both dropped twenty pounds, and we were already thin. Today I can see the severity of our malnutrition, but we had been raised to believe it was a shame to ask for help. It was forbidden to let people know that you were poor or struggling. We ran life so close to the financial edge that it only took an instant to fall into devastating circumstances.

The working poor in the suburbs are hidden. I waited until the middle of the night to grocery shop to avoid meeting people I knew in the store. I didn't want the neighbors to see our food stamps. The stores are empty at midnight and six in the morning, and it fit in with our daily schedule. I wondered, how many families faced our struggle and shame? How many families filled out mountains of forms and sat for hours to get healthcare, food stamps or assistance checks to survive, all while being degraded and faulted for being there? I had joined the unseen. I struggled filling out the paperwork and navigating through the red tape. I jumped through the hoops and ran through the bureaucratic maze to survive. How did other people make it through? How could a disabled person who cannot read gain access? How do the grandparents living on meager pensions keep their grandchildren out of foster care? What happens to the working poor who cannot support a family on a minimum wage? Jim and I were educated. Our poverty was hidden in the suburbs. Did we have others living next door with similar burdens?

Perhaps we waited too long before we waved our white flag. It took time for us to lay down our pride. We didn't want help; we wanted to do it by ourselves. We faced judgment and gossip from people we had called friends. On the other hand we were surrounded by the love of strangers. We did not take anything more than we needed. People talk about those who take advantage of the system, and I didn't want to be one of them. Mary from the hospital taught me it was a privilege to allow people the gift of giving. Someday we could repay their giving by giving to someone else.

There was talk behind our backs. What had we done to deserve Becca? People in our neighborhood and our church knew of our circumstances. We drove junk. We stood out. We had a large family. We would never be able to send our children to college. Our kids were doomed to a life of nothingness.

It's expensive to be poor. Everything costs more, from your car payment, to buying toilet paper. First, if you can meet the guidelines to own a home, the mortgage company charges high interest rates, the same for a car. Auto insurance companies charge more to give you the 'privilege' to pay monthly. Our homeowners and car insurance rating is not just figured with our driving record, but based on our credit rating, and even though we never had an accident our insurance increased as our credit fell. Our homeowners insurance was cancelled after the fire, and the next insurance company doubled our payment. We had not done anything wrong. The investigation proved the fire was a manufacturer's defect. I thought insurance was for accidents. It didn't cancel when you had to use it.

Driving junk is expensive, and our car was constantly breaking down. Jim learned his ten-dollar investment in the *Chilton's Auto Book* was the best money he spent. When a tire blew, he took a quick trip to the junkyard to find a used tire. Luckily the junkyard was walking distance from our front door. Jim fixed broken axles and serpentine belts. He changed head gaskets and starters. He replaced belts and transmissions. His least favorite was water pumps. Every one of our old cars seemed to have a bad water pump. Night after night he struggled to fix the car and do his homework so he could run papers the next morning before class. If the car was broken, we had no income.

One morning as Jim worked to get the brakes and axle repaired on the old minivan the bolt stripped. He forced the nut with all his might and the car jumped off the jack. His thigh was pinned under the tireless rim. He had moved quickly and without his speed he would have been killed. God had protected our family once again and Jim thankfully escaped leaving a chunk of his thigh in our driveway. The doctors covered it over, gave him antibiotics and a tetanus shot. He was told to stay off his leg for a week, but he delivered the papers the next day and continued on, without a word, to school.

We drove Jim's parents Plymouth Horizon with 200,000 miles on it. When that died we bought an old Dodge van for four hundred dollars. The rusty old van was a gas-guzzler, and as the paper routes grew, we often had to fill it every other day. Our vehicle was swallowing our profits. Jim's dream car was any car with a warranty and his goal was that someday he would fix a car because he wanted to, not because he needed to.

We lived one day at a time, and I bought only what I needed. Celiac's Disease prevented me from eating cheaply, and avoiding wheat, rye, oats, and barley left little option but expensive health food store bread or labor intensive baking. Rice flour and baking requires time and money we did not have. A tiny loaf of rice bread cost nearly three dollars a loaf. Our food stamps were not accepted at the health food stores where we lived, so to buy rice flour or bread I had to use cash or go without. Even when we got off the food stamps, we could rarely afford the cost to remain gluten free. Nathan, Ian, Marissa, and Matthew also reacted to gluten. Jim and Kristy were the only family members that escaped. I had inherited the Celiac's disease from my mother, and we had struggled to understand how so many in my family had been affected. Later, we would find out the reason when my dad was diagnosed with Celiac's and had been alerted by his anemia. Our family had won the lottery when two Celiac's married. The Celiac winners were four of my parent's five children, my five children, and my niece Kaitie.

I don't know how people who are low income afford to have food allergies. We ate rice and gluten-free breakfast cereals and I scoured the ads to find what was on sale. Some days we ate eggs, eggs and more eggs. Eggs are the most inexpensive source of protein and it was all we could afford. For lunch we made hard boiled eggs or scrambled eggs. For dinner we made deviled eggs or omelets with hash browns.

I cooked most meals from scratch and rice casseroles became a staple. We lived on our infamous Spanish rice casserole. I stretched a pound of hamburger by adding a can of tomatoes or spaghetti sauce with rice and a can of vegetables. This served as dinner for two days.

Living on nothing meant I could not take advantage of sales by buying in quantity like I used to. Planning ahead cannot happen when you live day to day. I only bought what we needed, when we needed it. I bought toilet paper when we were out and dish soap when it was gone with the little money I could scrounge up. Collecting pop cans on the paper route paid a nickel a pound, and a months supply of aluminum put $5.00 in the gas tank. I hoarded my food stamps, setting aside a small stash in case of emergency. I used coupons and dug through the grocery store bins for more coupons. The kids cut piles of coupons from the extra circulars that we had left over after assembling papers at the depot. Our extra coupons were dropped off in the store coupon bin, and the kids helped me search for whatever we needed that week. We always left more than we took. Coupons helped cut the cost of cleaning supplies, laundry detergent and paper products. It stretched the food stamps. My kids came to believe you could only buy cereal if it was on sale AND you had a coupon.

I was thankful to have heat, electricity and water after two months of boiling water on my electric stove. The medical requirements to keep our home at a constant 72° provided the key to an emergency energy order after November. No one could turn off our electricity or gas. Our earned income credit provided just enough money to pay the utilities bills in April, and we avoided spring utility cut off.

Jim became the lightkeeper. If the kids left them on, they lost their light bulbs for a week. Our two bulb ceiling fixtures contained one burned out light bulb and one 60-watt bulb to save pennies. He removed the light bulb from the refrigerator. We opened the curtains. Lights were a privilege you didn't take lightly. To this day, Jim freaks out when the children leave the lights on. To this day, I hoard food instead of food stamps. I have to have a well-stocked pantry and freezer in case of emergency.

We taped plastic inside the windows to cut the winter drafts and lower heating bills. We covered our bay window with a comforter. I applied for an emergency weatherization loan. The county agency caulked the windows, replaced the front leaking door, and blew insulation into the attic to help keep us warm and keep our expenses down.

I turned my thriftiness into a challenge. How far could I stretch a dollar? How little I could get by on? How little I could spend? How much could I save? What could I get for a dollar, five or ten? I kept a journal comparing the savings on how much I could have paid for it, with how little I spent. Instead of feeling bad about our circumstances, I became self-satisfied we were making do on so little.

The kids were well dressed. I made it my personal contest to make sure they did not stand out. My kids did not deserve to be made fun of, so I made sure they looked good to avoid even more bullying. Children can be cruel, and my kids were already taunted because they ate free lunch. Most of the kids could only eat part of the free lunch, the rest had to come from home, and it made them stand out from their food intolerances. It frustrated me that they were bullied for needing to eat. They did not need to be teased for not looking like the other kids. I used my sewing and garage sale skills to find or recreate brand name clothing.

When Becca was tiny, I did not have the time or money to buy or sew anything except for special celebrations. The few items of clothes the children owned were passed down from child to child, but Marissa could not use Kristy's hand-me-downs, as they were six years apart. Ian always wore Nathan's cast-offs, and by the time they reached Matt, they were worn out and full of holes. When Nathan outgrew his clothes, they were near perfect, but Ian was just the opposite. He was tough, always on his knees, and his clothes were stained and tattered leaving poor Matt with rags of bits and pieces. I knew the special sales days at Goodwill, but even that was too expensive. For a three-dollar pair of jeans we gave up one meal.

I shopped the salvage store where manufacturers' seconds, salvage and damaged clothes were sold at rock-bottom prices direct from the factory. This is all the stuff that is unusable to retailers. I had discovered it many years earlier, and my boys had grown up in Oshkosh seconds, irregular overalls and salvaged jeans. Now we were too poor to even buy off the salvage store racks. But twice a year they held a bag sale of clothing too damaged to put on the sales floor. Over a four-day period, boxes of torn, grease stained and broken clothes were dumped on tables for sale. The customer paid only five dollars a bag and I could stuff the bag anyway I wanted. I was hyped. I arranged for the nurses to stay with Becca, and put in a request that any unfilled shifts were staffed. I was on a mission and nothing was going to stop me. After the kids were off to school, Marissa, Matt and I were gloriously free to shop! The kids helped by packing the lunch boxes with snacks, drinks and a sandwich for each of us. We were on a grand shopping adventure to make a haul!

At the front of the store a dozen tables were filled with damaged goods, and it was replenished every hour or two when they dumped more boxes onto the tables. With my trusty scissors and seam ripper I was off. It was the one event of the year I could do something for our family's future. The bag sale gave my life hope.

I found Oshkosh overalls, sunsuits, pants and shorts. There were t-shirts without fronts. There were sweaters without backs. There were jeans with gigantic tears and holes. There were socks with slit toes. Our swimsuits and sandals came from the bag sale, along with a damaged designer handbag with a broken handle. I carefully removed the designer labels so I could sew them onto the new reengineered 'by Anny' clothing. I used skillful packing to stuff every centimeter of my bag. Each broken piece of fabric held a dream for one of my children. A couple of items could be sewn together to make a brand new pair of overalls or t-shirt. A damaged pair of cut off jeans became a hemmed pair of shorts for one of my growing children. A complete leg replaced a missing or torn leg cut from another pair of Oshkosh overalls. For the cost of the zippers my children had new winter jackets for years to come. Even buckles, buttons and inside pockets were recycled on different pairs of snow pants and overalls. Fancy knit collars and sleeve ribbings were precious jewels that provided the finishing touches on t-shirts that I could make in ten minutes with just the cost of the knit fabric.

Even the kids' socks and underwear could be found at the bag sale. Odds and ends of socks were paired up for repair. Six-year-old Marissa had an eye for detail and she was quite adept at finding the mates for the mittens and socks among the huge piles on the tables while Matt hung on my leg or played underneath. Every once in a while he rose squealing in excitement from under the table exclaiming that he had found his own matches. One time he even found truck mittens, and those mittens lived in my mitten bucket for years. I repaired them after I had repaired them, and repaired them again. They were a find Matt would not part with, and I am surprised they didn't go with him to college. The two little ones found that the tables contained 'treasures.' Marissa gathered up little girl pink purses, and odds and ends of costume jewelry and little girl trinkets, while Matt added his findings into a small bag given to them by the store manager to fill at no charge. I carefully filled my box with shoes to be sorted through later in the day. The next dump may contain the odd shoe or boot to 'almost' match. The kids happily wore two different sized designer boots or tennis shoes as long as they matched. No one could tell whether they had one size 2 with a size 2 1/2, besides two of my kids had one foot that was bigger than the other anyway and two different sizes meant a perfect fit! I found perfect sizes and perfect matches just right for who it was meant for. God showed me miracles even at the salvage store bag sale and I was thankful.

I went to the sale with a list of the kids needs, and within hours we had found everything we needed for the season. I dumped the odds and ends we couldn't find a match or a use for back on the table for someone else's blessing.

On the way home, I stopped at the fabric wholesale house. They carried the left over Oshkosh B'Gosh, Healthtex and other manufacturers surplus and seconds bolts of fabrics. I was delighted to find pieces of fabric that matched many of the bits and pieces I had packed in my bag of treasures. Unknown to the public, my kids sported one-of-a-kind designer Healthtex or Oshkosh attire. They went to school very well dressed, wearing outfits rebuilt out of the throwaways or recycled salvage garments. I figured they threw them away; they couldn't sue me for plagiarism. I wasn't selling them, I was just trying to keep my kids clothed, warm and accepted.

I reclaimed my life. Ann was back. In an afternoon of sewing while the nurses watched Becca, I stack-cut a pile of five or six t-shirts for each child. I produced the clothing like an assembly line as I sewed turtlenecks and seasonal t-shirts. I sewed shoulder-to-shoulder and side-to-side. My room looked like a colorful clothesline. The nurses were astounded; a grease-stained ugly piece of nothing was transformed into a real piece of clothing. One leg from this pair . . . a new front from this one . . . mixed with new buttons and buckles. Soon the conglomeration became a designer garment. It was fun to flabbergast the nurses with the healing power of my sewing machine.

They hadn't seen anything yet. They thought only surgery and medical equipment healed. Becca was soon decked out in pink bunny sunsuits, dainty collared t-shirts, and a dozen pair of little girl overalls. I darned holes, and covered flaws with ribbons, dainty trim and buttons. She was pretty in pink, rarely outgrew anything, and soon she was the most well dressed little girl in the neighborhood.

I still smile thinking back to those days, one day I was stopped at one of Marissa's modeling auditions and questioned about where I got her little Oshkosh jumper and blouse?

Umm . . . Should I say . . . . The little hot pink jumper was two put together, with a cast off collar on a matching piece of Oshkosh blouse material from the mill end store and a bag sale? I had even found the matching socks, by adding lace, and ribbons with a matching designer made headband. Marissa was one of the most well dressed children at her auditions and it all came from the healing power of my sewing machine, the fabric store, and bag of rags. I kept my mouth shut and Marisa's secret was safe.

The paper routes were not only a source of income, but also a recyclers dream. Our city's unlimited trash was placed at curbside the night ahead and as we went up and down the streets before dawn, the kids discovered a wealth of treasures. We recycled bright plastic Little Tikes toys we found at curbside. Using powder cleanser and a lot of elbow grease, the toys looked brand new. We found a plastic motorcycle with a broken front wheel, a free phone call to the manufacturer and a small payment brought a new wheel to our front door in two weeks time. A delighted Matt had a new vehicle.

Becca's skills grew as we continued to find her new large therapy toys, all castoffs at curbside. We found gently used bikes people threw away all because of a flat tire or broken chain. Marissa learned to ride bike on a hot pink nearly new twenty-inch bicycle, streamers and all, for the cost of a new link for the chain. Her fifty-cent bike lasted until she outgrew it and then it was passed on to another needy family. We were picky. We only chose the best of the best and only then was it brought home and refurbished. Things we did not need were passed on to others, and kept from filling the landfills.

My children learned this lesson well by example and today, full-grown they call me to brag about their finds. They are proud of their thriftiness and challenge themselves to outdo me. They have chosen life mates who enjoy this survival trait. Marissa calls about a 'great' piece of recycled furniture, or Nathan calls to tell me about his 80% off name brand shirt. I look forward to their bragging and phone calls.

Today I use my bargain hunting skills to help other persons in need clothe their children. I find happiness watching the surprised looks on their children's faces when they find themselves with new designer clothing.

▼

Over the years, as we healed, the Yurcek family understood the depth of difference between giving a hand out and a hand up.

My prayer is that someday the world understands too.

- 21 -
MILESTONES

No one knew Becca's prognosis for the future and we were warned that she might not survive. Many nights I tucked her into bed praying she would wake up in the morning. Her problems were so severe that the doctors questioned whether she had Noonan syndrome or not. They felt what she had was a Noonan syndrome mutation or something they had never seen before. The puzzle pieces of her complex issues had no answers or published papers. Becca was one of a kind. We fought the dark cloud following her through her babyhood. Our constant watching, early intervention and surveillance by the nurses, doctors, and therapists helped her beat the odds. I learned to use mother's intuition to monitor her fragile condition, and I listened to the little voice that told me something was wrong, preventing many crises.

Every milestone was celebrated as a victory of hope. We had no time to grieve for what could have been or experience the dashed dreams many families feel. We fought for her life every moment. We were too busy to feel sorry for ourselves. The fact that she was still here was a miracle in itself.

There are no calendars for exceptional children. Our children do things when they are ready and on timelines they create. Becca's baby calendar had stickers for all the early firsts; the first step, and the first words. For Becca those first stickers had no places to live during her first two years, they sat unused on its back page. Instead, the time was marked by a chronology of heartache and pain, dozens of doctor visits, hospitalizations, therapy appointments and surgeries. For a parent of a special needs child the baby calendar was a reminder of the normal celebrations our child may never have. It triggers heartache for mothers of children with developmental delays or disabilities. Thankfully, in time, we learned to appreciate each small thing Becca accomplished while other parents had the luxury of enjoying their children make each of their firsts. I realized I too had taken baby milestones for granted. Before Becca I didn't understand the long worked for victory they were for exceptional children and their families. I learned to never say never with my daughter; Becca proved the doctors, nurses, therapists and myself wrong time and time again.

In the beginning, she had little energy to do anything but breathe. Anything else overexerted and stressed her tiny body. Even something as simple as a warm, gentle bath caused her to be chilled and turn blue and left her needing oxygen and a two-hour nap.

Her first big milestone came after her open-heart surgery when she finally had the stamina to try to sit up just before her first birthday. Together, Becca and I proudly placed a sticker on her baby calendar! The rest of the pile of stickers waited until Becca was ready to do her other firsts. Becca passed her milestones long after normal children's, and each was a reason to celebrate. I had expected my older children to learn to grab fingers and drop toys. I expected them to roll over and sit up.

Becca gave us the gift of celebration and appreciation. Each day of survival was a miracle. Each new movement a time to rejoice.

Becca had her own style and did things in unique ways. She crawled on the backs of her fists to protect her hypotonic (weak), loose joints from pain and to gain leverage. Determined, she fisted up to two crawling movements, then her poor little brain got so mixed up she didn't know what to move first. We helped her move her little arms and legs across her body in a pattern . . . left arm . . . right knee . . . right arm . . . left knee . . . of movements so important to program her brain, but her little arms collapsed from weakness. We worked with the physical therapist on how to teach Becca movements, repeating, repeating, and repeating. She moved forward at age two by only a few feet, before collapsing. About the same time she learned to pseudo-crawl, she learned to pull herself up to furniture. She wanted to move by herself but was clumsy and unsteady and all of her two-year-old pictures have memorable goose egg headlights on her forehead.

By two-and-a-half, she cruised around the furniture followed by the six-foot tether of her feeding pump tubing. The boys lovingly teased her and told her she was a little dog on a leash. When the boys laughed, she giggled quietly and signed dog and arf.

Since she was fifteen months, Becca wanted us to know what she wanted. We had seen her frustrations with communication and so one of the nurses and I started teaching her from a Sesame Street Sign Language book. We were surprised to discover that Becca knew more than we thought. We found she had normal receptive language skills. She could point to items and show us what we asked her to find. By the age of two, she could sign eight colors. She knew the numbers through five and could identify half of the letters of the alphabet by pointing at them.

Her frustration with getting us to know what she wanted was eased when "want" became her very first sign. Soon to become "want book", "want eat," "want drink," want, and want, and want. Becca was good at getting what she wanted and we proceeded to teach her signs of politeness. She was getting silently greedy and we wanted her to understand manners. Please, thank you, and I love you soon became her favorites. She learned to sign all her favorite animals, colors, and numbers. By the age of two and a half she used over sixty signs. Becca was happy.

Becca's silence was disconcerting and she was nearly five standard deviations from normal speech and language on assessments at age three. The doctors ordered intensive speech therapy for her. Trying to get a washrag near her mouth was next to impossible. The speech therapist told us to place her in her high chair at the table with the family for meals. We gave Becca food, and for years she played with it, smeared it, and finally tasted it. She experimented with the flavors and textures, but never swallowed. We visited her speech therapist twice a week for two years to help her make sounds. The speech therapist finally diagnosed Becca with oral apraxia, a motor programming speech problem.

By the age of two and a half, Becca began to shine academically. At Courage Center, a Twin Cities based rehab facility for both children and adults with disabilities, she got her first chance to use a computer. We were blessed to be in a place with technology and innovative programs. Minnesota was a leader in the field. Becca loved the interactive preschool games and computer programs, and we discovered that she could problem solve and keep up with any game they gave her to play. When the nurse or I told her it was time for therapy at Courage Center, she made typing gestures with her fingers asking for "more computer." The therapists knew they could use the computer as a reward to get her to do the sensory and fine motor therapies that she hated.

At Courage Center, Becca went swimming for the very first time in warm water therapy pools. The water and exercise lessened the pain and strengthened her arms and legs, and she wanted to swim at every visit. She let us know what she wanted or didn't. She argued with the therapist in sign, "swim", "more computer" or "no play" when they wanted her to paint on the mirror with shaving cream. We worked for nine months just to get her to put one finger in the soft shaving cream without her having to wipe it off on a clean napkin. Keeping water out of her ear tubes became a constant battle. Her ears were too tiny for earplugs and the tip of her ears made it a challenge to keep any sort of ear band over them. Inevitably water seeped in, and Becca's ears got infected. The infection started a cascade of other problems. The antibiotic to kill the bacteria started yeast to grow in her ears, yeast that was already in her mouth and on her tiny bottom and the pain had to be immeasurable. When she did complain, we moved into action, usually landing at the physician's office or the hospital emergency room.

Becca was unable to make the simplest baby babble, the connections between her brain and her vocal cords were affected. We worked months to get an "mmmm" sound and for even more months for "bababa." We rejoiced when Becca finally made baby noise. She was silent at two and three. Then, sometime in the middle of her third year, it was like a little switch clicked and she figured out how to babble, and by four she was saying her very first words. In the beginning, she signed while she spoke. Then the signing slowly lessened, and by five she was talking in sentences. At six, she tested out of speech and turned into a motor mouth. There were days I wondered why we worked so hard as now she rarely ever shuts up. Becca was making up for the lost time.

We will never know if Becca lost her abilities when she coded or if she was never born with them. She walked at three and a half after years of practicing how to move her body. Her motor planning was impaired, and she needed assistance to teach her brain to be able to control her body by modeling the movements. Early on, a home-based therapist told us that because of the severity of Becca's motor programming problem she might never be able to print or write.

When Becca wanted to learn to color or print, we practiced each movement time and time again by holding her hand until she created it on her own. We did hundreds upon hundreds of circles, lines, and letters. Unbelievably, at six she wrote her name for the very first time!

We learned little Becca was often wiser than the rest of us. She made gains beyond anything we ever believed possible. She was a shining example of will and determination. If she dug in her heels, we learned there was usually a reason. There were reasons for everything she did or didn't do. There was a reason why she didn't eat and protected her airways. Years later, research revealed that some kids with Noonan syndrome have something called laryngeal and tracheal malasia that meant the muscles in her throat and larynx were weak. She was protecting herself from choking and aspirating into her lungs. A few other children with Noonan have had trachs because of that very issue. The 24/7 care, breathing treatments, precautions, slanted beds, and suction machines prevented Becca from having to be trached. And a trach probably would have killed her because of her recurrent staph infections.

She had already faced aspiration pneumonias from her own secretions when she had a cold. One of the nurses worried we could get in trouble when Becca was congested and feared that someday Becca might aspirate and be unable to breathe. We had the suction machine, but what happened if it went beyond the reach of the catheter at the back of her throat? The nurse shared the procedure to help Becca if we faced such a dire emergency. There would be little time to save her, and our normal procedures someday might be too late to make a difference. She must have had a premonition because her knowledge saved two-year-old Becca's life just weeks later.

Becca and I were home alone, and Matt was playing at the neighbor's. All of a sudden Becca inhaled the thick secretions created by her latest virus. Within seconds I realized that she was unable to move air and was turning blue. I ran from the kitchen to her bedroom for the portable suction machine and emergency bag. I held her face down drumming between her shoulder blades as she grew getting darker and darker. I quickly called 911, and though it was only moments, it seemed like eternity before they answered. Becca no longer fought for air, she was purple and limp in my arms. I felt her tiny heart barely beating her in chest. I knew I couldn't wait for the paramedics. She was dying. I placed Becca on the dining room table and threaded the suction catheter deep into her tiny throat. A clump of mucous came up the suction tubing. With the obstruction relieved, I blew puffs of air into her nose with the emergency ambu bag.

Becca began to breath on her own and by the time the police and paramedics arrived she was pinking up. The paramedics told me I saved her life. I knew I did not do it alone, it was a collaboration between the nurse's intuition, the doctors' and agency's orders for equipment and a miracle. I just reacted, and responded instinctively to the crisis. I did not think. I just did it.

After the crisis passed, I tried to tell myself that she was all right, and it was just another close call. But no amount of self-talk calmed the quivers of panic engulfing my body. It was a panic I had faced before, but suppressed by blocking it out when Becca's heart stopped for the first time. I tried to calm myself as my adrenaline rushed. My body was responding to the panic of nearly losing my daughter once again. A nurse joined me as we transported Becca to the hospital to make sure she was all right. Chest films showed her lungs were filled with tiny white mucous plugs, and she was given breathing treatments to unclog her airways. The doctor ordered bronchial drainage treatments every two hours alternating between two different medications in breathing treatments. For the time being, she would remain on oxygen and she remained off and on oxygen for a couple of months. Her chest films showed little improvement and her tiny lungs filled with the sticky goo. Yet, throughout it all, she continued to make progress.

▼

Becca's gains had a rippling effect. She constantly inspired us. My daughter had become my teacher. Throughout her pain she faced each day with a smile.

The day I came close to losing Becca without anyone to help me, I changed. I had handled facing life and death decisions on my own. I was no longer just a mom. I was no longer a rookie parent; I was a parent of an exceptional child, and I had joined the ranks of other warrior parents. Becca's near miss gave me a new confidence. I no longer needed as much reassurance from the nursing staff.

I began to trust myself.

- 22 -

DUCKS, RABBITS, AND PAPERS

With a leap of faith Jim returned to school. The paper routes were now our only income. Medicaid covered our children's medical needs while Jim and I went without. Jim never got sick, and I rationed my visits to the doctor and paid for my asthma medications out of our meager earnings. From the very first paper route of one hundred fifty papers we had taken on two more Monday thru Friday routes of nearly two hundred papers each. We increased our deliveries to include a Saturday and Sunday route when Jim returned to school, and that motor route was quickly growing from the original two hundred and fifty papers to nearly five hundred. The beauty of the motor route is no one had to walk. The papers were simply stuffed into tubes curbside. The kids and I doubled our earning ability when we added walking routes to the weekend routes. Soon we were delivering almost 3000 papers a week! We ran two cars from two in the morning on until we had delivered the last papers.

Seven days a week we delivered newspapers. The kids came up with their favorite joke "What's black and white and read all over?" They giggled in reply, "Newspapers, newspapers, and more newspapers." To this day, I can't look at a newspaper without thinking back to the days of the paper routes. We delivered over one half million papers before the sun came up over a seven-year time span. Jim and I alternated weekday mornings getting up at 3:00 A.M. to go to the depot to pick up the papers. Jim took Monday, Wednesday, and Friday mornings. I took Tuesday and Thursday. On the weekend we both got up, except when Becca was sickest or when there was no Friday night nurse. Then Jim did the Saturday morning route himself with the kids.

Jim had the heaviest of the burden for the first two years when he went back to school, and he rarely slept. He had always been a night owl, but now he needed to get up at 3:00 A.M., so we all went to bed by nine in the evening. I had the responsibility of Becca and the younger kids, and it was tough to be in bed by nine during daylight savings time and summer sunshine.

Jim and I each took one of the oldest kids with us to do papers. We developed systems to deliver the papers in record times. An adult took one side of the street while Kristy or Nathan delivered to the other. Poor Nathan was always stuck with me, he was stuck loading the vehicles, stuck with the walking route and stuck with all the hard labor. He never complained.

Weekday papers were spread thin and the kids ran the papers to the door while I quickly moved the van to deliver a paper to an isolated house then met up with the kids as they finished their strings of deliveries. My kids developed excellent map reading skills as they read the maps while I drove.

We paraphrased the motto of the United States postal service. Neither snow nor rain, nor heat nor gloom of night stays the Yurcek family from the swift completion of their appointed rounds. We delivered through rain, sleet, and mosquitoes, below zero Minnesota nights, hail, and thunder and lightening storms. We trekked through the northern suburbs with our loads of newspapers.

We made sure our customers woke up to their morning paper with their coffee. During the seven and a half years of delivering newspapers we kept a roof over our heads, food on the table, and the lights turned on in the Yurcek home.

Almost all of us have heard war stories from our parents and grandparents about how hard they worked and how far they walked. Our kids were with us, and they know the truth.

The Halloween blizzard of 1991 began as Ian trudged into the house with his five-pound bag of trick or treat loot. Becca was doing well, and it was a simple Friday morning route close to home. Jim and I left the kids home and ventured out to grab the papers at the depot four blocks down the street. Half way through the route, we realized the intensity of the storm and the insanity of continuing. We turned around and had to shovel our way out of the neighborhood to the main road. We barely made it back to our kids. This was the only time we didn't finish a route, but at least we tried.

The next morning we couldn't even get to the depot and this was the only time Saturday papers were not delivered in the newspaper's history. We walked to the depot in the deep snow late that Saturday and assembled Sunday's papers, too, then Jim and the boys worked thirteen hours on Sunday to deliver nearly 800 Sunday papers on our three different routes after a neighbor used his plow to make a single sweep out of the neighborhood. When they were finished they also helped the supervisor and the skeleton crews of carriers deliver the remaining routes when most carriers could not come in. My soldiers completed their day with a newspaper tally of almost two thousand papers. The kids and Jim got tips and hot chocolate. People gave them cookies, and one customer wrapped hand-knitted scarves around their necks. Jim helped shovel and pull out cars and he argued when he was given rewards for his efforts but gave in as the gas gauge was moving close to empty.

A couple weeks later, the carriers were given coffee mugs with headlines of the storm and the slogan, "we survived the blizzard of 1991." Thirty-six inches of snow had pounded the Minneapolis area and we had been more dedicated than the mail carriers. They didn't deliver Saturday, had Sunday off and resumed delivery on Monday after the roads were cleared.

It is easier to remember the hard work than live through it. We walked miles and miles to make sure each paper was delivered by the proper time to the proper location. We kept track of which customers got what paper, when they got it and where they wanted it to be. People wanted their papers in the door, on the step, in a paper tube or even on the front seat of the red car in the driveway. If their papers were not in the right places, the customer called in an error and received a free paper.

Some of our elderly customers filled their time with complaining, and we challenged them to a secret game called Satisfaction. No matter what, they wanted to get a free paper. We made it really hard for them to get anything for free. One of them upped the ante and required us to deposit the paper in his front door and not wake the dog who just happened to sleep on the other side.

▼

I took on that house.

I left the car running two doors down and snuck up the driveway. I carefully pried the storm door open and arf! Arf! Arf! I still woke the dog.

Ann 0 Dog 1

. . . he got his free paper.

▼

One morning the huge drunken client came storming out of his house screaming at us because Kristy woke the dog. He was shirtless and it was below zero. Kristy ran and locked herself in the car as he pounded on our windshield. Horrified I quickly came up to him and apologized, then I got in my car and drove off. That was the last time we delivered to his house. My boss blacklisted him unless he got his paper at a curbside box in the street.

We tried hard not to misplace papers, and the kids learned fast that any job worth doing was worth doing well. We knew some of our clients by name. Others we applied pet names to though we tried to be nice. We had Mr. You Don't Dare Step on the Grass, and Mrs. Garbage Can because that's where we placed her paper, and we had Mr. and Mrs. On The Kitchen Table. We actually went into their house and delivered it, because she couldn't bend over due to her arthritis and walker. Our children were given donuts, and candy, and cookies, and hot chocolate. On the holidays, we were surprised with crocheted ornaments, boxes of candy, tinned cookies, and gifts. Our loyal clients popped out to chat, and we took moments for small talk before continuing on our way. We walked. We jogged. Ian ran. We strained backs and shoulders with heavy Sunday papers. We sprained ankles from gopher holes and tripping on garden hoses. We took showers in automatic sprinkles as we quickly stuffed the papers under our shirts to save them. We had black ink hands, taped ankles, skinned shins and bandages knees.

Kristy, who became a softball team pitcher, got her practice throwing papers. She had knack for turning the most frustrating morning into a morning when we were all rolling in laughter. Kristy was strong willed and opinionated, so we argued, yet she also made the paper routes the most enjoyable. How she threw the paper towards the door and it landed on the roof I will never know. No one ever asked for their papers to be placed on their roof! Since no one ever asked for that landing spot. I had to pull the car forward, climb onto the roof of the mini van and shimmy up on the roof to get it down. We teased Kristy that she should never play softball, but Kristy didn't listen.

Some of our greatest memories would win viewing on America's Funniest Home Videos.

One morning Kristy came running back to the car screaming. She had walked up a sidewalk and discovered a mother skunk and her five babies. The newspapers took a direct hit from the scared skunk, and she dropped it. Kristy narrowly missed a tomato soup bath to deskunk her. The customer reported to our supervision that he needed a free paper because it arrived smelling of skunk and wasn't in his door. Kristy wasn't about to go back for round two.

We had close calls with raccoons, bird droppings bombed Kristy and angry dogs chased every one of us, yet no one ever got bitten, and nothing ever actually really got hit or killed in the thousands of miles we drove at dawn.

Four ducks staked claims to a yard, and Kristy loved to chase them causing them to fly. Whatever side of the street they were on, she was eager to harass the wildlife. One took off and flew into my windshield. My windshield cracked, but the tough little duck flew off to tell his survivor's tale. Deer darted out from brush, and I narrowly missed one or two, my heart pounding as the children watched them spring freely off.

But the poor Easter Bunny was not so lucky. I joked with the children that I was the mad animal hitter and I swerved right and left to avoid hitting the wildlife. One morning I joked about needing to go rabbit hunting. As I backed out of a driveway, Marissa screamed I'd hit a rabbit. Becca started crying and signing Easter Bunny. I stopped the car to examine the damage under the headlights. The only thing left behind was his tail. Mom had taken off the Easter Bunny's tail. I took the rap for the damage, but at least Mom didn't kill the Easter Bunny for Becca.

Scrawny Ian wanted to outdo his older brother Nathan by carrying the most Sunday papers and a Sunday paper could weigh four and a half pounds during the holidays. Not only were the papers heavy, they were slippery and cumbersome. Ian tried to carry ten. He was noisy and hell bent on being the fastest paper delivery person in the family. We'd pull into a driveway to make a delivery, and Ian would hop out of the van, take a couple steps backwards, and wail the paper at the door. The papers would hit the doors with a variety of crashes, bangs, and thuds. I was constantly trying to keep him quiet and not upset our customers. I held my breath as I watched paper after paper come near to break a window. Somehow he still managed to beat his older sibs. We made up rhythms of delivery . . .two . . . skip one, three, skip two . . . four skip two . . . two to help us remember the sequence. Block upon block, papers and more papers, seven days a week for nearly three years.

Matt could hardly wait until he could join in the delivery, and he rode with Jim in the back seat of the van in his Ninja Turtle sleeping bag. He was often awakened under a pile of tipped papers as Jim rounded a corner and he was always awake for the end of the route

Super America donut treat while Dad refueled. The kids cherished their trips to the gas station for a treat after a job well done.

As Marissa grew, she helped deliver papers too. Once after a rainstorm I heard a blood-curdling scream, and a blond Marissa came running back petrified to the car. The night crawlers and earthworms had come up from the earth to attack her on the driveway. She decided to walk on the grass from then on, and Ian, always the smarty, asked her where she thought the worms came from. Thanks Ian, now Marissa was afraid of the blacktop and the grass. She was also afraid of barking dogs, and shadows, and bees, and mosquitoes, and consequently she never turned into much of a delivery person. But she was one of the best when it came to assembling the papers at the depot. She and Ian could assemble hundreds of newspapers in as little as three hours single handedly.

At fourteen, Kristy went on paper strike. She wasn't going to deliver one more paper and we obliged. But there were conditions, the papers paid for the food, the house, the electricity and all the extras. She was entitled to a roof over her head, food and a warm bed, but the rest were all extras earned by the entire family. She could not use her electric curling iron, no electricity for her boom box, no rides to friend's houses, and no phone service because papers paid for those things. As long as she slept in at home, she went without. Her strike lasted a week. She grudgingly came back to help.

The paper business reached out beyond our family, and everyone got into the game. When Jim's parents came into town, Jim's dad became a paperboy. Jim and his father enjoyed the early morning hours talking and delivering papers. Granny who was a Registered Nurse watched Becca, and we let Matt and Marissa sleep in their own beds instead of the sleeping bags in the cars. The kids looked forward to waking up to the sweet roll treats and fresh fruit Grandpa bought for everyone.

When Kristy's friends slept over, they asked their parents if they could help Kristy deliver papers.

Our skills and reputations grew along with our routes. We subbed routes; and we took over downed routes, and we covered routes for people who went on vacation. The extra we made was often exactly the amount of money we were short for the week, or what we needed to pay a bill. We couldn't afford to turn down extra papers until after Jim got into Medical School and then we cut back on the weekday papers. I still subbed weekday routes and did most of it myself. Kristy, Nathan, and Ian took turns. Jim tried to catch up on sleep and watch Becca who was now more stable. When I got home at 7:00 A.M., he went to the university for the day while Kristy, Nathan, Ian and Marissa went to public school. I spent my days with Matt and Becca, doing housework and making the never-ending runs to doctor's appointments, therapy, and the pharmacy.

My children garnered a work ethic that molded them for their futures. One of the middle school teachers asked me how we had managed to raise children with such a strong work ethic. She taught sixth grade to our four oldest - Kristy, Nathan, Ian and Marissa. The paper routes were a gift, the gift of working together for a common goal – the survival and success of our family. Our kids learned from example and they understood what it took to do a job well. How many parents are fortunate enough to spend three hours a day alone with one of their teenagers? We worked and talked together. We enjoyed each other's company while tackling a less pleasurable task.

We worked side by side as we put papers together. They rode thousands of miles stuck in the car with Mom or Dad several days a week. Jim and Kristy talked about sex, and boys, and drugs. Nathan and I talked about relationships and treating a woman with respect. The newspapers taught us social studies and reasoning. Our children were well read on local, national and world events. They knew geography, politics, and business. Bright and opinionated, Kristy and Ian debated social issues. The car radio and love of music was a welcome diversion, and Jim quizzed the kids on who was the artist, name that song and what happened the year it was written. To this day the kids are experts on rock and roll trivia. We exposed them to all sorts of music from hard and soft rock to Christian music, from reggae beats to classical overtures. Some mornings we sang along to Becca's Disney tunes.

- 2 3 -
FUN

Riding the roller coaster of Becca's constant illnesses and the uncertainties of living day-to-day with a very sick little girl began taking a toll on our family and we needed fun times and recreation to keep going.

Jim won a VCR player for selling carpet so we rented tapes on Thursday night using their two for one special and watched them Friday evenings before going to bed early for the paper routes. Grandpa and Grandma recorded movies or kids shows for us from their cable. We set out the sleeping bags on the living room floor, and the nurses joined us with Becca and her medical equipment while we ate popcorn and drank Kool-Aid. We giggled and laughed. Becca signed 'more' when the movie ended because she did not want to stop, but 3:00 A.M. came very early, and the paper deliveries would not wait if we were to hold on to our reputation.

Being tied to home and trying to keep busy children occupied was a challenge, but being broke brought the ultimate challenge. Small miracles allowed us to have amazing adventures. Our church youth group provided activities on Wednesday nights. And each child could choose one community program per season for free for low income families. Often we had to say no to many of the things the kids wanted to do because the price was too steep. My kids were very fortunate to be included in a program called Sibshops at The Children's Hospital. The hospital hosted a Saturday conference, and while the kids met with other brothers and sisters of critically ill children, the parents listened to speakers about programs for their kids, the effects on the family and on siblings.

Other families get summer vacations, or trips to camp, or theme parks, but not our family. Even trips to the beach or pool were few and far between because Becca could not tolerate the heat.

But then there was Make-A Wish!

After my wish for Becca's half birthday party to borrow the camcorder, we were linked with Make-A-Wish. It was the parties from Make-A-Wish that offered a good side to having to live life on the coaster. When one family member has a chronic illness or disability it affects everyone and it was a welcome relief from the day-to-day pain for Becca, but also the pain felt by the entire family.

We were invited to the yearly pizza party in August held the same week as Becca's birthday. The restaurant and games were closed to the public so Wish Kids and families enjoyed a private party of food, games and fun. They provided unlimited tokens, and everyone played games and rode rides until the party was over. The kids ate their fill of pizza, and soda, and ice cream sundaes. Celebrities autographed shirts or posters. The Make-A-Wish pizza party was the highlight of our summer and it was exciting for my children to have something to tell their friends.

Every so often Make-A-Wish surprised us with free tickets to a Twin Cities event. It was fun to surprise the children with a surprise hockey, basketball, or baseball game or a trip to the wave pool. Taking Becca to a black tie gala benefiting the different non-profits turned her into a "little star."

It was challenging taking Becca out in public as we juggled her medical equipment attached to her ever-present feeding pump. At first, I felt uncomfortable with this different kind of attention. People stared. Others pushed their children away as if they were embarrassed by a child's curiosity. Eventually the Yurceks became used to the looks, and covered mouths, and pointing fingers. We smiled and waved at curious people and had fun. Instead of seeing the negative actions of people, we began to encourage the positive reactions of strangers. The more upbeat we were, the more people were drawn to meeting Becca.

Becca had a way about her and she melted people's hearts wherever she went. It was no secret she had disabilities. Her shining smile created an aura that affected people. She looked like a toddler fluent in American Sign Language. She seemed too tiny to quickly combine two or three signs to make her needs and wants known. It caught people's attention. No one could ever believe that she was as old as she was, and that created a conversation on its own.

We had been invited to a celebrity hockey game that included the TV anchors versus Twin Cities celebrities. The guests were Wish Kids and kids from The Children's Hospital. Tickets purchased by others raised money for families like ours. Jim joined us. School was a blessing that brought him back into the activities of his family. He enjoyed watching the boys run from player to player collecting autographs on their new t-shirts and programs.

Becca and Marissa joined the Vikings cheerleaders. It was amazing to see tiny Becca who had just started walking trying to keep up with the cheerleaders and being held in their arms. Four-year-old Becca came home with silver and black pompoms almost as big as she was as a gift from one of the cheerleaders. She was made an honorary Vikings Cheerleader and she gave Marissa a pom pom so they could play cheerleader at home.

In the lobby Marissa, Kristy and Becca danced along with the band. I cried in joy as I followed her everywhere she went tethered to the six-foot tubing that connected to the feeding pump housed in her purple and green Barney backpack. The nursing agency had secured funding for a portable pump so we could take Becca with us and it provided freedom during the warm weather months when

Becca was the healthiest.

Becca watched the kids who were dancing carefully as she tried to figure out what she was supposed to do. Then in Becca style she danced while the Make-A-Wish photographer followed the tiny tyke with glasses and brown ringlet curls.. . .Click . . . Becca at twenty pounds. . . Flash . . .wearing eighteen-month size infant clothes. . . .Click . . . She made quite a sight dancing with her sisters, and the clowns, and the cheerleaders with her red clown nose given to her by the clown patrol. The crowd circled her and she felt like she was the star of the evening.

Becca was just starting to say a few words and didn't venture to say anything beyond the doors of our home, but then a clown joined my two daughters, and soon Marissa and Becca were both engaged in a giggling conversation. The night was a miracle, and Jim and I smiled contentedly as we looked in the back seat at the Tiny Titan who very quickly fell fast asleep for the forty minute ride back home.

- 24 -

MED SCHOOL

Jim had two semesters behind him as a student and the newfound confidence was apparent. He was happy and had new life energy. Everyone who knew Jim saw the difference. Best of all, he was an involved father, and the kids loved it. He didn't have time to vegetate on the couch. He was no longer working all the time as he had been for so many years.

It was nice to look over my shoulder and see my husband and his little daughter with piles of textbooks and picture books. He and Becca snuggled together with their heads buried in paper and pages. Becca was becoming a daddy's girl. As she stabilized, her home nursing hours were cut back so Jim watched Becca while I cooked dinner or washed clothing. I was glad the days of juggling laundry baskets while carrying a three-year-old attached to medical equipment were behind me. Doing housework while watching Becca required great energy and careful strategizing. Jim made my job easier.

Jim was back to the man I had fallen in love with. For years he had buried himself in his work and now he had time to be a parent. Jim ferried the children as a taxi driver. He wrestled the boys on the floor and taught them to snap towels. He helped Matt put back the bikes he had taken apart and egged on Marissa in her theatrics. He did his homework while Marissa did photoshoots and watched football games with Ian as he tried to study. Jim had fun with the children. He wired them up before bedtime and then picked them up and threw them on their mattresses. The children adored having Dad!

Our days began early and we took turns with the paper route. Whoever got to sleep in was in charge of the kids, listening for Becca's alarms and doing her four and six o'clock neb treatments and medications. After the routes we rushed to get ready for our day. I got the kids ready while Jim showered; then he dropped the middle school kids off at school and I took the younger ones to school after the nurse arrived to avoid having to take Becca out.

Jim worked hard and achieved straight As for over a year with nothing but hard-core sciences. He was thinking about applying for Medical School. He'd have to pass the Medical School exam to apply and everyone who'd taken the test said it was the test from hell, besides costing two hundred dollars. We borrowed the money from Jim's parents, and he spent hours reading the self-help MCAT books.

The day of the exam finally arrived and my younger sister, Gretchen, joined him in taking the test. The day was long and I went to Mom's with the kids to quit thinking about Jim, my sister, and testing. So many times we had faced crisis after crisis when my life was filled with fear, and uncertainty.

What if . . . What if . . . I told my thoughts to quit! There was nothing I could do to change things anyway.

Jim came home and announced he had gotten himself into Medical School! My father told Jim that no one could know he or she did well, but Jim ignored the remark.

After dinner and dessert we took the kids home and put them to bed. Later we discussed what my father had said. His remark hurt Jim. He felt as though he had never met the approval of my parents. He was not good enough. It was a long wait for the test results, and Jim called many times to check if I'd gotten the mail.

Jim had been right, his scores were astounding. He was at the top of his class. He had scored in the ninety- eighth to ninety-ninth percentile of all those applying. I could not wait to tell Mom the great news, but Mom advised me not to tell anyone in the family as it might make my sister feel bad if she did not score as well.

▼

The second year of school flew by.

Jim studied, applied for Medical School and we hoped he would get into the University of Minnesota. He applied to the three Medical Schools in Minnesota: Duluth, the Mayo Clinic, the University of Minnesota and also applied to Medical Schools in the surrounding states. Moving with the kids, especially Becca and all of her medical problems, was scary and seemingly impossible to me. Becca's pediatrician offered to write a letter of recommendation. I called around to different state parent support groups to find out which states we could safely take Becca to and get adequate services.

We needed to stay in the Twin Cities for Becca. We had the paper routes here. We had our house and our credit was trashed. Very few families who have family members with catastrophic medical conditions survive financially, much less make it through Medical School with six children, one of them medically fragile. Everyone said it was impossible.

▼

It looked like Jim had a chance of a spot in Medical School. Transcripts were expensive and the application fees stretched our floundering budget so I typed the applications with Becca on my knee. Our earned income tax credit arrived just in time to pay off the late house payment with enough left over to apply to Medical School.I said a prayer as I sent off Jim's application to the University of Minnesota Medical School. Jim asked his parents to help him buy a suit for the interview. He hated to ask, and he vowed to someday repay them. Thc applications went in the mail in October.

It was January before we heard anything. Jim was denied an interview at the University of Nebraska and we received a kind letter of denial. Then two weeks later, he received a letter inviting him for an interview. He and his mother drove to the University of Nebraska and during the interview one of the questions they asked was what Jim was going to do if he did not get into Medical School. Jim walked out to his mother and told her steadfastly "I will be in

Medical School next year" and he bought t-shirts from the University of Nebraska for all the children.

Ian to this day is a fan of University of Nebraska football.

At the end of January, Jim got an interview at the University of Minnesota. Interviews usually last less than an hour and Jim was there for over an hour and a half. The deans were impressed with his transcripts, impressive MCAT scores, and his straight A's in science classes, especially in organic chemistry and biochemistry.

It was the day of the annual bargain bag sale and I was shopping for clothing treasures for our family while Jim was at school. He came home, picked up the mail and discovered a big envelope from the University of Minnesota. He knew a denial letter was only one page like Nebraska had sent him so he figured he was accepted from the weight of the envelope! From there Jim went to the bag sale to find me.

He greeted me with the saddest look I'd had seen in some time and told me he'd heard from the UofM.

My heart sunk, I was so sure he would make it.

Then he smiled and I jumped on him hugging and crying.

He then went to pick up Kristy from school and handed her the letter. She couldn't read it because she was too emotional so she handed the letter to her friend who proceeded to read it aloud, "You have been accepted to the University of Minnesota Medical School Class of 1997." Kristy screamed and since Jim was still in the car she didn't have a chance to jump on him too.

Jim had two more interviews lined up for other schools and he called and cancelled them. Life did not have to change. We did not have to move. Becca could keep her doctors. The kids could keep their friends and schools. Dreams could come true.

Medical School started in September, but Jim called, asked about early admittance for gross anatomy and was accepted. That was a great class because it was taught by the Dean of Admissions and Jim enjoyed conversations with Dr. Donald Robertson. Jim's acceptance into the early entrance program allowed him along with a select few to start in June.

Jim applied for a student loan of fifteen thousand dollars to cover tuition. The Medical School expected students to study and not work. He could borrow eight hundred dollars a month to supplement our paper route money. We were going further into debt, but when Jim was a doctor we could pay it back.

Jim, a doctor?

Those words seemed strange.

▼

Jim used to be uncomfortable in the NICU. He couldn't clean up vomit when the kids were sick. He passed out from shots and lab draws. Now he was training to be a doctor!

Jim thrived in Medical School; the dreaded Anatomy Cadaver lab was his favorite place, and it was Jim's topic of conversation with Kristy and Ian. They poured over the anatomy slides with their father, and the grosser the story, the better. Marissa buried her head under the covers, gagging and squealing for them to stop.

When the other medical students arrived in September, Jim was offered a position as a teaching assistant for fifteen hours a week at ten dollars an hour for the first semester. I cut back the weekday paper routes and eventually gave them up most of the time. I still subbed, and we handled the weekends, but now we could sleep about half the mornings.

We were exhausted, but it was a good kind of exhaustion.

We were digging out.

- 25 -
LIFE GOES ON

The Yurceks rolled with the flow. We accepted change at a moment's notice, not because we wanted to, but because we had to. We knew the stress did not last forever; sooner or later life always settled down and smoothed out. We faced the roller coaster life of a catastrophic illness each and every day, this was our normal, and only families who have walked our walk can understand its uncertainty or how we manage to cope. The doctors were pleased with Becca's progress. Our appointments were becoming fewer and fewer.

Becca graduated from her apnea monitor. Then she graduated from her suction machine. And finally she graduated from her oxygen. As each piece of medical equipment left our family celebrated and this mom silently said a prayer that we would never need it again. The equipment was a technologic safety net, and now I was even more on my own.

New firsts for Becca arrived. At three she started walking and she spoke a few words. She had her first IEP, (Individualized Education Plan) which included occupational therapy, nurses, paraprofessionals and school buses.

Twenty-two hours a day Becca was attached to her feeding pump with two one-hour breaks. She was nearly four-years-old, and she now attended half-day school with the nurses. A little orange short bus came to our door to pick her up in the morning and deliver her and her nurse back home by noon. We had placed the feeding pump and its case into a brightly colored character backpack for durability, and it hid the pump from view. Everywhere Becca went the fancy Barney or Little Mermaid backpack followed. The backpack changed as Becca's obsession changed from one cartoon or Disney character to the next. The nurse carried the pump backpack; while Becca carried a second on her wee little back very proud of the school papers she brought home to hang on the refrigerator. School gave Becca a daily break from Mom and home.

Nursing was slowly being cut back. With the portable feeding equipment we were out in the community in the fall, summer and spring. Only in the winters were we now quarantined.

Marissa had entered a contest when Becca was in the hospital with her heart surgery and won a modeling contract with a prominent agency in the Twin Cities. I finally had time to let Marissa model. She won jobs filming commercials for McDonalds, Mattel, Duplos, and Country Kitchen. She was perfect as the Wedding Fair flower girl and looked like a fairytale princess on stage with her strawberry blond ringlets. Marissa only needed me for driving; she had confidence beyond her years and at nine was a veteran at handling her appointments with her agent. Even so, the modeling and acting gave her valued alone time with her mom.

After school Becca joined Marissa and me in downtown Minneapolis for auditions. One day Becca caught the attention of the casting director for a spring Target print ad while Marissa was at an audition. Marissa was shocked to hear she did not get the print ad, but her little sister did and Becca was not even there to model!

Little Becca was a mini star in her pink size two-toddler outfit, glasses, dark brown curls and new hot pink Zippie Quicky wheelchair. Soon Becca hung on ten-foot posters at Targets coast to coast. She landed another job for Target, but her career was short lived when they pretended to hit me over the head with a balloon as a practical joke and Becca broke into tears. That was the end of her modeling career, but the end of Becca's career meant Marissa could have alone time with Mom at auditions again.

This mom was proud of Marissa, but mom's always think their children have talent. Soon offers arrived for auditioning for amazing full-length movies. We could not take Marissa to Los Angeles, New York or Chicago because of Becca's health and our financial circumstances so she had to decline the offers. She joined a community theater and acted whenever she got a chance.

Matt started afternoon kindergarten and for the first time since he could remember he had alone time with his mom. While Becca was in school in the mornings, he helped me with housework, and we played Batman, zoomed Hot Wheels cars and built imaginary projects with his Legos.

Kristy was now a high school freshman and was excited to make the Varsity football cheerleadering squad. Jim took the boys to the football games, and when weather and Becca's health permitted, Becca came, too. The cheerleaders had all fallen in love with little Miss Becca, and Becca loved the attention. She used her sisters practice pom-poms and was made an honorary cheerleader by Kristy's best friends.

At one football game, Becca was in the front row of the stands between Jim and me attached to her feeding pump imitating Kristy's cheers. The stand was on a concrete slab ten feet in the air where we could see Kristy and help cheer the team on. As Becca happily cheered along, a group of kids came running by and knocked Becca off her hypotonic legs, and she went flying. Jim grabbed her ankle as she slipped between the seats of the bleacher into the opening to the ground. Everyone around us gasped, Jim held her dangling nine feet in the air upside down by her tiny ankle. Nathan reached down and grabbed the other ankle and together they carefully hoisted her back to safety. Jim made the best catch of the day – the Spring Lake Park Panthers lost 7 to 0.

We knew we could no longer take Becca to the games, after the close call. She was still much too fragile and uncoordinated. The bleachers were unsafe, and she couldn't see from the grass. Jim took the kids alone, and I stayed with Becca at home. Kristy and her cheerleading team changed their practices to our house to practice cheers with Becca. She wore an oversize Panther sweater that hung to the floor. Becca was still a cheerleader even though she was banned from games. She mimicked the girls with her blue, white and red pom-poms and those moments of happiness are forever etched in my memories. I am not sure who had more fun, Becca or the teenagers. Perhaps it was I who watched in awe, my Tiny Titan being accepted and loved.

▼

I had always worried about saying the right thing at the medical visits because I didn't want to be second-guessed by the doctors about my care for Becca. As parents we are judged for everything and veteran parents had forewarned me to use prudence around professionals. Use 'caution', they had whispered in the halls of the NICU. And 'use caution' continued to haunt me. We lived in a fishbowl. It was bad if we were over involved, yet, if something happened to our child under our care we could be found medically neglectful. We could easily be viewed as looking for attention, not competent, or overreacting. I kept my place on the hierarchy ladder. I learned the art of getting Becca's needs met without telling the doctor what to do. It had to be their idea. I was the parent on the lower rungs. I used the nurses to maneuver when I couldn't get what Becca needed. I was very careful. It was a game of cat and mouse. The nurses and I knew that it was the professionals who were given credibility, rarely the parents. It didn't matter that we lived, loved and cared for the child twenty-four hours a day; they read the charts while we read the child.

I was tired of watching my daughter suffer from gagging and retching. It was pathetic to see her sweating and shaking. It scared me as her heart raced and pounded in her teeny tiny chest. The nurses and I had discovered that whenever we stopped Becca's pump she was a different child and when we were not feeding her she was not sickly or stressed.

Becca had not seen the gastroenterologis since she was in the

NICU at three-months-old and the nurses finally convinced the doctor that Becca needed an assessment. I made sure Becca's most experienced nurse accompanied us for credibility when we told the doctor our concerns. We threatened him that he needed to listen, or he could feed her for a week. Somehow I found the courage to tell the doctor that her feedings were making her sick.

The GI doctor looked stunned by my demands for help for Becca. He listened as the nurse, and I explained the horrific stress Becca had to live through as we struggled to feed her. The doctor was concerned and said this should have been looked at long ago. She should have been seeing a gastroenterologist since her discharge from the NICU. Somehow, the NICU had dropped the doctor and with so many others it got lost in the depths of her gigantic medical charts. He arranged for testing at The Children's Hospital the coming week.

▼

I will never get used to the uncertainty of the waiting. Once again I waited while Becca was under anesthesia. I tried to stay busy while I kept my eye on the door for the surgeon to come through. When the gastroenterologist summoned me to the consultation room, I immediately knew he had found answers.

In the consultation room he picked up a red dry erase marker. He began drawing pictures, Becca's intestines were inflamed, and he performed biopsies. She was pooling at the base of her esophagus, and things were not moving down through the Nissan into her stomach. He carefully diagrammed this in red and green. That was why she was getting so many aspiration pneumonias. He stretched the opening. He showed me exactly where in his drawing. Hopefully this would prevent the pooling and stop the pneumonias. He showed me how in green.

It hurt her to try to eat and by refusing to eat, Becca was protecting herself from pneumonia. Because she would not have the pain, hopefully she would want to eat. He smiled and continued drawing. Further down he found polyps in her intestines. He drew an X where he had removed them. The biggest finding was that he had fixed her malrotated intestines. The pyloric valve that opens into the small intestines was wide open. Everything dumped into it and emptied in seconds. The surgeon explained that she was having an adrenalic reaction to being fed too fast.

I was stunned.

How could that be?

Becca was on a feeding pump drip at two ounces per hour.

He sat down and explained that with all the inflammation throughout her intestines she needed a very specialized formula. People with Noonan syndrome have impaired lymphatic systems. This had affected Becca's intestines. We had already tried dozens of formulas with no improvement. I couldn't believe there were more formulas than we had already tried. We learned she absorbed certain kind of fats better than others, and we needed to avoid long chain fats because she could not break them down. He smiled.

Becca's doctor had listened. I was relieved and I thanked him for his thoroughness, I loved that he had treated me as not 'just' a mom, but helped me understand the complexity of Becca's GI abnormalities. We had hope that Becca didn't have to continue to suffer and I had something new to try.

Becca thrived on the new formula and within a month she was a different child. She was no longer sweating. Her hair grew in and was no longer sparsely scattered on her head. It was thickening up, looked shiny, and felt soft. She gained strength. She had energy to move and everyday was something new.

Within a year, Becca's blood counts were getting closer to normal, and for the first time in her life her high white count had dropped and her T cells were functioning normally. Her immunity for upper respiratory infections, and autoimmune markers remained at lower levels, but all in all we had a much healthier little girl.

I finally had time for activities for the boys. Matt and Nathan went off to friend's houses. Ian played junior football. Running the kids from place-to-place was a happy reminder of normalcy. Becca attended Wednesday night activities at church, feeding pump and all. She had fun with our church's Cubbies program for three- and four-olds. Every Wednesday she spent time doing arts and crafts, playing with other children, and earning Cubbies badges to put on her vest. The nurse or Kristy joined her so she could practice independence from Mom. She struggled to recite short memorized Bible verses. When her speech failed she resorted to signing. It was something to see her sign and speak with normal preschoolers and be fully accepted. The church made accommodations to accept her, and in return they witnessed a miracle in progress.

We were no longer isolated by being home quarantined with Becca. We walked to the park with friends and the neighborhood children eagerly pushed Becca in her little hot pink wheelchair, arguing about who got to push next! Kristy or Nathan followed Becca through tunnels and mazes of the playground equipment, all the while keeping the feeding pump and tubing safe and untangled. When kids asked about Becca's differences, we explained simply, and our answers satisfied their curiosity. Parents rarely asked unless they had a close relationship with a child with special needs. Their silence and looks no longer mattered to me. I watched neighbor children gently push my tiny daughter on the swing. She amazed me. Everyday she progressed further and further. She scurried up slides and crawled through tunnels.

Not long ago the doctors told us she would die. They told us she would never do what other children did normally. They told us there was 'little hope' for Miss Rebecca.

So I had believed there was 'a' little hope!

Hope? Yes, it was a little hope and a lot of faith and as much love as seven Yurecks could muster.

Our Becca was smiling in the sunlight. Her brown curls were blowing behind her as she chased her brothers and sisters. They were all happy. I felt like I had cried a trail of tears over this Tiny Titan for the last four years. Becca had changed me. I watched my daughter, and I cried tears of gratitude knowing in my heart and mind each day was a gift, a gift of love and a gift of family. Each day was a miracle of its own.

- 26 -

JUST ANOTHER KID

Jim and my children were now all in school. Becca was gone half days and after so many years with children and medical crises I had time. Perhaps it was a hint of what empty nest might be like. Whatever it was, I felt like I didn't have anything to do! I was used to operating in overdrive and our budget needed help. I had too much time on my hands. Yet with Becca still struggling sometimes, I had to be able to drop everything in a moment's notice to focus on her issues. What could I do? The answer popped into my head. Do what you do well. I love children. I love caring for children. That's it! A friend asked me to watch her daughter, and I said yes. I could stay home, be with Becca and make a little extra money.

I watched Michelle who was a year younger than Becca in the late afternoons and into the evening while her mother went to work. Michelle joined our family for homework, dinner, baths, and family time. Becca was barely twenty-five pounds soaking wet and Michelle was a little roly-poly. They were bathtub bathing buddies in opposite size swimsuits. They were movie partners and playmates. Becca and Michelle became best friends. Michelle became a role model for Becca, and Becca grew as she played with and watched Michelle. My neighbor and best friend, Sharon, started staying home when her younger daughter Shannon was born. Shannon and Matt grew up together, and now that Becca was stable I was finally able to go out and visit. Sharon, and her day care kids became Becca's playmates. On good days we went walking and swinging on swing sets. Becca joined the day care children in birthday celebrations and holiday events. She was mesmerized and quietly analyzed each little thing another child did. We set Becca on the picnic table in the day care room as three and four-year-olds giggled and romped and played. She watched them eat and drink, and in time she put small bites of the snacks to her mouth too. She had a sippie cup like the other kids and she took miniscule sips of apple juice. Stuck her little tongue out in pride, and then choked and gagged. She wanted to be like the other kids. She kept trying.

Sharon's day care was full and neighbors and friends continued to ask her if she could care for their children. Michelle was working out well in our home, and when another neighbor needed care, I decided to apply for my day care license. I was worried that I might not be able to get one because of Becca's history. I wasn't sure if her doctors would clear her to have more children near her. I was still a wimp when it came to doctors but I finally found the courage to ask Dr. Wineinger and the nurse about the idea, and they agreed that it was a good one. There were, however conditions. 1) If Becca became sick more often I had to promise to quit. 2) All the children coming into my house needed to have flu shots in the fall to protect Becca from influenza. 3) Hand washing, toys and surfaces had to have stringent cleaning protocols. 4) All family members needed physicals.

Becca had two years of early intervention preschool, plus being around Sharon's day care children, and she'd had no stints in the hospital from normal colds and viruses. Medicaid covered the costs for all of us to have physicals. It had been a couple of years since I had a checkup, and Jim had not been in since we were first married and now Kristy was nearly fifteen-years-old.

Kristy had packed up Marissa's Barbies, telling her that she could no longer have them in their room. Kristy and Marissa were at war. Their room was tiny, and Kristy, a highschooler, did not want her little sister hanging around and she manipulated Marissa by threats of abandonment. One night a crying kindergartner showed up in my bedroom choking back sobs trying to tell me that Kristy was going to move to Disneyland and be Minnie Mouse and we would never see her again if she didn't do what Kristy wanted. We needed to separate the two. Kristy needed her privacy. Marissa needed her toys back and unpacked. Jim and I finished taping and sanding the last two unfinished rooms in the lower level. Jim laid the carpet that had been rolled up and waiting since the insurance settlement for the fire arrived. Marissa's room and the family room were finally finished.

I began equipping the family day care room by utilizing the early morning empty hours without children to visit garage sales. I still had all of Becca's baby equipment; her high chair, booster chair, and Port-A-Crib. I found a second Port-A-Crib for $10.00 with original tags on it, a second high chair, car seats, and a potty chair. The kids went through their toys to see what ones they didn't mind sharing. Any toys they would not share needed to stay in their rooms. We bought shelving at the outlet center and a craft store was closing and offered eight foot shelving for $15.00 a section. Jim unassembled the units, moved them home and put them all back together.

The room was taking shape with cast offs from others. A scratch and dent kitchen countertop was placed upon a scratch and dent base cabinet and at another store I found the matching upper cupboard missing its hinges. For a couple dollars I had a food preparation, crafting and paperwork area.

I loved being able to garage sale again to find the best of the best for as little as possible. In less than a month, I found a Fisher Price table with five chairs. I was so excited, but I was still short one. While subbing a paper route, there in the trash was the very same table and another chair, the children slid down in the car because they did not want to be seen. I asked who was going to see their mother taking the trash before the trash man took it, after all it was 5:00 A.M.. With a little elbow grease, bleach and cleanser it looked as good as new. I now had the full set! I had Fisher Price learning toys and Little Tykes riding toys. I completely outfitted a tiny toy kitchen.

I was ready for inspection. Sharon gave me a copy of her rules. Jim made sure the house was up to code, he put fire proof sheetrock under the stairs and he finished it to store the extra toys and supplies so each toy had a place. My day care room was organized.

Marissa offered a corner of her new room on weekdays for quiet time in a Port-A-Crib for a napping baby. We took the crib down on weekends so she had her whole room to play Barbies or practice her homemade plays.

My license was approved!

I had a new career that allowed me to stay home with Becca and make money using my talents. I loved the kids. My first kids were medical professionals' children: a one-year-old boy whose mom worked for a clinic not far from our home, a brother and sister that came part-time, and finally a baby. The day care filled quickly but I had to be selective because of Becca. With Michelle, I now cared for six children beginning at six in the morning and ending close to eleven at night. The days were long but manageable.

Money was easier and we were off assistance. We could pay our own way, and it felt good. We were making it! As time went on I increased the number of children I cared for and I was able to buy my own health insurance for our family even though they wouldn't cover Becca. Our life of situational poverty had disappeared even with a medically fragile child. Her government waiver and social security checks provided for much of her care. I had business tax write offs, and we fell under the ceiling for the programs. We were a family of eight and we could now use deductions for day care use.

Sharon and I joined forces in the mornings, and our groups of children played outside in one or the other's yard, or we walked to the new playground down the street. What a site! A dozen little children walking single file next to the curb, looking like little ducklings. Mama Sharon and a stroller headed up the flock I brought up the rear with my double stroller with Becca. Becca and the kids played when she was home; I had the freedom to get her off to the bus along with the two brothers who arrived after kindergarten and first grade. Becca, Mike and James were all less than a year apart. I now had eight children I cared for. My license and reputation were in good standing, and I was offered a group day care license, which meant I could care for even more children each day.

I needed another vehicle if I was to manage all these children legally and safely. I spied a car lot filled with Ford Econoline Vans that seat fifteen. Our credit had been destroyed, and we were just climbing out of poverty. I wondered if finally we could qualify for a decent vehicle again. All the debt had been in Jim's name. We had put the new income in my name; maybe I could get a loan on my own. With two weeks of income, I saved a thousand dollars for a down payment. I walked into the car lot to look at vans. Then I applied for a loan for a big red van and I was shocked to find out that not only did I qualify, but it was a business expense! I couldn't believe it! We were the proud owners of a two-year-old Maxy Van as my kids coined it. It fit all my kids and it could carry even more papers!

I was surprised at the referrals for my home day care. The letter 'Y' should be at the bottom of the list on the county daycare alphabetical referral sheet. Yet when someone called needing daycare for a child with special needs, I often got referrals. It seemed as if I was the first on their special needs list. One day I was sitting rocking a baby when a call came in from Tammy, a mom who was looking for childcare for her four-year-old daughter. She was returning to school and having trouble finding someone who would allow her to have a later schedule, allow her guide dog in, and was flexible enough to wait eight weeks for reimbursement to start from the state agency for the blind.

The mom and I talked a long time, and I invited her to come out and a take a 'look' at my day care. I felt foolish for my poor choice of words, and apologized.

She told me not to worry. In time Tammy and her daughter became an integral part of our lives. Tammy and Jacqueline became Becca's and my best friends. Tammy inspired me with her determination to face obstacles. She began her day being picked up in a small bus designed for people with special needs that she had to schedule each day and that first bus took her to the county line where she had to catch another bus since the buses for persons with special needs stopped at the county lines. To get to school she left two hours early to not be late for class. The routine was the same for her return—four hours of traveling on County Travelers just to attend school. The County Traveler brought Tammy and Jacqueline to my driveway where I ran out to pick up her daughter. The traveler picked Jacqueline up after dinner, well after the other children were gone. I made sure Tammy's darling little four-year-old was all ready for bed in her pajamas. Often scheduling flukes stranded Tammy at the county line, then Jim swung by from the university to bring her home from the women's college where she was training to be a physical therapist. Tammy always apologized for the inconvenience; she didn't need to apologize for the system's failure to get it right.

Jim became a part of my daycare. One-year-old Taylor ran to "Dim" with outstreched chubby arms and remained snuggled in his lap while Jim studied. Jim talked and played with the other little children and they loved when he was around. Jim got to play 'Dad' to a whole crew of munchkins and I am not sure who was having the most fun. The big 'kid' or the little kids.

The next referral was a grandmother who had been told I accepted kids with special needs. With over the dozen places she had called she had received no for an answer and she was relieved she had finally found a caring place. When she explained Kim's needs I wasn't afraid of caring for her, it was no big deal. She had just gotten her feeding tube out, and she was on special formula and ate baby food. Kimberly was three, had spina bifida, was paralyzed, was non-verbal and one of her arms was twisted and contorted.

I told the grandmother I dreamed of that eating day for Becca.

Kim needed catheterization to pee and I was not afraid to learn to help Kim. Grandma and Kim's mom trained me, and Kim was soon a part of my home and family. Kim was silent when she arrived and she reminded me of Becca as she studied the other children while they played. Her tiny little head with blond ponytail and wire rimmed glasses watched each move intently. Her bent arms and legs remained still.

In time Kim scooted on her little tush to be in the middle of everything. She pointed for toys she wanted to play with and another child would gently hand them to her. Becca responded without speaking and by signing to Kim. They created their own non-verbal system of communication that was a secret from all of us. Soon the two of them were giggling at jokes and shenanigans that only they understood.

Sharon and I held combined holiday parties. Sharon was great with supervising kids. I was creative and loved to teach. She watched the little ones while I did crafts with the older ones. We made Halloween piñatas as a group. Santa Claus visited all eighteen children who were dressed in red and green elf collars and hats from my sewing machine. After the kids were down for their naps or resting Sharon and I shared a glass of soda or late lunch while talking together on the phone to prepare the schedule or lessons for the next day.

With the purchase of the van, I was able to take a couple of Sharon's kids to preschool along with Jacqueline. All I needed to do was tell the little ones it was time to get ready, and even the one-year-old came carrying his shoes. The older ones helped with the little ones and within five minutes or less we were in the van, buckled up and ready to go. They all knew the system and we were prompt and efficient. The kids knew to hold each other's hands. They knew who was the buddy to whom. In the summer and on school vacations we took trips to the zoo, museums, and parks with each of my older kids assigned responsibility to a younger child.

Nathan spent hours building Duplos with Kim. He entertained Mike and James. He was a born babysitter. Ian was the gym teacher and organized ball games and obstacle courses. They played rounds of dodge ball in the backyard or climbed on the massive wood play structure that Jim and the boys built from scratch. Marissa played dolls and house with the little girls. Kristy helped with Kim when she was around.

Kim thrived in my day care. Soon she was stacking Duplos with her previously useless arms and hands with skilled expertise. At four-years-old she began saying a few simple words. At five she pulled herself to her feet with her arms at the side of the toy table on her paralyzed legs. I was moved to tears. At my house she was just another one of the kids and she challenged herself to be a part of everything. Because of Kim's successes they qualified for a stander and then a walker with braces. I helped Grandma have courage to speak up; Kim secured a communication device to help her get her needs met. Little Kim was happy – she was understood and mobile.

The county-generated paycheck for Kim and the state check for Jacqueline paid our insurance and van payment. Our day care participated in the federal food program to feed the day care kids. My own kids qualified for school free lunch under our income eligibility. I stretched the grocery money by using coupons at the grocery stores from the recycled newspapers from the depot. I went through a dozen rolls of paper towels each week. We bought a freezer from another garage sale so I could buy in bulk. I had little time to shop for lessons and craft supplies, so I found mail order preschool lessons with crafts delivered to the door each week. Each week we received an exciting package of new things to do.

Like Jim, I had a newfound confidence. We were self-sufficient and it felt good to stand on our own two feet again. Better yet, it felt really good to give back to the community. No more food stamps for the Yurceks! All the children at my daycare were learning about giving, sharing, and acceptance. I was helping Becca, Kim and her family, and Tammy and Jacqueline.

When Becca was sick, the nurses' aides who had now replaced the nurses cared for Becca upstairs. The rest of the time, Becca, like Kim was just another kid.

- 27 -
PAY BACK

Life was never easy, but it was much easier than when Jim and I were starving to save food for the kids, living without heat and hot water, and with broken down junk cars. We were content albeit very busy. We knew the roller coaster never stopped long before it picked up more passengers for another go around.

Each of my children was miraculously matched with another capable person with unique interests and gifts. They had that special someone to confide in or spend time with. With their special someone they could forget the stress and uncertainty of living life on the roller coaster. I thanked God my parents and extended family had arrived just when I needed them most. My sister Martha had moved into the Twin Cities a few years before my parents and my brother and his wife a few years before that. My aunt and uncle and cousins were cornerstones of the church where I had spent much of my teen years while my dad was working on his doctorate.

Our family had never had it very easy; especially when Dad was a full time student with four kids and another on the way. People had come to help us and I knew how important extended family was to my children. People from our church brought in meals a couple times a week. At thirteen I cared for my younger siblings as my dad struggled to juggle school and four kids with a bedridden wife.

Mom's last pregnancy was difficult and she was bedridden to keep my littlest brother Tim. In 1971, my mom, a teetotaler, was given IV's of alcohol to keep the pregnancy.

My dad's mom came into town from the farm and I loved my grandmother. She was one of the missing piece in my life puzzle. She shared stories of our family history and I learned we had a heritage filled with hidden surprises. We were related to President Rutherford B. Hayes and his teetotalling wife, Lemonade Lucy. I inherited my grandmother's gifts of creativity, and we spent long hours talking about books, arts, crafts and designing. She proudly told me about creating stuffed Disney characters after seeing the movies in the 1940s with which she won first place ribbons at the Wisconsin State Fair. I was the only grandchild that could touch the perfect condition box of 64 Crayolas that Grandma kept on her craft shelf. She painted paintings, sculpted seashells into ornamental figurines and designed elaborate Barbie clothes for me when I was little. We designed together. She had shelves of dusty old books that made me sneeze, and I loved to cuddle up with one under old patchwork moth-eaten quilts in the rickety bed in the old farmhouse. Grandfather stayed on the farm and always had a box of Cracker Jacks with a prize for us. We called him the Cracker Jack Grandpa.

Most of my time growing up my mother struggled with not feeling well. Her heart had been affected by childhood rheumatic fever, and doctors were confused by her ongoing fatigue and gastrointestinal problems. Even the famous Mayo Clinic had no answers to help her. Then the year I was twenty-two, just prior to Nathan's birth, Mom learned she had Celiac disease and perhaps her heart problems correlated with that. The next year I was diagnosed along with five-month-old Nathan. Nathan had been hospitalized as failure-to-thrive. I was nursing him and starving myself. Both of us changed our diets. Nathan was placed on a specialized formula. I stopped eating wheat. Our family soon discovered many of us were affected. Doctors were baffled. Why so many family members? My siblings Gretchen, Tim, and Dan were all diagnosed. My niece Kaitie and Marissa, Matt, and Ian of my crew all had to remain gluten free. The answer lay hidden in my father's gene pool. It was discovered he was anemic while he gave blood. Cancer was a concern, and then by chance the doctor found Dad had Celiac disease too. We won the celiac lottery. People ask Mom how did you two ever get together? Mom answers, "that God knew before we met that someone needed to know how to feed and take care of my husband, Alan."

The life lessons of my past were available when we needed them. As a child, I had learned to handle adversity. I knew what it was like to be different and struggle to walk when my knees wouldn't hold me. I knew what it was like to have respiratory problems and not have the energy to be able to breathe. I had constant stomachaches or queasy feelings because I had Celiac Disease and didn't know it as a child. I didn't know what it was like to be Becca, but my own experiences gave me insight. I had been seasoned for this journey. Our family had grown up just like the old woman Alice had told me at Becca's dedication. We understood that life was precious and often way too short to worry about the little things. We were blessed by our adversity.

▼

Jim enjoyed school. My day care was fulfilling. The kids were in activities and doing well in school. Each day Becca was learning more and more. We spent time with my parents, and my siblings, and their families, and my children adored them. Becca was now able to enjoy spending time with Grandma and Grandpa, too. My mom still babysat my niece, Kaitie, who was only nine months older than Becca and the girls enjoyed playing together despite Becca's disabilities.

Mom, who also has Celiac disease became a baker extraordinaire at gluten free baking of cookies, cakes and snacks that I did not have time to make. Her gluten free angel food cakes were better than store bought wheat ones.

While Dad was at school, my boys hung out with Grandpa. Grandpa was the fun guy. He was an inventor and had been a college teacher. He took the boys to the airplane hanger and he had the boys help him build and drive unique bicycles, go-carts, and minibikes. He let my boys be the helpers as he built prototypes of projects from wood or metal for people from across the country. My boys were in heaven, wheels galore.

In the back of my mind I knew that the roller coaster seldom stopped for long.

▼

My sister Martha had graduated with her Master's degree and was working in the health care field in management when she was diagnosed with ovarian cancer - stage three. She was rushed to surgery and immediately began intensive chemotherapy. Martha had fought for Becca and out of her fight came the new discharge procedures. It was my turn to be there for Mom and Dad as they watched their daughter fight cancer. Martha told me that she had to beat it. She would fight. Her role model for living was her little niece, Becca.

The same church that had been there when I was a child and continued to rally around my family with Becca now went to work to help my sister and my parents. The spirit of the never-ending prayerchain picked up another member of my family in its arms. We were survivors. Martha nearly lost her life to the chemotherapy. Her type of ovarian cancer is usually a death sentence.

We celebrated her last treatment on Valentine's Day after four and a half months of intensive treatment. Five years later my nephew, Eric, was born on Valentines Day. After the cancer Martha had found love, married, and had her miracle son and then a second son she named Eddie. Doctors cannot explain the miracles. She should not have been able to have one baby, let alone two. Eleven years later she remains cancer free.

We were reminded of the sanctity of life with Martha's close call with death. We had learned to believe in miracles, Becca and Martha were here to prove it.

I had always been afraid of what could be, and day-to-day uncertainties. We had faced death with Becca and Martha.

▼

Sharon and I spent everyday sharing our day care children. Jim and my children continued to do well in school. Sharon had gone off on St. Patrick's Day to day care licensing training. I was putting Becca to bed when I received a panicked phone call from Sharon's daughter Tonya. Her dad had picked her up from school and he asked her to drive home because he was not feeling well. Once home, he had gone down to Sharon's day care room to watch TV and collapsed on the floor. Her little sister Shannon tried to help her daddy up, but he wouldn't wake up. Tonya cried. I ran, chasing the ambulance to respond to the panic-stricken phone call.

Sharon had been concerned that week that Tom was not feeling well and could not convince him to go to the doctor. Tonya had called the next-door neighbor who was an EMT who called the paramedics as he ran to the scene. I filled them in on his history and tried to calm the two girls. I tracked down Sharon at her day care class, and told her to come home because Tom was sick. I stayed with the girls; praying for guidance to know how to help them cope.

Sharon arrived home and they were still doing CPR waiting for a family member to agree to stop heroic efforts. I figured it was better to hear it from me than from a stranger that her husband was dead. Sometimes God asks you to do something you never thought you were capable of. Somehow I found the words to tell my best friend that her husband was gone. Tom was buried leaving behind two young girls, with no insurance and no savings. A devastated Sharon had to learn to move on for her daughters.

I was freshly reminded about the preciousness of life. I renewed my vow to make each day count. None of us was guaranteed a tomorrow. My nightmares that haunted me after Becca's birth resurfaced. I had to face death, not Becca's, but my best friend's husband. To this day on March 17, I begin my day calling my friend from wherever I am to offer support and say I love you. Her days are still filled with kids and laughter, and she is now caring for a second generation of day care children. Sharon has found strength out of adversity, her heart remains filled with caring.

Through life's crises we find those who help us. They care in many forms, for many reasons. We just have to see them through our grief and fear. It is true. Every cloud has a silver lining. I have seen time and time again my past comes full circle to create a miracle.

- 28 -

Celebrations

Some days moved by slowly; others flew by. Everyday I hugged my daughter I knew it was a miracle. We had survived two years of critical care with Becca, two years of undergraduate courses to get Jim into Medical School, and now two years of Medical School. It was going by fast and Jim only had two more years to go. He was starting clinical rotations and was ready to see hands-on patients while his daughter wanted to be free of hands-on care. At age six, Becca Yurcek fired her nurses. She told them that Mom could do it. She didn't need them, and Mom didn't need them either. I could do it myself, and she wanted me, and me only. She had had enough of the nurses that came and went. The only one she now missed was Grandma Zoe.

Our family joined forces to save money for a road trip to attend Jim's sister's wedding in San Diego. His parents had always been there when we needed them, and they had offered to help get us there, but we declined and wanted to do it ourselves. The kids picked up pop cans for a year for spending money. We took on extra paper routes. The eight of us, and our dog Brady, piled into our new used air-conditioned mini van with Becca's medical equipment, our clothes and a packed cooler. We were bound for an American adventure. We drove through South Dakota and the Badlands. We visited Mount

Rushmore. We drove up the mountains in Colorado, and Jim and the older kids climbed the mountain slopes and skipped stones in mountain creeks. We crossed the plains of Wyoming and the barren deserts of Nevada. We rode through Death Valley to California. The girls sang, and the boys complained as they tried to listen to the sports.

We spent two days at Disneyland while Becca's favorite Disney characters greeted her. Sitting in her little pink wheelchair, she hugged Minnie Mouse and then we went searching for a hug from Pocahontas, her new favorite. I had dreamed of the day that I would get to take my children to Disneyland and we were really here. I watched my kids laughing and Becca shining. I bought souvenirs before we left for home and gave each child a new Disney t-shirt and Disney mini notebooks from the bottom of my suitcase. They set upon a mission to see who could capture the most autographs. We kept our eating budget down by eating cereal in the room and sandwich meat, cheese, chips and fruit along the way. Once a day we ate at Mc Donald's or Burger King from the dollar menus and surprised the kids with ice cream as a special treat.

We drove down to San Diego for the wedding. Jim's entire family was there for a family portrait. The girls were in their best dresses; the boys were in their shorts and knit polo shirts, and Becca wore a little cream satin dress. She looked healthy in the warm California sunshine. We had done it! Our family had a much-deserved vacation from all the work and crises of these past years.

Jim and I walked along the ocean beach while the kids played in the sand. We watched little Becca as she sat in the shallow ocean water as the waves nearly pushed her over with their power, but the Tiny Titan refused to tumble. The kids romped and chased our dog Brady in the sand while we sat next to the bonfire watching the sun go down. It was picturesque and romantic, and Jim and I reminisced as we watched our children.

The waves of adversity had not swallowed up our family. We had survived against their force. We found strength we never knew we were capable of. Becca pushed us beyond what we thought were our limitations. She had not let the Noonan Tsunami waves drown her.

We celebrated Jim's parents' wish of all their children being together while we made our children's dreams come true. No one did it for us. We did it together, as a family, with hard work and determination. We watched the kids riding the waves on their boogie boards. When they fell, they got up back on their boogie boards and tried again. We had done the same. Wave upon wave had pummeled us, and we fell many times. We just kept keeping on and so had Becca.

With our trip behind us, we were back to life as usual. We were busy with visits to the doctors, and schools, and kids, and day care kids and lest we forget . . . more and more newspapers. The next two years flew by and soon it was a time for planning ahead for our family. I had been used to living one day at a time. It was hard to think ahead, but we needed to. Amazingly Jim was getting ready to graduate from Medical School. Where did the time go? He busied himself studying for his final board examinations. In July, after his graduation in June, at long last he would be starting residency.

Jim was honored with a scholarship from the Minnesota Medical Foundation. The foundation sent a professional photographer to take pictures of our family for their annual report. Jim was a different kind of medical student, and they asked us if they could tell our story. Out of his tiny daughter's frail condition, he had found a calling and a mission.

He had told me he wanted to be a pathologist, but the day he came home from his first day of surgery rotation, the look on his face told me that he was to be a surgeon. I had told him that he needed to do a short residency, three years at the max. But I had to change my mind. If Jim had put in all the hard work, why lessen his dreams? As the surgery rotation proceeded, he became more and more determined. Finally, one day he announced that he wanted to be a surgeon if he could get into a surgery residency. Primary care slots were plentiful, but only the highest achieving medical students received the much-coveted specialty residency slots, especially a surgery opening.

I called the state programs for kids with disabilities to find out which states had the best services to be able to meet Becca's needs. There were only three residency programs in Minnesota, and two of them required a couple of added years of research that Jim could not afford. That meant we had only one residency program in Minneapolis. Jim and I worked on filling out the lengthy applications between putting the kids to bed and getting up early to deliver newspapers. We were taking on more routes, even on weekdays to be able to have the money we needed to be able to pay for traveling and hotels for Jim's upcoming interviews for residency. With only one option in Minnesota it meant we most likely would have to leave our family, the doctors and the support systems that had kept Becca alive and move out of state. The kids would have to leave schools and friends. The kids were uncertain about leaving everything they knew for Dad's training. I tried to reassure them that this was an adventure. Just as our trip to California was an adventure. And soon we were on the road to interviewing for a residency in Detroit, Michigan.

We were on a residency adventure to the east. We drove through Wisconsin and on to Chicago. We crossed the tip of Indiana into Michigan. We drove through the night, and Jim changed into his suit at a rest stop along the way. I dropped him off for his interview in the morning just as my very hungry children were awakening. We didn't know our way around Detroit so we stopped at the nearest Mc Donald's in the inner city. Ian noticed that there was a group of men talking quietly and hanging near the restroom. They were dressed in dark hooded clothing and were packing guns. He loudly told the rest of our tribe about the guns, all the while excitedly pointing. My girls looked horrified. I hurried the children out to the car while the little man of a million questions continued to talk loudly about never seeing a real gun before and telling his siblings where the man had quickly hidden it.

I found a mall not too far away, and we browsed the stores, while Ian loudly stated that they had green grass in December and there wasn't any snow and that meant it was warmer in Detroit than in Minneapolis. I felt like I was a stranger in a strange land in the heart of Detroit. I never let the kids out of my sight as I continued to listen to their commentary. Barren empty houses were boarded up with cheap and poorly attached plywood. The public school we passed was surrounded by barbwire. Metal bars were placed on store windows. This was no place for our family to go. Jim finished his interview early in the afternoon. He told me the interview went OK. I told him we are not moving here!

Jim drove to the outskirts of the city, and then I took over. I drove down the interstate and passed through the town of Kalamazoo, Michigan. I knew that Jim was awaiting an interview for a residency slot in that city, so Nathan and I braved getting off the highway to see the town. We went touring while Jim slept soundly. This town was not too big and not too little. The schools were similar to the schools in the suburbs of Minneapolis. I said a prayer that he did not match in Detroit, and he got an interview in Kalamazoo.

▼

Kristy had stayed home alone to study for her senior finals. She was graduating early to work full-time to save money to pay for her college. Kristy and her giftedness had always been a challenge. High school was too easy, and she had learned to slide by. Schools don't have the resources to deal with a child who can multiply five numbers by five numbers in kindergarten, and she was dumbed down to the level of the other kids. Her grades and her lack of enthusiasm for school were costing scholarships, which she desperately needed. Her ACT scores were her only salvation. Kristy applied to the College of St. Catherine's, an all women's college and she was accepted on probation, with financial aid and a small scholarship.

Jim took a weeklong trek alone to interview at nearly a half dozen residency programs across the Midwest. His first stop was Kalamazoo and he was hit with a snowstorm as soon as he entered Michigan. He had to stay an extra day because the freezing rain had turned to blinding snow and now the freeway was closed. That evening he and another interviewee were treated to dinner with the other residents and the program put them up in the Radisson for the night. The day of the interview Jim helped start a resident's car, stayed the night and then drove to interviews in five other Midwest cities from Ohio to Missouri.

We waited to see where he would be placed. Jim's qualifications and a computer seemed to be deciding our lives. The med students rank their preferences, and then the residency programs rate the students they want. Jim filled out his rankings, and we waited to get the news where life would take us. We had little control; we would go wherever we were led, knowing we would make it through as we had before.

We gathered for a party with my sister Gretchen and Jim's med school class for the passing out of the envelopes containing where we would be going for the next few years of our lives. One moment in time would change the course of our lives, just as that moment eight years earlier when Jim decided to go back to college instead of remaining bitterly struggling in poverty and hunger. We had made a choice then to make a change and strive for a better life for all us. Now life and an envelope was handing us a new path.

I barely breathed as I watched Jim open the envelope. I prayed silently, I don't know why as the decision had already been made, but talking to God and prayer had become a normal part of who I am.

Jim said Kalamazoo!

My jaw dropped. My heart skipped a beat. I gave Jim a big hug. Jim's hard work had landed him a residency slot in surgery. But for Jim to train the next step required us to move out of state. We would move away from family. We would leave the security of everything in Minnesota for places unknown. I had to remind myself what I told the children about adventure. Maybe if I said it to myself enough, I'd be convinced too.

Anxiety from the force of change engulfed my body. I prayed. *"God you've taken care of us in the past, I am trusting you will in our future."* I had wished we would have been able to stay in Minnesota, but if we had to move, I reminded myself that Kalamazoo was my second choice.

▼

Becca's appointment with her cardiologist confirmed that miracles could happen. Over the years the thick walls of her heart were slowly improving, and the final appointment with her cardiologist gave me news that I had dreamed for. Becca's heart showed no remnants of her cardiomyopathy. The walls of her heart looked nearly normal on the echocardiogram. As I left the hospital I was beside myself with joy. I lifted Becca from her wheelchair and hugged my daughter tightly. I was on top of the five story parking ramp, gazing up in the sunny blue sky, the fluffy white clouds floating in the air.

"Thank you!" I yelled at the top of my lungs.

God had mended my daughter's heart and I continued drawing out my words to the heavens. "Becca, you are 'just' a kid. And I am no longer 'just' a mom. You have taught me immense lessons. I look at myself, and I like who I have become. I am confident and compassionate. I can be assertive without being too scared. I find happiness now in the small things. I am ready to give to others who are starting on the journey of being a parent of a child with Noonan's or some other illness or disability. I have learned to listen with compassion because of the road you took me down. I no longer feel less than the professionals."

"Becca, you and I are partners in your care. It takes all of us together to survive. You have taught me much my teeny Tiny Titan. I have learned to advocate for the rights of the disabled. I have letters to prove it from the governor to our state senators. I have learned to fight for programs that are being cut because of lack of funding. I never want anyone to fall as far as we had to. I love you, love you, love you, Becca."

▼

From that moment on, Becca's heart has beat strong and well. Well, at least most of the time.

▼

I didn't care if people on the streets stared up at the ramp wondering about the lunatic yelling on the rooftop. I had witnessed a miracle. Seven years ago, I cried from this very same parking ramp. I cried out to the heavens a promise to my daughter. I promised to love her for as long as we had her, accepting that someday she would leave me. From that promise we had found love. We found a new life. Jim and I and our children understood that everyday was a gift. And it was all because of Becca. How many people get the chance to live and love well? How many people learn to focus on the present instead of chasing after the daydreams of tomorrow? Becca showed us the fragility of life. Each second, every minute was precious.

I renewed my promise to the heavens. I would give back to others all that had been given to me. I would make each day count. I would love Becca for whatever it takes of me, not just for Becca, but also for our entire family.

The months of getting ready for Jim and Kristy's graduations flew by. We had to sell our home. We had to get Becca's medical records. We had to work hard to save for the six hundred mile move.

It would be difficult to leave our family and friends who held us up during this eight-year journey. I would miss the doctors, the nurses, the hospital, and the other professionals who helped Becca. We would start all over in a new house, in a new town, and in a new state. Becca trusted life. She trusted that things would work out. I had to believe like my child. God will provide. He always had.

▼

Surgery residency was not an easy undertaking, but we were used to hard work. We could make it. Jim and I talked about his and Kristy's joint graduation party. It would be a party to celebrate success. We would celebrate accomplishment and ending. We would celebrate a new beginning. We wanted to thank everyone who helped make this day possible.

We had to invite everyone.

Jim and I had fun trying to remember each person and what they did when. Becca's nurses and their families would be invited. We couldn't forget all Becca's doctors. And how could I forget Mary? We had our extended family and all our neighbors. We couldn't forget the people from church who prayed through the night for our daughter's life and were there over and over again when we needed them. We had all the people from the newspaper depot and our route jobs. And the kids had friends and families who were important to them. And of course my day care families and Sharon's day care families had to be included. Somehow all of us because of Becca had intertwined in a community built on love.

Santa! I sighed, we couldn't invite because we still had no idea who so skillfully and secretly blessed us.

The more Jim and I talked, the more excited we became. Well, at least, I became really excited. I love parties, and holidays, and celebrations. A celebration of an end of schooling, an end of Medical School, but most of all, it was a celebration of gratitude for the journey. After six long years of schooling, we looked forward to a paycheck. It wouldn't be large, but big enough to make a difference for us. A paycheck, a benefit package, and maybe someday a savings account or a retirement plan. Becca will finally have insurance. We could be real people again.

We had so much to celebrate, the people who we have become and the lessons we have learned. The good times and the bad times, some that were only known to Jim and me. We would of course celebrate the completion of Jim's education from Medical School and Kristy's graduation from high school.

Jim is not the only one deserving of a diploma. This party would serve many purposes, dual graduations, and a way to thank the people who provided support. Without them we would not have made it.

▼

We did not do it alone. Our families, our community, our church, the vast numbers of people who were needed to help Becca.

We all did it together!

▼

I wrote of our journey as a thank you for our community. The story was for the local paper, and I made the editor promise to not publish it until we were already on our way out of state.

▼

We look with hope as Jim and I and our children continue on life's journey. We are a strong family united by adversity. We were blessed with so much, especially our Tiny Titan, Becca, our miracle.

During the past seven years we had learned some of life's most important lessons.

- *Anything is possible if you can dream it.*
- *If you can believe it and follow your heart, amazing things can happen.*
- *And most important of all was never. . .never . . . ever. . .never give up on hope.*

Becca gave us the gift of realizing that loving well today is what truly matters.

There is no guarantee of a tomorrow.

Welcome to the
Yurcek Family

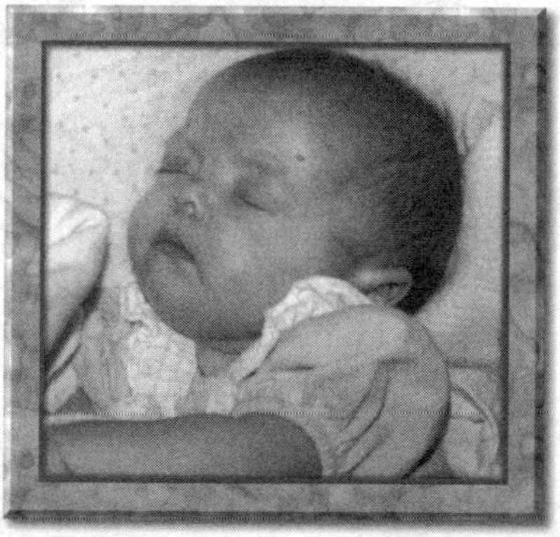

On August 3, 1989
Rebecca Nicole
joined our family
and life as we
knew it
changed.

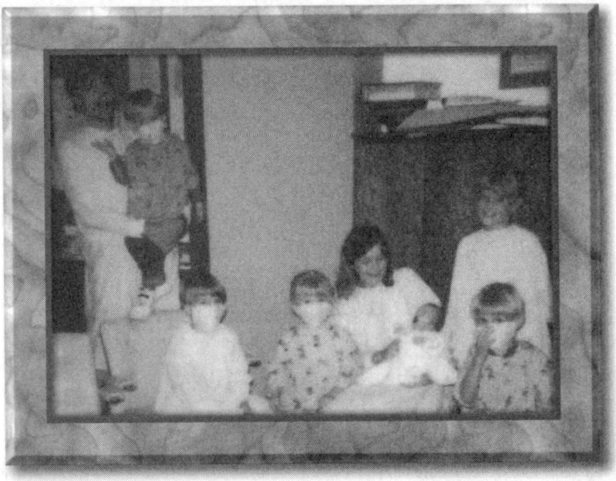

The Yurceks

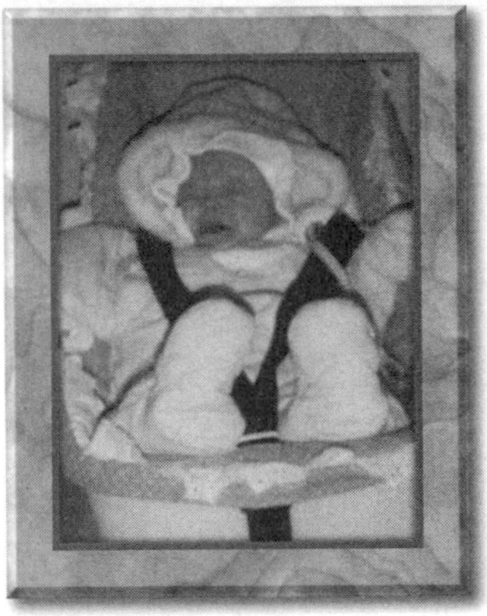

Going home

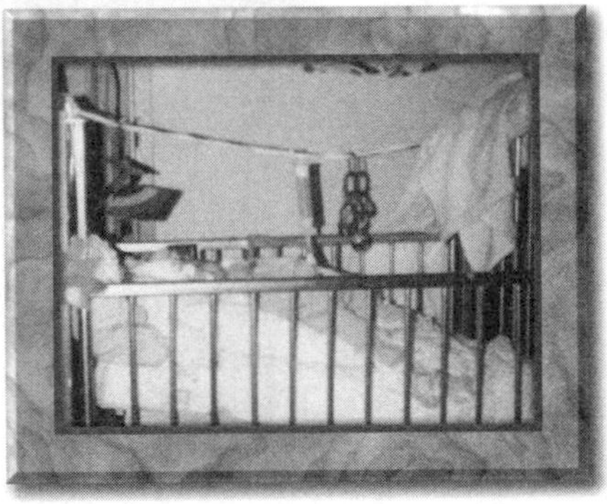

Children's Hospital

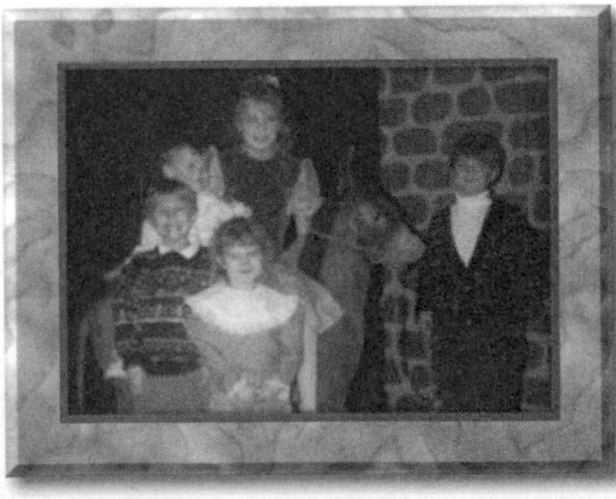

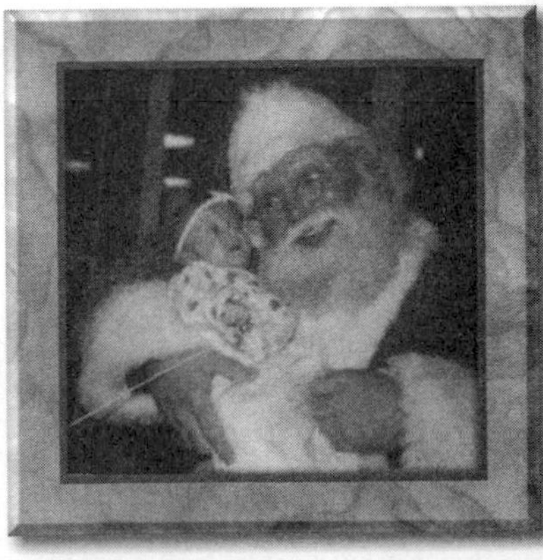

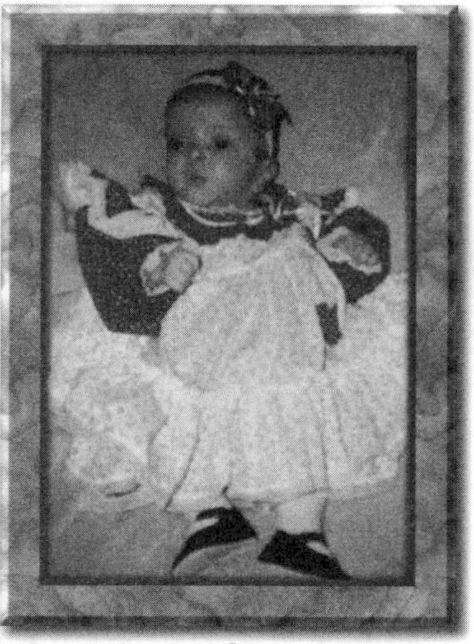

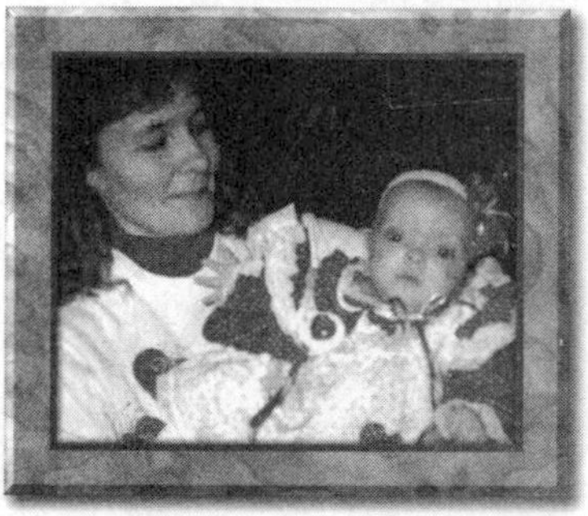

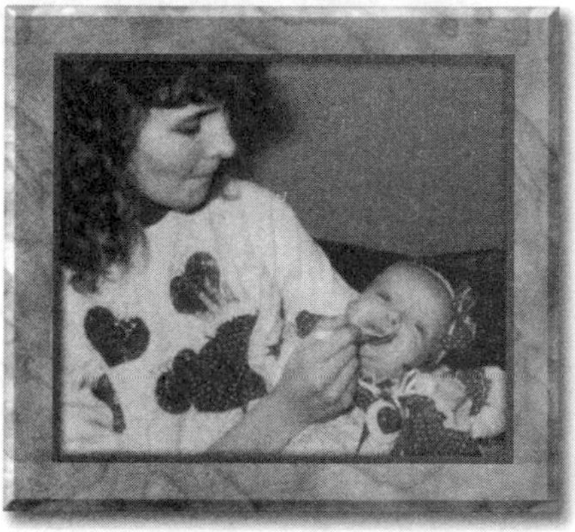

Hearts of Hope

Special Thanks to Make a Wish!

Matt was the perfect Lion and Becca made a darling Toto

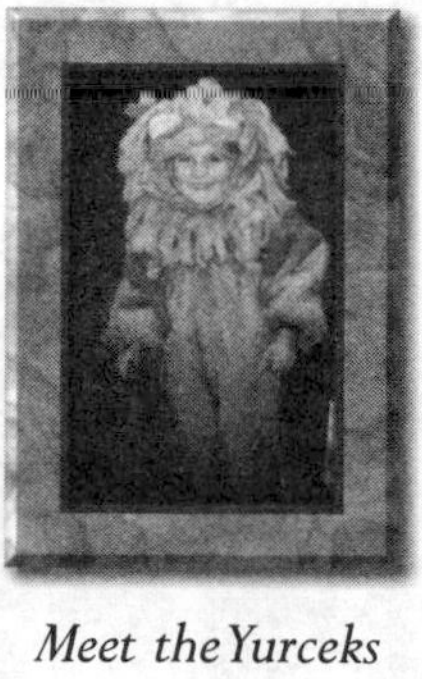

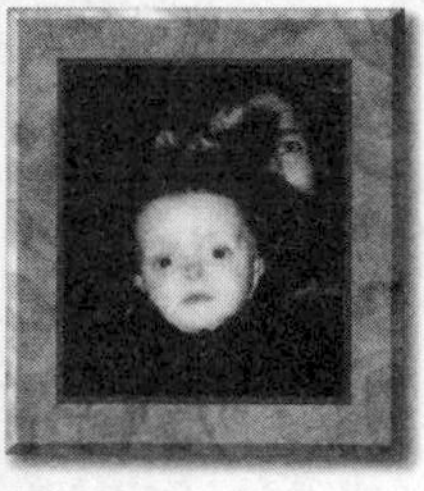

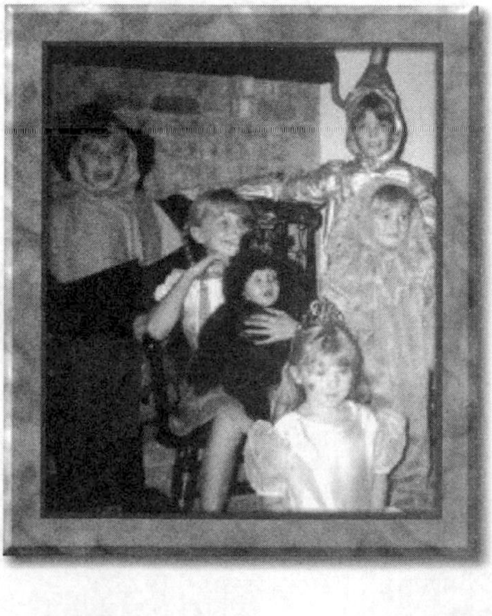

Meet the Yurceks of Oz

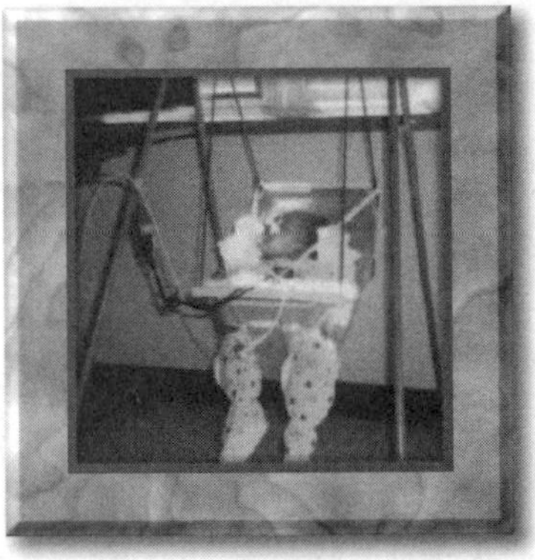

Intensive Care Becca -
After heart surgery

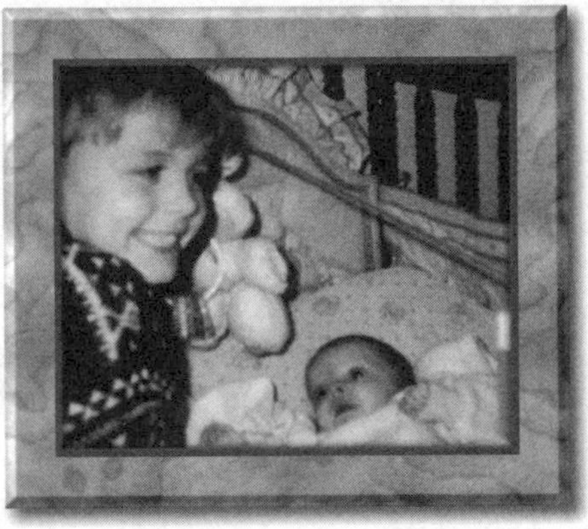

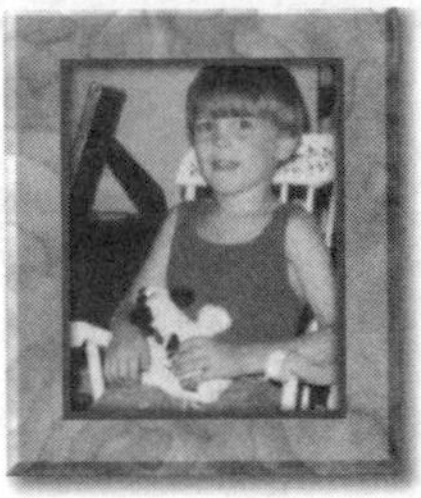

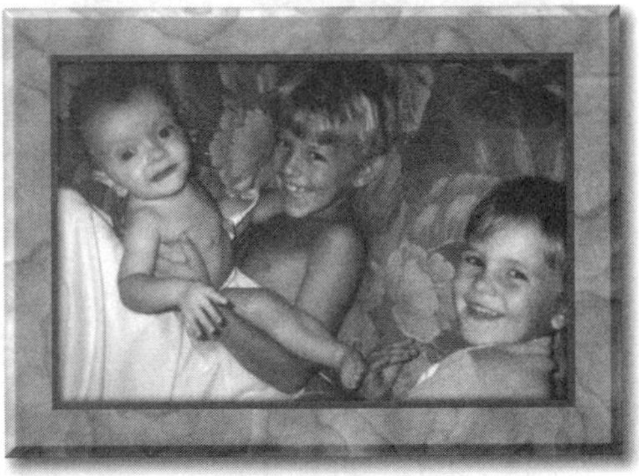

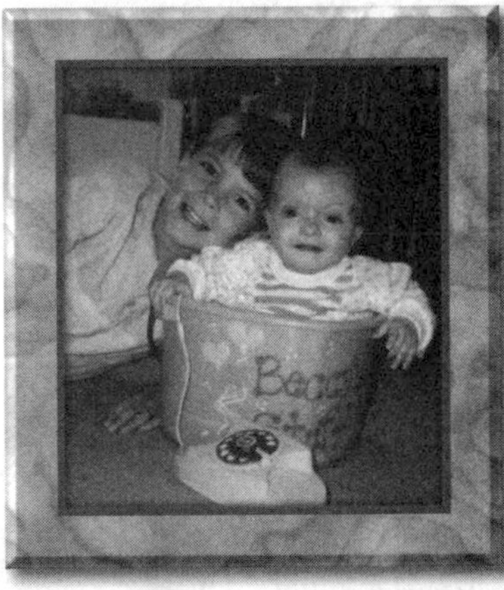

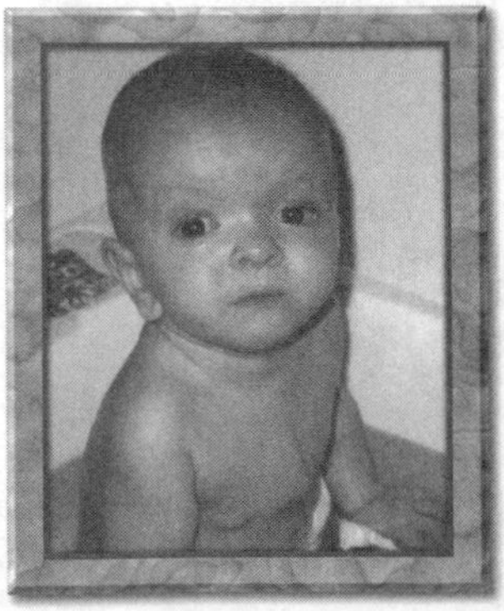

Becca - Age 1

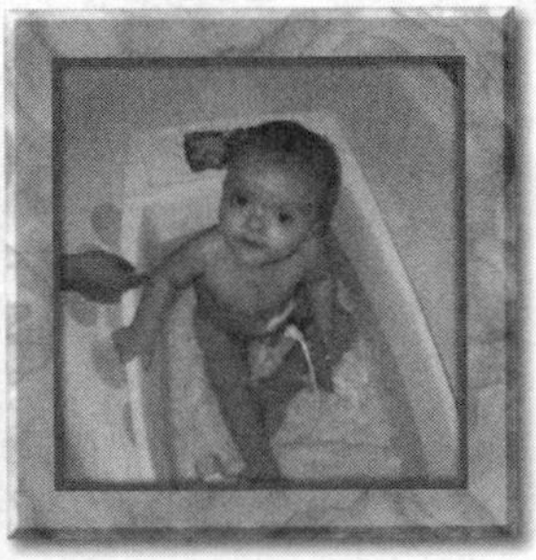

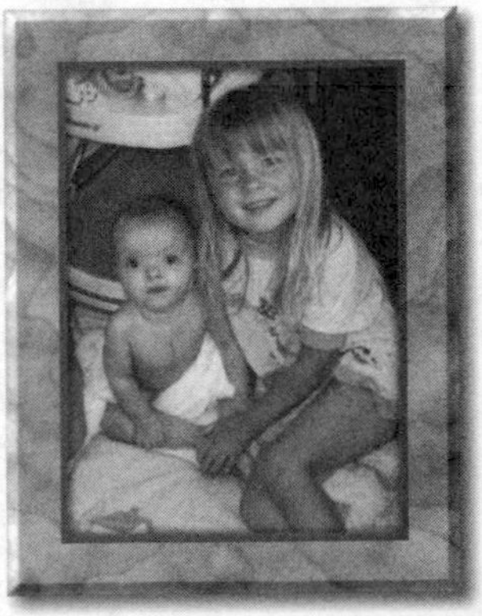

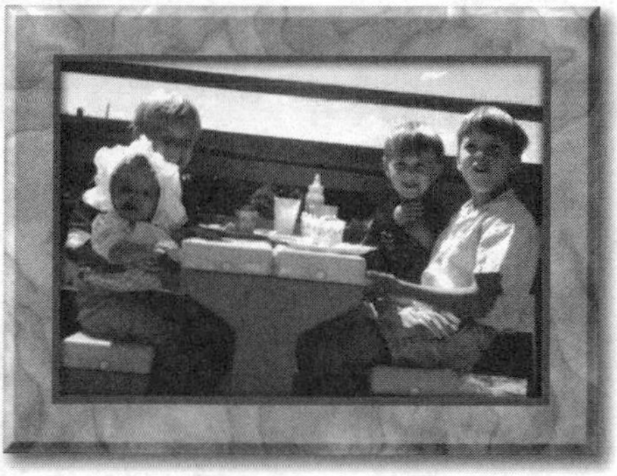

Becca - Age 1

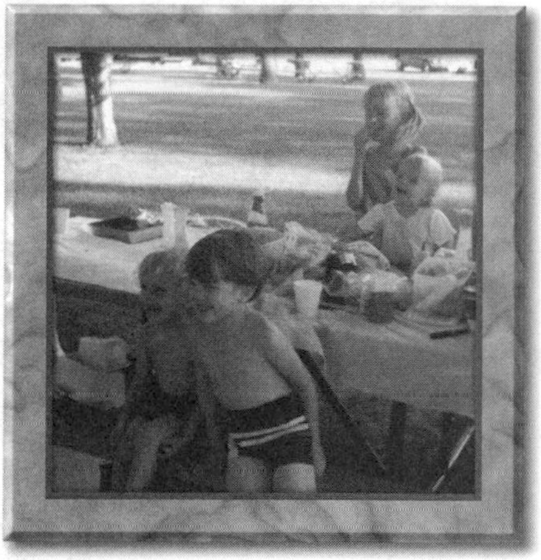

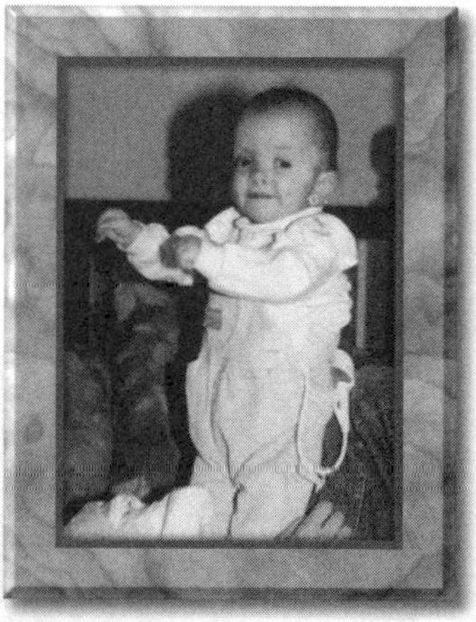

Becca - Nearly 2

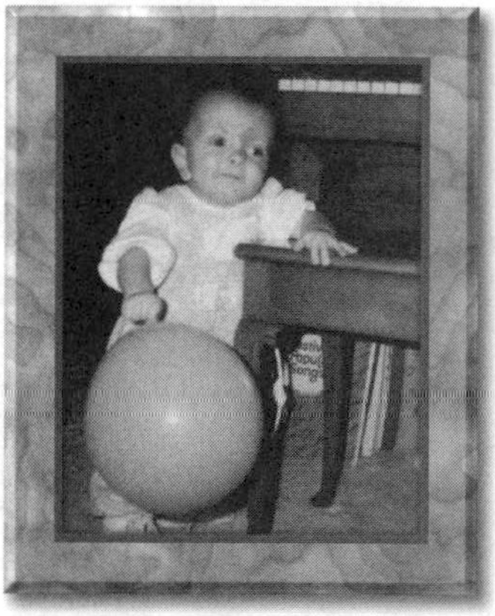

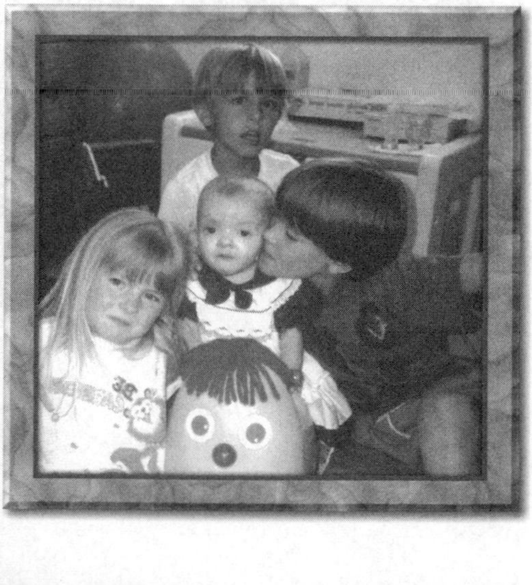

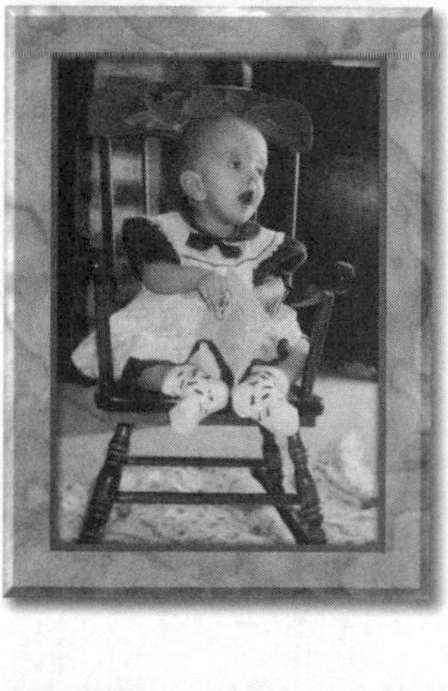

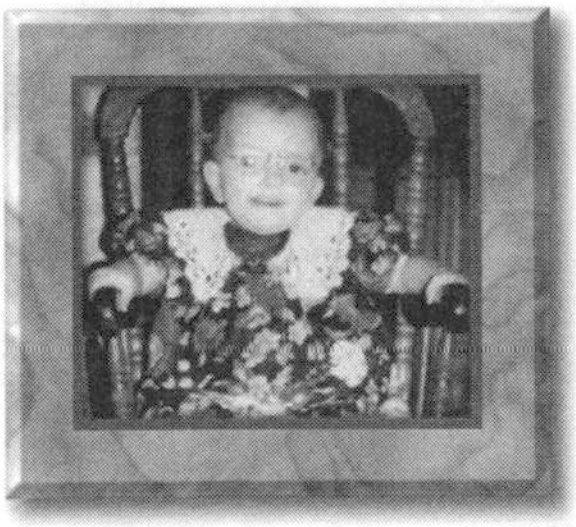

Becca - Age 3

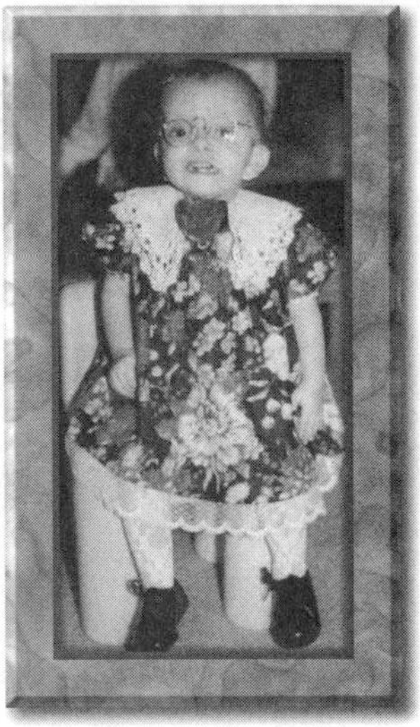

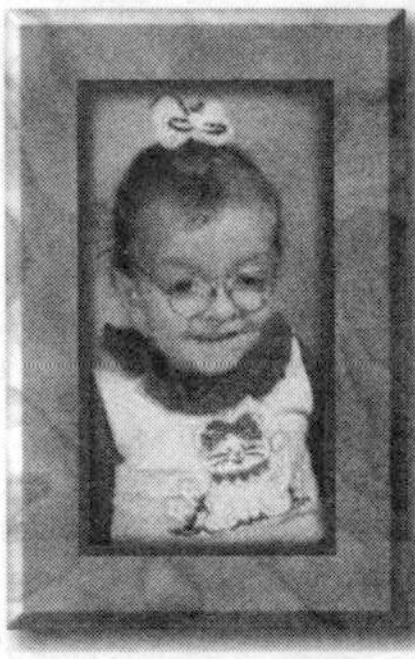

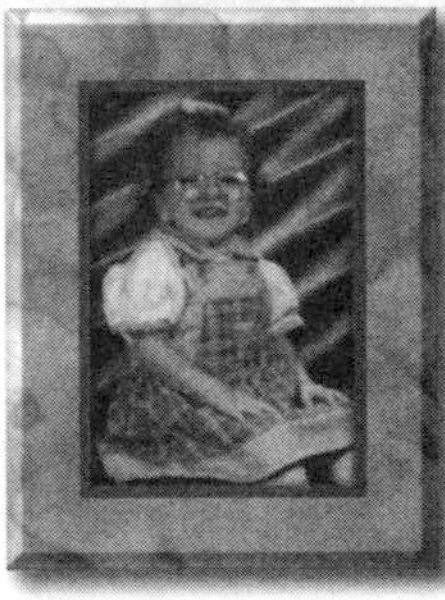

Becca - Age 2

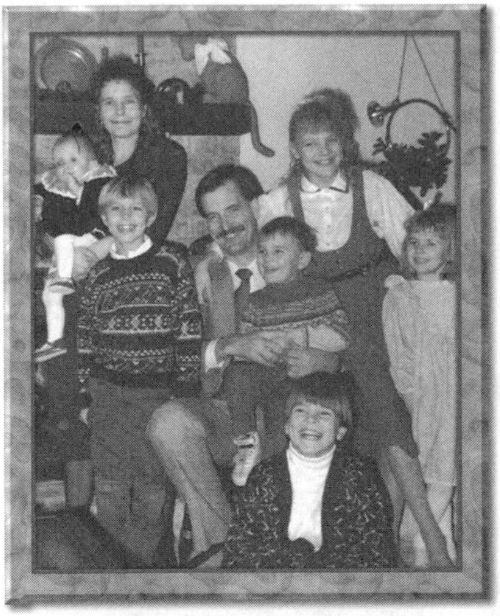

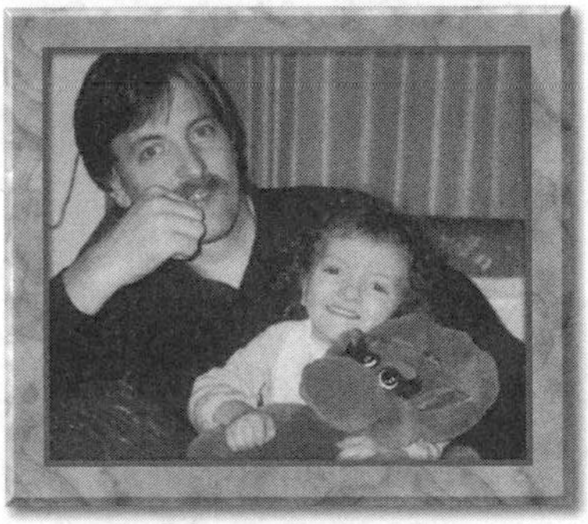

Daddy & Becca - Age 4

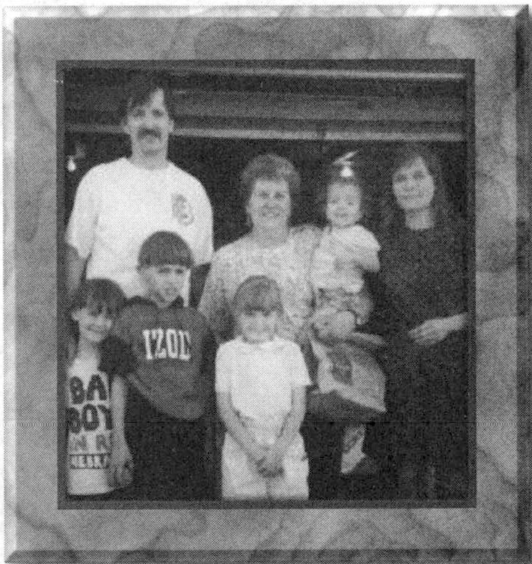

Grandma Zoe

Special Thanks to Caregivers Network!

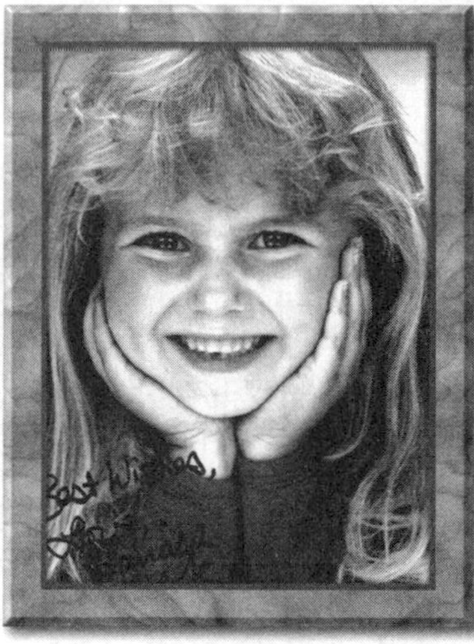

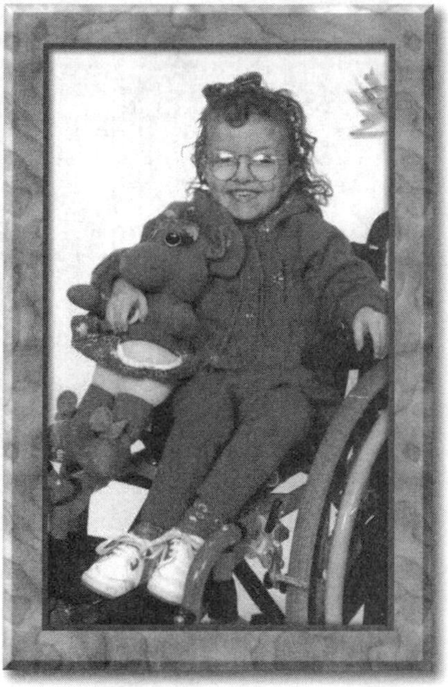

Our models

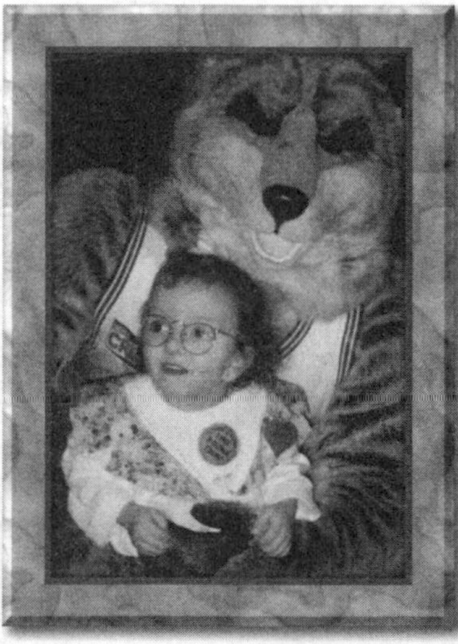

Becca and Crunch
Age 5

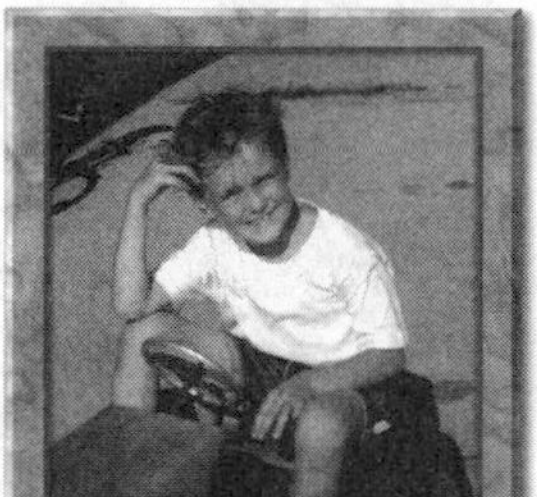

Matt and wheels

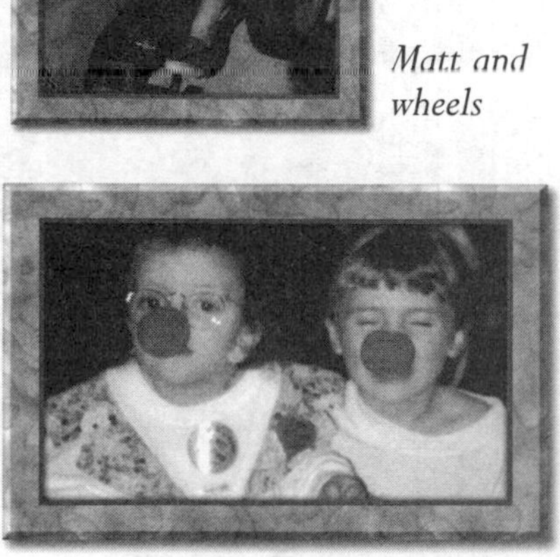

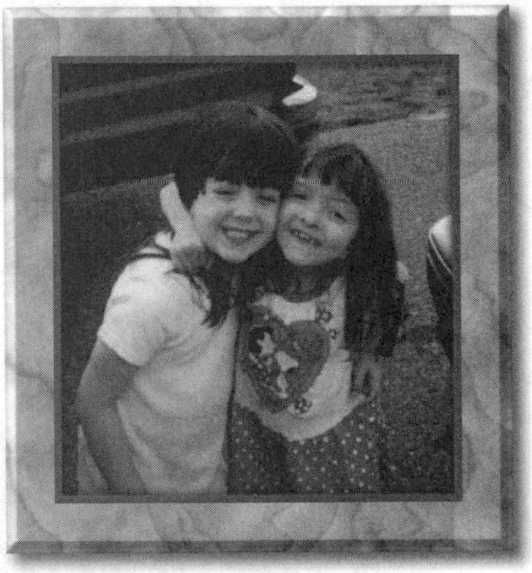

Best friends - Becca Age 7

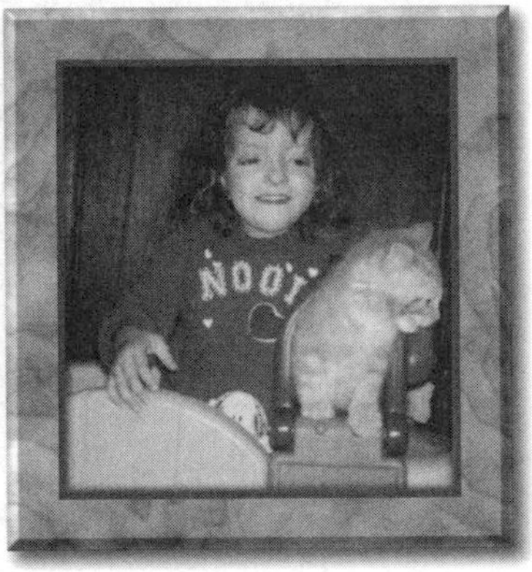

Josey & Becca - Age 6

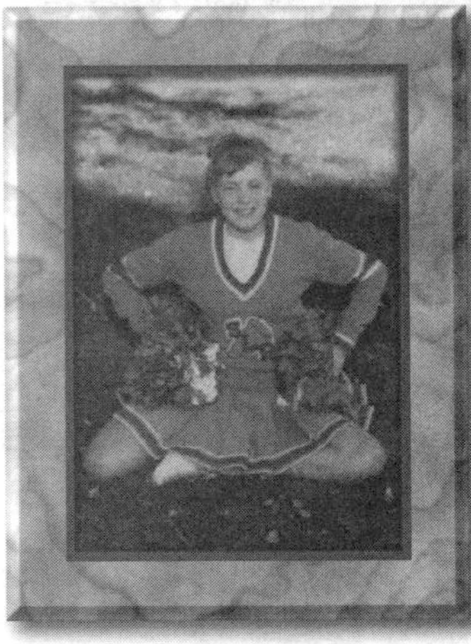

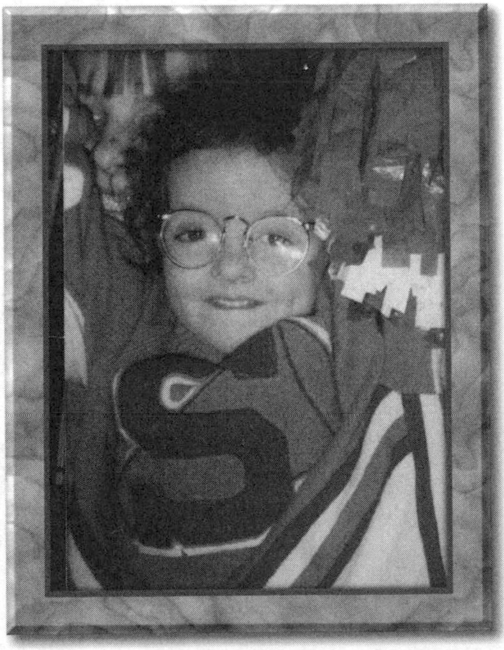

Team spirit - Age 6

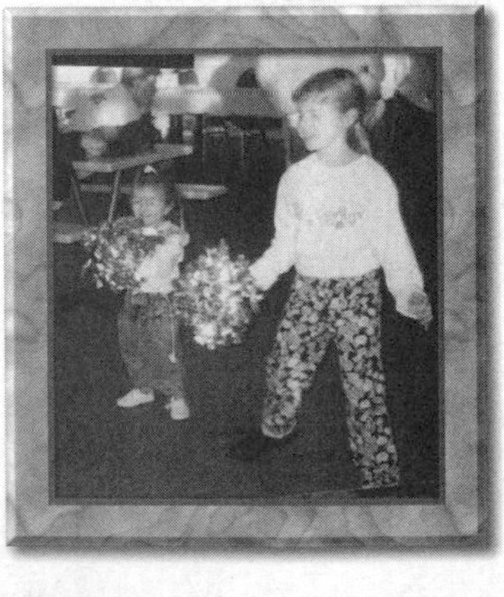

PART TWO

MIRACLES BY THE DOZEN

Part Two - Miracles By the Dozen

- 29 -

THE ARRIVAL OF SOMEDAY

We had become survivors. We were now moving on to a new place, a new life, and after seven years a new and very different Yurcek chapter. Although this part of our story began in *Part One – The Gift*, I have purposely left it out to appropriately begin *Part Two – Miracles by the Dozen*. Let me back up in time, to a few months before Jim graduated from Medical School . . .

▼

The ad for an adoption fair stared at me from the stack of papers on the table. I promised myself someday we would add to our family when Jim was finally a doctor. Remembering back to the promise I had made so long ago, I committed that someday I would turn our struggles into something positive. We had learned so much with Becca, we knew we could help another child with special needs. I felt it was something we were supposed to do. Jim's dream was finally being realized and now the heartstrings of my childhood were also pulling on my heart. I had grown up devouring stories of large families and the book the *Family Nobody Wanted* was my all time favorite. Published before I was even born, Helen Doss had opened my heart to adopt a child. Someday our home would be the place for a child nobody wanted. So much had been given to our family because of Becca. I promised to help another. Now that Jim had explored his dream, perhaps it was time to begin exploring mine.

I remembered the children in the NICU who had no home, not even a foster home. The place they lived was filled with multiple caregivers, bright lights and stark walls. Their only family was the doctors, nurses, and therapists. Some were sick like our Becca and their medical conditions were just too much for the families to handle, others had no home because of substance abuse issues. These children jittered, shook and screamed from withdrawals. Some curled up in little balls and detached from the world. Others scrunched their tiny little faces, their little bodies withering in pain. I promised as I watched those wee ones, someday I would be there to give back. Someday . . . .

Without a second thought, Kristy and I visited the adoption fair. We paged through the nearly one inch thick catalog of children waiting for homes. Most were older kids, or siblings. Many were children of color. The faces affected Kristy. She had a special place in her heart for little Kim at my daycare and she asked who would take care of her when Kim's grandmother died from cancer?

I assured her that Kim's aunt and uncle were planning to become her parents. Kim was a lucky little girl who did not have to go into the foster care system. Kristy insisted these kids needed homes. Our family had talked about sharing with others, but I told her not until Dad was done with training.

At dinner that night I told Jim and the other kids, about my dreams as a child, and my promise to make a difference. It was settled, Jim and I signed up for the adoption classes.

Jim was finishing his final year of Medical School and had time in the evening to devote to learn more. We would attend adoption classes together and the older children would watch the younger ones.

At the very first class, we found ourselves in a room filled with a dozen diverse adults. Each person and their reasons to adopt was unique and special. There was a middle aged Hispanic couple, two older African American women, a couple of middle aged single women, a female couple, two young couples, a single man, and another middle age Caucasian couple. In time we found ourselves leading the group with our knowledge of parenting and our unique experiences with children who had differences and special needs.

At the very first class, the instructor proudly talked about a set of six siblings she had recently found a family. This family would adopt all six children who had been living in different foster homes for the last five years. This family would bring these beautiful African American children together.

The picture circulated around the room. What struck me was how connected they appeared with each other in the pictures. These children were different from many of the kids in the waiting children book at the adoption fair. Their eyes had spark, while many of the pictures Kristy and I had seen had eyes with vacant stares, or showed sorrow, or worry. I had seen that look often on the abandoned babies back in the NICU. My heart said they had hope.

The oldest boy was a thin, middle teen, but his eyes told of wisdom beyond his years. His posture showed he was the protector and caregiver. He sat next to a girl about age eleven, I looked longingly at the little girl, her look was different from the others. Of all the children she appeared to have been lost in the struggle and looked a little slow. The next two boys seemed to be six and seven with a cute little brother with a big huge smile who was maybe five. A beautiful teeny-tiny shy-looking girl smiled coyly among her older siblings. She looked like a toddler, but we learned she was almost five. They were a beautiful family.

The children's story was heartbreaking, they had lived through domestic violence, drug abuse and neglect. These children had been separated for nearly five years and monthly visits were their only connection to each other. Jim and I heard the statement. "The couple that was adopting them had never parented any children," and we looked at each other shocked.

On the way home, Jim and I questioned the wisdom of combining inexperienced parents with six children who weren't even used to living together. How could this be a proper placement? Were they that hard up for parents? Were they thinking with their heads or with their hearts? Parenting children with special needs was exhausting and required expertise. These kids already had so many strikes against them, and would need so much. It didn't make sense to either of us.

These children didn't need rookie parents. We had six children and we knew what it took. This was a special needs transracial adoption and these kids would come with emotional baggage. Someday we would be able to afford to adopt. We knew that even with our skills we would be challenged with such a tribe. Maybe someday the right baby or little family would be waiting to join our home.

We told no one of our talks about these children and we finished our eight classes. We determined that someday we would adopt a medically fragile child to add to our family and we would use the knowledge we had learned with Becca to help that child thrive.

Jim finished his final months of Medical School and we planned for graduation, and a new chapter in our lives.

It was Unmatch Day, the day we anxiously hoped 'not' to receive a phone call by 5:00 P.M.. Jim hoped for a surgery residency opening. At 4:00 P.M. in the midst of parents picking up their children at my daycare, I received a call from the adoption worker from the county. I put the call on hold and hustled a four-year-old out the door with his parent. She was wondering if we were interested in adopting a sibling group. One of the social workers that led the adoption classes had called the adoption workers from our county asking if she would call us and see if we were interested in adopting. As she described the children and their story, I soon realized that it was the siblings from that very first class. I told her that in two days our lives would be changing, then without hesitation said that if we matched in the Twin Cities we might consider it. But if we had to move to one of ten other places, this was not the right time.

She got me to agree to see the print out on the children, it seemed crazy that she was calling us about this sibling set when she knew our story. She knew we had six kids. She knew one had special needs. The social workers in the class knew we were delivering newspapers as our source of income. They knew Jim was a medical student. Why us? How could this be?

Less than an hour later, at 4:55 P.M., Jim called me to play a joke- the phone call of dashed dreams. All the medical students who did not get a match were to get a phone call at five o'clock so they could scurry to find an open residency slot A phone call on Unmatch Day would be devastating for anyone. The phone rang. I jumped. My heart sank. How could it be? Jim was at the top of his class. He blew away his entrance exam scores. He did well in Medical School. Maybe it was because he was so old. Jim was almost forty and residency for surgery was grueling. On top of that add six kids, one chronically ill.

He laughed.

I told him he was not funny and we talked as the clock ticked past five o'clock and we knew he had matched. Only then, I let him know of the strange phone call from an adoption worker offering us siblings who needed a home.

He said, "It's the six isn't it?"

How did he know?

He said he just knew and what did I say?

The flyer arrived two days later, the same day we learned we were moving to Kalamazoo, Michigan. The flyer tugged at my heart. I called the worker at my county to say the timing was all-wrong. We had to sell the house, find a house, and move to Michigan. She would pass on our decision to the worker.

I felt obliged to call the social worker from training and explain our circumstances. As we talked, she understood. I told her we might be interested once we settled in a year or two, and we knew we would adopt someday when Jim was through his surgery residency. Someday we would be there for a waiting child and I did not want to close the door.

She talked about the kids, their histories, and the fact that the agency had to identify parents. Termination of Parental rights was being appealed for the second time, and because of court technicalities they had to start over. The kids lived in three different foster homes, separated in pairs. The mom's attorney's arguments were that no one would keep them together. The littlest girl had been in foster care since she was two-months-old and was now nearly five. This seemed to be the family nobody wanted.

For the next several days Jim and I talked about the insanity of thinking this was possible. We had to move to Kalamazoo in two months. Every time we found reasons why we couldn't do it, the social worker called unexpectedly with the answer to the question that we had only asked each other. Our hearts were being moved towards the adoption with serious reservations.

We had to sell our house. Our house sold in a record three days. We had to find a house in Kalamazoo. We drove through the night to Michigan and checked into a motel to sleep for an hour before meeting the realtor. We left Nathan in charge of the kids while we spent the morning and afternoon in a flurry touring houses. We saw twelve houses, and most were small and needed a lot of work. The first house made me wheeze from mold and I ran from the house with my inhaler in hand as Jim finished the tour. The next house was being remodeled and never finished, it was a mess. It was large enough, but we would not have enough time or money to make the necessary repairs. The rest were too small to fit six children, let alone twelve. Twelve! What were we thinking?

The very last house was located in a part of the city we were told had the best schools. We were surprised as the car pulled up to a well-manicured white split level with glossy black shutters. The shiny red front door greeted us. In the house, we found two bedrooms on the main level, and two good size bedrooms in the lower, and a small office. The office was big enough to convert to another bedroom. There were two full bathrooms, plus a half bath in the hallway off the living room. That meant five bedrooms and three baths, a downstairs family room, a good size living room with an eating area and a tiny kitchen attached. It was just right for all the children! There was a big back yard that had a swing set with a slide and a chain link fence to protect the dog. It even had a basketball hoop on the driveway and a sidewalk for the smaller kids to ride bikes. In less than a day, we had found the perfect house for a family of fourteen.

The price had just been reduced by $15,000. The residency program in Kalamazoo helps residents buy their own homes with little money down. Jim had been matched to one of the only programs of its kind. I had argued with Jim before we left that this couldn't be true. Our past eight years had taken a disastrous toll on our credit. The $110,000 was still above the bank pre-approval of $107,000 and I could still not believe we were even approved for any house loan.

We picked up Mc Donald's, as the realtor wrote up the offer. I took our patient children to the pool and Jim fell asleep. The following morning we woke to the news that the owner rejected our offer and our hopes were dashed. An hour later the phone rang with news that both the seller's agents and ours wanted us to have the house and they cut their commissions to make up the difference.

The realtor made arrangements for us to bring the kids to see our new home and sign another purchase agreement. I took pictures of every room, and the kids ran through the house claiming bedrooms. The house passed the kids' stamp of approval and it reassured me they would be all right with our move. After signing the purchase agreement and writing a check for the down payment, we had just enough cash to drive home. In forty-eight hours, we had driven 1,200 miles and bought a new house. We spent our house payment to get there, but with our Minnesota house closing only a month away, we could pay it back. It had all worked out in less than a week – two houses – one sold, one bought. By Monday we were back home exhausted, and went back to work.

I brought the film in to be developed at the film store and I called the adoption worker to tell her about the house. We scheduled the home study and began to complete pages and pages of questions. It seemed unreal.

The home study left no question unasked. We were examined, assessed and put under a microscope. What types of kids were we comfortable to be placed with? We said we would not take kids with severe emotional disturbances. We would not take kids that would act out. We would not take kids that put other kids at risk. We had to think of the well being of our current children. We had to think of Becca and all her needs. So Jim and I set solid and clear limits with the agency about what we could and would handle.

Our background checks were complete because of my daycare license. The kids needed physicals for the home study, but with moving they needed to have a check up anyway. The ICPC interstate placement paperwork was approved and I began making whirlwind visits to the children's three different foster families.

First I was to visit with Detamara and DeShawn's foster mom. I was surprised when I answered the front door and there stood little Detamara who had tagged along. I could not believe that she was already five. She was tiny like Becca and her hair was beautifully done. Her foster mom explained to me how to keep it up. She made sure I understood which products to use and how to style it. The next day, I met Detamara and DeShawn's preschool teachers.

I visited DJ's and Shay's (Delonsha) foster parents. The foster parents told us the children were well behaved and didn't present any unusual challenges. Shay liked to help the foster mom around the house; she was in special education and had an IEP like Becca.

My parents questioned our sanity. They were worried about us, but we felt that this was the right thing to do. The coincidences were too great and this was our calling. If God was leading us to do this, He would open the doors. Through the years with Becca I had learned to trust what I was led to do. This was a big decision, seemingly impossible and probably crazy, but if God wanted us to do this, He would lay the path, and make things happen. I just had to trust and have faith. My parents shook their heads bewildered.

We had the gargantuan party of our dreams when Kristy graduated from high school and Jim graduated from Medical School. Now it was really time to meet our new children.

We would spend ten days off and on with them. The first day Jim and I met the kids as a group at the two middle boys foster home near the university. Delonzo was seven and Deangelo eight and they stood waiting on the stoop of the brick row house. Grandma Dorothy was a veteran foster parent in her seventies and the boys were her final placement. Shay was twelve, and was shy and awkward. We were introduced and she ran off to play with her younger brothers. Her facial features showed she possibly had some sort of syndrome, but none was listed on the paperwork, other than she had a developmental delay. It was DJ's fifteenth birthday and he was off at the mall celebrating with his friends. We would meet him the next day. The last foster mom arrived with the two youngest. Detamara looked up and smiled slightly. She seemed to recognize me from her previous visit to our home. DeShawn was precious; he ran up to Jim and jumped into his arms the moment they met, calling Jim, Daddy.

The small townhouse was crowded with all the adults, the foster care worker and five lively children. The kids needed to wear off some energy, so I suggested we walk to the corner park and play with the children together. We watched the interactions between siblings. It seemed that the foster care separation had not affected their love for each other. They were siblings in every sense, including arguing. The two-hour visit flew by, and we said goodbyes until tomorrow.

This next day the kids were delivered to our home. The guardian ad litem brought the oldest two, the foster care worker dropped off the two middle boys and the foster mom delivered the two youngest children. We introduced the current Yurcek children to the future Yurcek children. Kristy broke the ice by introducing herself, then Ian, and soon the rest of the kids made their introductions. My kids took their hands and led them off into the house, and soon they seemed like old friends.

DeShawn bounced affectionately from person to person. Detamara silently followed the tribe hanging onto my hand for dear life. The kids were all very polite. The boys seemed to hit it off immediately. The girls were distant. Detamara left my side and began to follow Becca around like a shadow. Shay tried to interact with Marissa but seemed unsure how to act, but in time the girls seemed more at ease with each other.

The ten days passed quickly. We visited the zoo and went to our favorite parks. Some days we simply hung around home. I didn't want to give the impression that everyday was a holiday. I wanted to see how they interacted with each other at home in everyday activities. A family friend invited us for a bonfire and barbeque at their home and the oldest two kids spent the night to help us move.

The next morning was moving day, and that evening Jim and I and our current six would leave for Michigan. The plan was for our new children to join us once we were unpacked and settled.

DJ and Shay helped us load the moving truck along with Jim's parents and sister and brother-in-law. DJ loaded his new birthday boom box unto the truck. Grandpa told us later that he overheard DJ telling Ian that if his boom box was on that truck that meant we were really going to be his family and he would be going to Michigan. With the boom box loaded, we said our goodbyes to DJ and Shay. Sue, their guardian ad litem picked them up to drive them back to their foster home. We loaded up our six children, the dog, and the cat into the moving caravan and drove off to the next chapter.

This new chapter had now added the family nobody wanted. Perhaps it was impossible and crazy or nuts, why us? We were led to them. I don't know why, but the doors had mysteriously opened and all the barriers had been moved. I had been told homestudies take months. In a record four weeks time, the home study was done and we were approved to be parents for the six new children. The interstate paperwork never moves smoothly, it was done immediately. Our house sold and we had money leftover. Then unbelievably we found a home to fit the fourteen of us on residency pay that was ready and waiting. If the kids were meant to come with us, I prayed that God would provide. The doors kept opening and we faithfully followed.

We were now two families moving on to new lives, coming together as one in Michigan. We were merging two families together like on the Brady Bunch. Both families understood adversity. We had both faced hunger, loss, and pain. We both had struggled, but we were all survivors.

- 30 -

NEW KIDS ON THE BLOCK

The whirlwind started when we arrived in Michigan. Jim had a week to prepare to start his residency. We unloaded the moving truck and found new places for our belongings. Within days we received a phone call from the private adoption agency to update our home study.

The Michigan workers arrived, and they asked us questions about the new children and to see their records, but we had none. We told them we were not allowed by Minnesota law to see the records on our children because confidentiality laws kept them hidden in Minnesota. They couldn't believe we had no paperwork. In Michigan families are given copies of the records and can view the files. We told them we had been allowed to ask questions of the foster families, but they had told us very little. We were seasoned enough to understand that childhood neglect would have an impact on their development. We knew that the children would come with some problems, but we had been reassured that these children did not have any issues that endangered others, they did not act out sexually, and they were not severely emotionally disturbed. Those were our criteria from the questionnaire asked by the home study worker back in Minnesota.

The worker shook her head. She asked if we really knew what we were getting into? I had no idea why she seemed so concerned. I had read books on adopting hurt children, I thought I was prepared for the bumpy road to attachment, and we had been told these kids were not severe. Trying to reassure myself, I left her concern alone.

We took some of the money from the sale of our home, and replaced the hodge-podge furniture we had left behind. We needed nearly everything. Our furniture was a collection of early garage sale and bargain thrift store finds. It was not worth moving and with the wear and tear of children it was in need of replacement.

It was fun shopping, I found a used table and chairs and added new benches to slide into our dining area. The new arrangement would squeeze in ten of us. The plastic Little Tykes table would hold the smallest of the children for the time being. We found a new couch, loveseat and bedroom set for Jim and I at a clearance sale, along with three sets of bunk. We had purchased a loft bed from my brother for Marissa, and Grandpa and Grandma had sent twin beds with box springs that they no longer needed. Now every member of the family had a bed.

Since we were doubling our family I needed more of everything. The social workers arranged for money to help with the cost of the new children's furniture. I bought eight more place settings of silverware, to add to the eight Mom and Dad gave me for my birthday. I color coordinated the towels and sheets for each room, pink for Becca and Detamara, mint green for Shay and Marissa, blue for Deangelo, Delonzo, Matt, and DeShawn, and tan for Nathan, Ian, and DJ. I had replaced my broken sewing machine with a new embroidery machine and I monogrammed the towels and washrags for each of the kids to keep them straight. My red fifteen-passenger daycare van converted to our family vehicle. The MAXI-Van was big enough to hold our new entire family, and we 'thought' we were ready.

We would begin life with the children as their new foster parents and then move on to adoption. We were aware that this was a legal risk placement, and everything could be overturned based on the outcome of the termination of rights appeal. A legal mistake could force the return of the children to their drug-abusing parents.

Kristy had already returned to Minnesota for work and college.

It was hard to say goodbye to my daughter. She was old enough for her independence, but torn about leaving or staying with the family. She sobbed as she left and I held back tears while I prayed for her safety. The first phase of my mothering of her was complete. No longer would I be there to protect her. I had to trust that we had prepared Kristy to stand on her own and now we would be six hundred miles away. My heart ached for Kristy. She was now starting college at the same college Granny had attended to become a Registered Nurse.

Moving to Michigan was a new start for everyone except for Kristy who had always dreamed of independence. I felt like we had abandoned her in Minnesota without her family and sending her back broke my heart. I missed her, she was my helper, she was the big sister, and she was leaving her very special little Becca. Now that we were so far away I was apprehensive even though she would have the long distance support of our family. Her cell phone became her connection to us but it wasn't enough and there were days when loneliness took its toll.

Kristy buried herself in school and work to soften her loneliness. I worried about her. Then her rusty secondhand car broke down on the freeway coming from school in the wee hours of the morning I knew we were needed even more. Helping Kristy buy a car from long distance was an adventure, our credit was ruined and we were little help with getting her into reliable safe affordable transportation. Granny and Grandpa came to the rescue.

Kristy's two jobs provided her the income for budgeting a two hundred dollar a month payment, but that was it. When the car dealership sales person tried to take advantage of a pretty young woman, Kristy turned around and walked out when the payment was ten dollars too high. They called her back and she got the car off the new lot with the payment under her budget.

▼

Our house soon felt like home. The deadline of July 28 and the arrival of the new kids was coming fast. In driving through Kalamazoo I was delighted to see the town had a very diverse population. It would be a good setting to raise a transracial family. Word spread like wildfire about their impending arrival. Matt's friends parent leaked the word of our family to his next door neighbor who just happened to be a news reporter for our local CBS affiliate. The news reporter landed on our doorstep wanting to tell the story while the kids and I were in the process of freezing twenty pounds of blueberries. We had discovered Kalamazoo was in the heart of fruit country. It was lush, and green, and temperate because of Lake Michigan.

They told the story about the upcoming arrival of the children on the five o'clock news. They wanted to come with us to the airport but Minnesota social services wanted to keep it private. I promised the news channel that they could have a story when things had settled down and we had approval.

Then we were off to the airport to bring home almost ALL of our kids.

▼

The Kalamazoo International Airport was tiny. We watched our children walk off the tiny commuter plane up to the gate. They were finally here. The kids ran up to each other like old friends and we now had eleven excited children ages five to sixteen busily chatting, while we herded them towards the baggage claim area. Grandma Dorothy had sent Deangelo and Delonzo with two huge duffel bags as big as they were. DJ and Shay had two boxes and two small bags and DeShawn and Detamara each had a small box. We claimed children, and their luggage, and set off for home.

In the middle of the excitement the social worker pulled me aside to tell me that we had a small problem, Shay had just gotten her period. Marissa, Shay and I left the teens and the younger kids in the care of Sandra the social worker at home while we went to Target for supplies. The store was only five minutes from home, and I hurried to not leave the social worker with my tribe of children for long.

Our new neighbor from across the street and Sandra met us when we pulled into the driveway. Something was wrong. The neighbor was angry and she pulled me aside and explained to me that the youngest boy had grabbed at her twelve-year-old daughter's chest and tried to reach up her shorts. DeShawn was only six, but that was enough of a red flag to put me on alert to watch him carefully.

I apologized, but from that time on she wanted nothing to do with any of us. We had not made a good first impression on our new neighbors.

We had stayed in contact with the children and their foster families during the month while we prepared for their arrival. We had heard that DeShawn had cut the computer cord at school before the end of the school year. I bought the book *Adopting the Hurt Child* by Greg Keck before we left Minnesota, and the book prepared me or so I thought about what to do to help my new little boy attach to our family. I thought I had learned the red flags of a detached child and what to watch for. Little did I know the comfortables were out to get us?

The boxes and bags were moved in and Sandra, the kids and I spent the next few days exploring Michigan. We romped and played on the shores of Lake Michigan in South Haven. The beaches were busy, and knowing where every child was, was nearly impossible. Watching the six younger children and trying to keep my eyes on five teenagers was a challenge. I was used to children who listened and came when I called. With Sandra's help, I managed to keep everyone in sight. What used to be a joy-filled day at the beach filled me with anxiety as I tried to manage this tribe. The kids were having a great time, but not Mom.

The kids buried each other in the sand. Detamara was petrified of the water and wouldn't even get her toes wet. She sat quietly and shoveled sand. Becca floated in her pink Little Mermaid life jacket while DeShawn tried to dunk her. Shay was a fish and didn't want to get out of the water, while Marissa suntanned on the white sandy beach. Deangelo and Delonzo chased each other, while Nathan, Ian and DJ surfed the waves.

We had packed two-dozen sandwiches, a bag of apples, and a huge cooler of drinks. The food was demolished by starving children and teens who immediately announced they were still hungry. After dropping $25.00 on ice cream we took my tired, hungry and sunburned children home.

I was naïve and I learned several things that day.

First, children with African American heritage can get just as sunburned as fair-skinned children. I had asked Sandra if anyone needed sunscreen when we arrived at the beach. I didn't know and DJ laughed at the thought. He assured me that dark skin does not sunburn while I lathered the sunscreen on Nathan, Marissa and Matt who had inherited Jim's fair skin. In my whole life I never had sunburned with my olive skin, but Jim, on the other hand, turned as red as a boiled lobster, so prevention of sunburn was part of my beach routine. I brushed off DJ's laughing and believed Sandra when she said that they did not need lotion. Poor Shay burned the worst and she remained two-toned from the peeling for the rest of the summer.

Second, I learned that a shopping cart full of food was not enough to even dent a beach lunch. And third, it was going to take eyes on the back of my head and sonar to keep track of my new charges. My children seemed to lack structure and self-control. Sandra snapped a picture of myself and eleven of our twelve children on the shores of Lake Michigan for our new family photo album.

Two days later, after the kids settled in, Sandra returned to Minnesota. She had completed her delivery of the children to our care and had met with the new agency who would be supervising our foster care placement and impending adoption.

▼

I quickly learned I had to develop a routine for everything from getting up and eating to going to bed.

Everyone was finding his or her place while I worked on organizing the house. The teen boys Ian, DJ, Nathan slept in one bedroom, and the four youngest boys Matt, Deangelo, Delonzo, DeShawn slept in the downstairs bedroom on two sets of bunks. Detamara and Becca shared their pink bedroom on Granny and Grandpa's twin beds. And Marissa and Shay had a loft bed and a single bed underneath in the office bedroom next to the family room.

The little ones played in the fenced backyard and sidewalks, while the older boys played basketball on the driveway. Our dog ran and jumped and played in the backyard.

We were all settling in and getting comfortable.

I took special care to unpack each child's belongings privately. I thought it would be a special time of bonding. The two middle boys were prepared for the start of the school year. Dorothy had made it easy, everything was carefully folded and washed and she had even planned ahead for the start of school. You could tell she had really cared about my boys and had spoiled them with all they owned.

DJ and Shay weren't so lucky.

DJ had a few items and I knew he would need a few more things to start school. As Shay and I unpacked her box, she became upset because many of the items in the box were not hers. They were the rotten cast offs of her foster sister, and she told me all her good stuff was now stolen. Only a few things in her box were usable, and the pieces of clothing that were, did not fit her. Her total inventory of clothes consisted of two pair of underwear, two pairs of socks, one pair of jeans, a robe and pajamas. She had no jacket. She had two dresses and the outfit she arrived in. Shay needed everything and we needed to go shopping.

Shay pulled out her prized "Welcome to the Family" notebook I had put together and given to the social worker. Then she showed me the photo album of the foster family that contained pictures of her and her siblings on family visits, and a picture of her mother. She shared openly and tenderly. She lovingly put her Bible and stuffed animals gently on the shelves and returned to her box.

She burst into a torrent of tears when she discovered her Tweety poster glass frame was broken in the move. The poster was the last birthday present her mother had given her in March. I tried to reassure her and told her that we could fix it with new glass, but she was inconsolable and pulled away. There was nothing I, nor anyone else could do to comfort her and she cried herself to sleep.

I was even more disheartened when I opened DeShawn's and Detamara's small boxes. Everything was unusable and it smelled of mothballs. DJ volunteered to take the boxes to the dumpster.

All the poor littlest ones had were the clothes on their back.

Becca and Detamara were the same size and I put her into Becca's pajamas while Delonzo shared his pjs with DeShawn who drowned in them. All DeShawn owned was a toy robot and a color book while Detamara had an empty purse with her name on, and a well-loved brown bear.

My heart broke for them.

The following morning we were off to the store and I let each child pick out a new toy. Thank God for the small clothing allowance from Minnesota and the house closing check. With clearance racks and frugal spending we were able to outfit eleven children for the summer and the beginning of school.

▼

Birthdays are special days for Yurcek children. The birthday child got to choose dinner and I looked forward to starting the tradition with our new children. We celebrated Becca's eighth birthday five days after the children arrived, and Detamara's would follow six days later. It would be fun to introduce them to our traditions.

We had a family party for Becca with gluten free cake, ice cream, and her requested pizza dinner. Chef Nathan created four regular family sized pizzas, and one gluten-free homemade pizza for the celebration. Everyone seemed to have a good time eating.

▼

The next morning Becca fought me in the bathroom while I prepared to give her a bath before church. She pushed and shoved me away and tried to stop me from taking off her pajamas. It made no sense, as Becca loves water and baths. She loves to pretend to be Free Willy or Shamu in her bathwater. As I pulled her pajamas off I discovered that she was covered with gigantic bruises. The largest bruise covered her whole chest. Becca's bruising was something we were used to as she had been diagnosed with a bleeding disorder, but this was severe. I felt sick to my stomach, and I ask Becca what happened. She told me that DeShawn came into her room and beat her. Then he stuffed his robot into her private parts. She was torn, and bleeding. I was sickened, and horrified. I was panicking as I called Jim to come look at the bruises.

I wrapped Becca in the towel and called Sandra at an emergency number she had given me before her departure just days earlier. Becca at eight finally weighed thirty pounds and was thirty-six inches tall, the same size as most three-year-olds. DeShawn was two years younger than Becca, but he was much bigger and strong, even though tiny himself.

We were in new territory we had never even imagined and Jim and I realized that DeShawn had to be watched every second. We lectured him about hurting Becca. I spent the day playing musical bedrooms as I moved little girls into big girls rooms for protection. I could not have DeShawn near Becca without supervision so I moved Marissa in with Becca and Detamara in with Shay. We installed a locking doorknob on Marissa and Becca's room.

We didn't believe that little Detamara could protect Becca or visa versa. Detamara later revealed that she had awakened and discovered DeShawn with a pillow over Becca's face smothering her to keep from telling on him. Detamara bit DeShawn in the leg and he retreated back to his bedroom, saving Becca's life. Behind the scenes Detamara and Becca learned they could count on each other - both girls had suffered abuse at DeShawn's hands and they did not ever want to see him again. The girls watched over each other and they formed a bond of protection that we didn't understand until later.

It was only one week after placement with us and we were already scurrying to find a therapist who could work with DeShawn and help us help him. I knew from my reading that he had probably been molested along the way and I asked the new therapist for help finding a special therapist for him. She pulled out a list of qualified therapists, and I asked her whom she would recommend. She circled the first, second, and third choices, and amazingly one that stood out was covered under our new insurance carrier that Jim received through his residency. Her name was Colleen and I placed a panicked phone call to her and she agreed to meet on an emergency basis.

In the first appointment we discovered we had a very severely disturbed child. He told the therapist blow-by-blow of how he planned to wait for the house to become quiet, of sneaking into the girl's room, and how he hurt Becca without remorse. He had plotted to take Becca's birthday away from her and the only thing making him angry was that he was caught. I was told to watch him every minute, He was not to be trusted and he could never be alone with the girls.

The more I watched DeShawn, the angrier he became. In less than ten days, he left a path of destruction everywhere. I caught him in the bathroom naked horsing around with the other boys and they told on him.

Deangelo disclosed that DeShawn tried to climb onto his bed during the night, and he had knocked him down from the top bunk forcing him to retreat to his own bed.

Matt told us DeShawn had also tried to climb up onto his bed and Matt pushed him down. DeShawn retaliated by breaking all of Matt's prized toys.

Once again we played musical bedrooms. This time we moved DeShawn away from the downstairs bedrooms, upstairs with the older boys. He would be right across the hall from our room and this made him furious.

The more we watched him, the more dangerous life became. We had to watch him day and night and when he wanted to play outside with the other kids, he could not play unsupervised. If one of the older boys or I was not outside, he could not play. He let us know that he hated it. He broke doors. He broke the mirrored closet doors in Jim's and my bedroom. He smashed the hall mirror in a rage. He peed everywhere. He would tell me no, and then pee at my feet. He peed down the heat registers and his 'pissive' aggressive behavior flabbergasted me. I later learned that this was not unusual behavior for traumatized children.

I caught him trying to sodomize the dog and now the dog growled every time he came near. The cat disappeared and hid from him when he walked into the room. After fourteen days of barely sleeping and some nights sleeping on the floor in front of the girls' door as a sentry, I called a meeting with the social worker, therapist, Jim and I to discuss that we could not safely keep him in our home.

The adoption agency made arrangements for a thirty-day out of home crisis placement. As the time wore on, I realized this was more than we could handle. We could not risk any child's further abuse, and we told them that we would not adopt DeShawn. We were told it is policy for siblings to remain together. The social workers ordered us to continue visitation and because we were not their legal guardians we had no say about visitation.

The two little girls were very afraid of DeShawn, and after every visit with him we saw more problems. Becca no longer slept in her own bed. She moved into our bed and we struggled to get her back to her own bedroom. Detamara withdrew and screamed "Don't drown me!" when I bathed her. As visitations continue Detamara shut down completely. She no longer spoke and she quit using the bathroom. The therapist met with us and wrote that it was no longer in the girl's best interest to visit DeShawn at this time.

The boys however, still wanted to see their brother, and when a weekend sleepover was planned my uneasiness worsened. I called Sandra in Minnesota and questioned if it was appropriate to spend the night. I told of the attempted visits to the boy's beds by DeShawn. I was told this was just innocent play. I had no say and the boys were to visit their brother.

After the sleepover, now even my boys were acting strangely. I knew my intuition was right when Deangelo later told me that the littlest brother was scaring them. He told of DeShawn's inappropriate play. He shared that DeShawn was threatening to "shoot them when he grows up if they told anyone."

The excitement of the upcoming first day of school was a welcome relief from the trauma of the loss of the dream and DeShawn. We found happiness in buying backpacks, school supplies and picking out our first day of school outfits. The kids happily unwrapped pencils and erasers from store packaging and stuffed their backpacks while I tried to get copies of immunization records to enroll our newest kids and then headed off to the immunization clinic to get kids shots who needed them to start school.

With a mountain of paperwork I was off to enroll ten of my eleven children at four separate schools. We were 'getting ready.'

▼

Getting everyone ready for school took routine, structure and careful planning to get everyone clean, showered and out the door. My oldest five left in the first wave, Shay and Marissa were off to the middle school, Nathan a junior, DJ a sophomore, Ian a freshman went off to the high school. They looked handsome and proud as they walked off together to a new school. The new school jitters were alleviated because they had each other.

The five younger ones got up an hour later and gave the water heater a chance to recover from the first set of morning showers and bathroom regime. With everyone in their new outfits, backpacks in tow, we loaded up in the big red van for the first day of school together. Matt, Deangelo, Becca, and Delonzo's elementary school was only four blocks away, but because Becca could not walk that far without her wheelchair, I always drove.

Detamara was bussed from the elementary school to the Young Five's Kindergarten Readiness Program. Luckily, her Minnesota school papers arrived and we found copies of her special education assessments that made it easy to get her help. With an August birthday, she would have been one of the youngest in her class and she needed time to adjust with all the recent changes and allow her time to catch up. We held her into the Young Fives' instead of starting kindergarten.

- 31 -
In The Trenches

Adjusting to life with both families in a new place was similar to the roller coaster ride I had ridden with Becca. It was a balancing act at its best. I juggled to keep things from sinking, and enjoyed the highs that kept the hope alive. The trauma of losing DeShawn set the stage for the children to lose trust. The hope and promises to the children of keeping them together and being their forever family were broken. They longed to be able to trust us, and needed that trust. Yet, trust would no longer come easily.

We would have to work to prove we could keep our word.

When we adopted the kids, we promised them along with the social worker a 'forever family' and already their brother was gone.

Who would be next?

Our new children came from a chaotic background with limited parenting. They were not going to allow anyone to get too close, especially new adults. DJ had been their parent and guardian and they knew little of trust. We were warned that it would take time for them to adjust, and now that bonding and attachment would take even more time.

▼

The fall brought school, structure, and homework for eleven, and now dinner for thirteen. Groceries, groceries and more groceries. Six boys, three of them teens and five of the children did not know how to be satisfied. Even when they were full, they kept eating. A couple would eat themselves sick. I could not keep food in the house, not just because of the amount needed to fill every meal, but also because of the sneakiness. My children, because they'd been neglected, often hungry and at times starved did not trust food would be there when they needed it so they hoarded everything. Groceries for this tribe challenged my budget and frugalness to the max and it seemed any budget I tried to set continued to be blown away.

My first meeting with our new local doctor was because Delonzo was all stopped up. He had eaten the entire container of dried Quaker Oats he had hidden in his bedroom. When the dry oatmeal hit his GI tract, it swelled and no laxative or quantity of prune juice helped. The pediatrician and my husband's colleagues brainstormed on how to get him unplugged. Finally, after a week of a swollen tummy and cramps he was relieved. Then within days he was back to food hoarding. Unlike my other children who learned lessons quickly, Delonzo only got sneakier. We found forty-eight ounces of different frosting containers in his pillowcase and thirteen neatly folded flat empty cereal boxes were under his mattress. He slept in the crumbs and denied he did anything.

It didn't matter he had been caught red handed.

He still answered, "It wasn't me."

Delonzo was not the only one hoarding food. I found remnants of snacks anywhere anything could be stuffed. There were traces of hidden goodies in the underwear drawers. I found things under switch plate covers, in pillowcases, and behind, in, and under furniture. I even found snacks stuffed into the toilet roll holders in the bathrooms. I knew it was not only Delonzo, because he continued to hide his snacks in the same places over and over again.

In time I understood why they stole food. DJ and Shay talked about the lack of food in the home. Their mom and the little kids' dad sold their food stamps for drugs and alcohol. They had been starved much of their lives with their parents. DJ was the breadwinner of the family. He was resourceful; he had shoveled snow to buy boxes of cereal that they ate with water. DJ had become an expert pickpocket to get the food they needed to survive. The kids ate condiments that DJ had stuffed in his pockets from the fast food restaurants.

The counselor from school showed me the drawing that Delonzo drew showing when he and Deangelo ate grass because they were so hungry. Shay and Detamara did not ask for anything. They just stole it. When offered a cookie or a treat Shay politely refused, then when my back was turned she grabbed the entire package and hid it. As time went on, the extent of their neglect was exposed and they began to trust us.

Shay was like the wind blowing, one-day compliant, the next defiant. It was like we lived with two different girls. Marissa shuddered and remained kind, but inside she was struggling as she was seeing behavior behind 'mom radar' I never witnessed. The wrath that went on behind my back did not help in attaching to the family. Even when everything looked like things were smooth on the service, they were being undermined in the corner. In Minnesota, Marissa had been the little sister and a sweetheart who played in her pretend fairytale world, especially when Becca needed care. In our new family, she rose to the occasion and played a new role that was forthright and determined to manage whatever she could behind the scenes. She was blunt and direct as she orchestrated and nudged inappropriate behaviors into a resemblance of normal. Marissa was called to guard duty each time I went to the bathroom or left the room. She had replaced Kristy as the drill sergeant, a common role for one of the siblings of a large family.

Being the sister in control of the new crew built up her acting skill to an even higher level and put an incredible burden on my teenage daughter who we required to be kind even when she wanted to kill them.

Shay seemed to be the new kid who adjusted the best and she was always talking about being happy. In fact, Shay at twelve was always talking and she was rarely silent. Everything that popped into her mind she said when she was in a talking mood. She talked easily about her foster home and her biological home. I had been told to be patient and when they were comfortable the kids would open up. Shay seemed comfortable from the start. Shay opened the doors of understanding the circumstances that led to child protection removing them from their parents. Still Shay concerned me.

From the beginning she did not know how to do much for herself and she needed to be prompted for everything. Getting her to take a shower was like encouraging a stuck mule and she even needed cues to brush her teeth. What didn't make sense was that she would not sleep in her bed. At night I tucked her and Detamara in, and in the morning Shay was always curled up on the floor by her bed inside her blanket. When quizzed, she finally disclosed she was used to sleeping on the floor. The bed in their home with their mom was a single pee-stained mattress and all five kids shared it with a single blanket. The other kids told me that Shay had gotten mad at the stinky mattress and had taken a knife to tear it up.

I lost sleep thinking about the horrors and wants of my new kids as they were revealed. I realized that the five years in foster care had brought them far. The four oldest children luckily had spent the majority of their time in the same foster homes offering them stability. Detamara and DeShawn were not so lucky. We found out that they had been removed from their first home for substantiated physical abuse against DeShawn. Previously, we had been told they were moved because the foster parent was too tired to care for them.

This was the first inconsistency in their history, and it would not be the last. Later we learned that we'd been told many lies and that much of the children's history had been omitted, but the history came within the children and could not be erased. DJ and Shay helped us to understand. Things seemed good for Shay; she wanted to be in our home. Her delays were apparent, but she had insight into things some of the other children didn't.

Shay liked to help and she loved to set the table and do laundry. The laundry room became our Mom, Shay and 'no one else' talking place. She'd set herself upon the never-ending pile of laundry we christened Mount St. Yurcek. The high pile for thirteen seemed always ready to erupt. We laughed as I told her to keep down the growing pile. Our laundry room therapy sessions revealed her life history and painful struggles at school.

Table manners at our house were atrocious, and one day Shay ate in such a hurry she resorted to eating spaghetti with her fingers. We worked on manners with all the children, and finally we got through a meal without being "grossed out" as Ian put it.

It wouldn't take long to discover that DJ had his own set of problems. He was unsure whether he wanted to be adopted and Shay ratted him out. He claimed he only came to Michigan to make sure his brothers and sisters were OK. His foster parents didn't want to adopt Shay, but they wanted to adopt him. He had made a plan to make the adoption fail, so he could go back to Minnesota and be adopted by his foster parents alone.

DJ didn't like to be second in command. He had always been the parent. He was the one who provided for his siblings. He was not going to allow me to be in charge of 'his' siblings. DJ spent his days trying to get out of the adoption instead of fitting in. He became best buddies with Ian and defiant with me. He picked fights with patient and gentle Nathan.

DJ told me later that he had nearly been missed by a shot as he walked to school by an abandoned crack house a block from the foster home. The gangs ran the neighborhood, and it was not safe for kids to be outside to play. Shay also filled me in that the foster parents would not adopt him because he was too noncompliant. He'd disappear for hours with friends.

I called the guardian ad litem to find out if the adoption story was true. She told me she had huge concerns about the lack of structure and the chaos of the foster home. It was Nathan's birthday when I made a phone call to the social worker in Minnesota and she revealed to DJ that if he didn't want to be adopted by us, he could return to Minnesota but not to his former foster home.

DJ was angry when he got off the phone with Sandra. He slammed the phone onto the hook, near the kitchen. He had been watching Ian mess with Shay.

Ian was horsing around with Shay and giving her a hard time. When Ian walked in to get his after school snack he got in DJ's way. Ian didn't know the reason for the attitude and refused to back up, after all he and DJ had become buddies.

DJ felt he was protecting his sister like he always had. In less than a minute, Ian got blindsided with a punch to the nose that contained fifteen years of built up anger. Ian's nose was pushed sideways and loose in his face, the blood poured onto the floor. DJ started screaming, he was sorry. He cried with his face in his hands and was inconsolable.

Jim screamed at him trying to push buttons and make a dominant male statement, but DJ maintained control and refused the challenge. Ian was in crisis. Both boys were losing it. At least Jim was home. I ran for towels and ice bags for Ian.

The other new kids cowered with fear. Nathan and Marissa looked angry and worried. Marissa took everyone downstairs to play Monopoly in the family room while DJ said over and over again that he was sorry. He told us in a quivering voice that he did not want to be like the kid's dad. He did not want to hit people. He did not want to hurt people. He did not think he was capable of being like that.

In a stern voice, Jim told him that hitting anyone that hard could kill them and after the age of sixteen he could be charged as an adult and he would be locked up for life. Right now we could press charges against him for assault on Ian.

DJ promised over and over again that he would never hit anyone ever again and DJ kept his word.

Jim and I, took DJ and Ian, and headed off to the emergency room leaving Nathan and Marissa managing the home front. Jim had made DJ come along to see the aftermath of his anger. I faced the security guard at the hospital who quizzed us on what had happened. I explained it was an argument between two brothers. I didn't want my next visit to be with some police officer to discuss the domestic violence that had now erupted into our home. Another ghost of one of my kid's past was being relived in our family.

DJ held Ian's hand throughout the examination.

The doctors gave him the fifth degree about the nose, and a plastic surgeon was consulted. They bandaged Ian's nose and gave him painkillers and I was not sure that it was only Ian who needed them. I was seriously thinking I might need one or two of my own and I made the choice to each a chocolate bar instead. Ian was scheduled for surgery the next week, and we took DJ out of school to watch the whole procedure. It was his job to hold his brother's hand as both boys shook before surgery. DJ was going to be there to comfort Ian when he woke up. DJ was banned from this year's basketball team because he took Ian's opportunity to play away by his anger. Whatever Ian could not do, DJ wouldn't be able to do either. When Ian needed nursing care, DJ was his nurse; soda, pillows, retrieving the remote, getting a snack, doing Ian's chores, it was 'all' DJ's job. We knew that DJ needed to make restitution for his crime; he found himself a job to pay for Ian's surgery and doctor bill co-pays that the insurance did not cover. DJ held up his end of his sentence, and after six months was released for serving the entire consequence. His word remained true. He never thought he was capable of the violence of his biological family and promised to never do it again. He held to his promise and soon began to open up. Through it all Ian and DJ became inseparable and true brothers.

▼

Our first Halloween was a mixed up holiday, and I soon discovered my children's childhood ghosts would haunt every holiday. The kids readied themselves with their costumes and Becca and Detamara were the cutest Eeyore and Tigger anyone had ever seen. The boys were Scream, or their father. Three of the boys dressed as doctors with head covers, lab coats and scrubs, and Jim and Becca's stethoscopes. Shay wanted to be a witch. A trip to the fabric store, supplied a big hat and a piece of black satin for a cape. The evening of Halloween we met with another resident and his family, and the die-hard trick-or-treaters scrambled for goodies.

Detamara was scared of the all the scary costumes and decorations. We carried Becca who was too tired to walk. We brought the little girls home early with only a few pieces of candy in their pumpkin buckets. Shay was overwhelmed and wanted to sit after an hour.

The boys arrived home when the neighborhood lights were finally turned off to begin the infamous Yurcek candy swap. Halloween has always been Ian's favorite holiday of the year, and he prides himself with the title of Candy Champion for capturing the most candy. Ian tipped the scale with an amazing twenty-one pounds of loot. Everyone traded their candy for ones they liked better. The kids with Celiac disease traded their wheat candy for other tasty morsels they could eat. The kids took pity on poor Becca and Detamara and filled their plastic pumpkins. We divided up the remainder of our leftover candy for those who had little. The kids sorted, counted and admired their prized treasures and knew exactly how many of what each had. After the games, the candy was stored back into their pillowcases and each child cleverly hid their own candy before heading off to bed to protect it from candy marauders.

In the middle of the night we woke to the sound of Delonzo throwing up the contents of two hundred ninety five empty candy wrappers. His entire bucket of candy was gone and the multi-colored 'barf' was absolutely disgusting. We shook the pile into a trashcan, removed the bedding and pulled out a sleeping bag for our pathetic little son. Maybe this was a good lesson on limits he may remember.

But we soon discovered Delonzo had just begun his candy rampage. Ian's twenty-one pounds was disappearing at an alarming rate and DJ's private stash followed. Once again all the candy wrapper evidence was in the little thief's bed and the boys wanted to throttle Delonzo. Reminding the boys of our no violence rule spared their little brother from his big brothers wrath, but they wouldn't let him forget, and for weeks he made their beds and picked up their rooms as a consequence. No matter where the candy was hidden, he or someone else stole it from the others. I couldn't wait for the loot to be gone, Marissa was angry at Shay, the boys at Delonzo, Becca at Detamara. The candy wars continued until there was not one piece left! When we intervened with the boys, we gave Delonzo next year's Halloween consequence. He had to hand over all his candy as restitution for the stuff he stole the year before. The next year Delonzo made good on his promise and went trick or treating for his brothers. Even then DJ would not get his candy, the dog lifted his leg on the whole duffel bag of his sugary treasures.

The stories and horrors of Halloween became memorable firsts. Ian took the little boys' trick or treating when some bully popped out of a dark corner and stole Deangelo's nearly full bag of candy. A fast and agile Ian took him on and the middle school bully was no match for a high school big brother looking out for his little brother. Ian demanded the candy back, and after a struggle, returned his younger brother's candy. From that day forward, Deangelo had a new bond of trust with his older brother and Ian was his hero.

Our first Thanksgiving was a memorable moment. Kristy and her boyfriend, Brian, made the trip from Minnesota to Michigan. We were thankful, I had all my children under our roof for the holiday. Our combined family was coming together as we began building new family traditions. Everyone chipped in as we cooked for fourteen. But, the holidays were a mixed blessing, there was excitement in being together, but there were feelings of loss of everything we'd left in Minnesota. We had always celebrated with my extended family and I missed them. For the new kids, my middle boys missed Grandma Dorothy, while Shay and DJ dealt with issues of holidays they never had. We made up new traditions to fill the loss.

The day after Thanksgiving became our tradition of our *Great American Shopping Day Challenge*. After we ate our feast, we scoured the Thanksgiving paper's ads. We plotted our strategy and planned out a budget. Jim and I set aside Christmas money out of the house sale proceeds to pay for our first Christmas as a family. We rose at 5:00 A.M. for bargain hunting of the loss leaders and all the free stuff. The game plan was mapped out on the dining room table and the 'who got what, when and where, and what time' was plotted on a giant piece of tag board.

The oldest boys were stationed at Best Buy, Jim at Circuit City, Kristy and I at the mall. The entire plan of attack was to get the prized item at a ridiculously low cost. Brian slept in and babysat the younger children and by the time the kids awakened, the bags were piled high in the living room. My next challenge was to find hiding places, a difficult task since the kids knew more places to hide in the house than I did, and the kid sneak-factor had skyrocketed.

Years later, I finally learned to outsmart my even sneakiest children, I price matched the ads at department stores on Thanksgiving Day and then I put it all on layaway and let the store hide it! I carefully hid the layaway receipts in one of Jim's medical books and put it back on his library shelf. I had one-upped and outsmarted my children and I felt content with my secret.

It was hard to say goodbye to Kristy and send her back to college. Kristy was lonely and torn leaving home and her tears broke my heart, but I had to be strong and not to let too many tears fall. Our newest children knew the deep pain of losing people they loved. No matter how much they went through, they still loved their biological and families. I shared about missing people we had to leave behind, trying to reassure my moping children. I told them that those we love are always with us in our hearts and memories no matter where we find ourselves. Kristy, our grandparents, Grandma Dorothy and DeShawn remain our family no matter where they or we live. Family is for always.

The subject of the kids' parents was a tough one, and I tried not to judge. I let the children lead the way on how and what they needed to cope. We weren't allowed to see our children's histories, but the histories were imprinted into our children. In the beginning, the two-page placement history was all we knew, as time wore on the children slowly unraveled the threads. Each little piece they shared gave us a small cluc to all thcy wcnt through.

There were many restless nights I struggled after they revealed pieces of the sordid past. I could not fathom some of the history they shared and lived through.

Susan, the guardian ad litem from Minnesota supported us because she believed we could help them better if we had more information and this eventually got her into trouble. But she was right, without her we did not know how to help the children. Susan told me that DJ was the caretaker, and Mom's keeper and protector at the grand old age of ten, Deangelo the bright one, DeShawn the cute one, Delonzo ignored, little Detamara the beautiful one, and Shay, well Shay got the brunt of her mom's hatred.

She told me of the first time she met the children. They were excited and greeted her with smiles and laughter, except for Shay. Eight-year-old Shay sat alone in a corner. Her hair was tangled and matted and she smelled of urine. As she looked up with her severely crossed eyes, she didn't smile. Susan said, her heart hurt to look at Shay; unloved and uncared for.

She saw the pain in that poor little child. Rejected and ignored, Shay was hidden from the authorities and at eight it appeared she had never been to school. DJ told me their mom was afraid Shay's appearance would raise too many questions. So Shay came into care unparented, unkempt, unwanted, rejected, and unloved. In years to come we learned many of the words she used to describe Shay mirrored their birth mother's psychological assessments.

How could parents tie their children with extension cords to a pole in the basement and whip them? The boys talked of the time their dad lost his temper and threw the television on the head of their two-year-old cousin who went to the hospital and was permanently brain damaged. The hospital workers were told the TV shelf fell over on the poor little guy. DJ hated his step dad and became his siblings guardian angel. He called the police when the parents were high, and drunk, and arguing. He ushered the children out of the house before the authorities arrived so they wouldn't be found with their beaten and bloody mother and risk being taken away. The well-rehearsed plan to keep away from the prying eyes of child protection worked and kept them together for months and years.

In time they shared the fateful day when the authorities came to remove them. DeShawn and Detamara were already in foster care. They had been removed at Detamara's two-month check up when the doctors discovered that both babies were suffering from starvation and dehydration. Detamara was born with cocaine in her system and weighed less than her birthweight. DeShawn at seventeen months weighed the same as he had at four-months-old. His dark hair had turned red from malnutrition.

Their mother had not complied with the orders of the courts, and was refusing treatment. When her support check came on the first of the month, she went on a weekend drug binge selling their food stamps for drugs and alcohol. She violated the court order to stay away from the kid's dad and the two adults went on a weekend binge. When the authorities arrived to take the children, DJ ran and climbed into a nearby tree. They lured him down by offering him and his brothers and sister ice cream. The police officer helped him out of the tree and led the kids away. Shay screamed as she was placed in the police car with her arms and legs flying. They loved their mother and they didn't want to leave her! This was their home!

The kids never got their ice cream.

Their mother had put the fear of authorities into them and she and the children moved often from place-to-place to outrun case-workers. The boyfriend followed them as they jumped from one county to another and then back. I shook my head, finding them was not rocket science. If they really wanted to find them, all the authorities needed to do to know her whereabouts was to cross check the lists for food stamps.

▼

Our family's first Christmas together arrived.

My new children had been separated by three foster homes and Detamara had only lived with her siblings for the first two months of her life. They had never been together at Christmas so this holiday season was important and it would set the stage for the traditions and remembrances to come.

Our living room was packed with presents and everyone dressed up for our Christmas Eve tradition of finding the lights. I was not brave enough to take all of them to the packed Christmas Eve service. Detamara had such trouble going to church it was not worth the trauma and sleepless nights that would follow. We left Nathan, who was seventeen, home to play Santa, and put the remaining packages that had been hidden at our friend's house under the tree. He filled the pathway in the living room with five brand new bicycles he had secretly put together in our neighbor's garage. Jim and I were amazed at what we were able to get bargain hunting and price matching and for the first time in a very long time we got to spoil our children. DJ, Shay, Deangelo, Delonzo, and Matt were all getting brand new bikes!

Their excitement shook the walls of our home. Jim and I watched with amazement as our ten children tore open packages. We missed Kristy who could not risk driving the six hundred miles on icy roads and was spending Christmas with my family.

Shay stayed off in the corner with her packages. Jim and I watched Shay as she tenderly opened each one. She placed her new CD player and headset onto her ears and stood up to make sure we noticed and then she retreated to her room alone.

The children took their bikes out on the sidewalks in December to try them out. All the kids were thrilled, surprised and spoiled. The tiny living room was filled with laughter, wrappers, boxes and toys of all sorts. The cat and the dog tunneled under the mountain of empty boxes and wrapping paper while the kids searched for their footballs, dolls, games and electronics. Detamara's wish for a tool bench and toys with buttons came true. Detamara had been grounded from buttons after we discovered all the remote controls in the house missing, and were found underneath her covers. DJ and Ian sported their new basketball shorts and shoes, while Nathan was excited to get his traditional Christmas Lego set. Marissa had new clothes and her wished for musical CDs.

Once the presents were unwrapped and the excitement over, the discussions and sharing switched to empty Christmas pasts, and old pain surfaced. They cried. The boys missed Christmas with Grandma Dorothy and her extended family. DJ and Shay mourned the Christmases they never had.

Soon many of the new toys were broken to the point of throwing out. Unlike the care of things our first family had, nothing was taken care of by the second. I ached at the hard work and money now wasted. Each broken toy came with a crisis of someone who took it, broke it, or stole it. I was the referee and detective to sort out who did what to whom. Somehow we survived the aftermath of the holiday minute-by-minute. I couldn't wait to get them back to school, and forget about Christmas. They wouldn't let us spoil them.

Stealing was a constant problem. The rule became, if its not yours, don't touch it. Just ask. But some of the new kids rarely asked. They did not want to have anyone tell them what to do or when to do it. They did not want help from anyone. Little did I know that having things too good would be the downfall for our family. It was the comforts that always seemed to get us. The kids sabotaged the success and happiness they didn't believe they deserved.

So we worked on simple rules with constant schedules. Homework was done at the dining room table. There were too many kids to manage this on my own, so I setup a system of homework buddies. The middle schoolers and high schoolers were home forty-five minutes ahead of the younger five. By the time the younger ones came in, the older ones were well into their work, and they helped the sibling they were buddied with to do their homework. I paired DJ with Deangelo, DJ's math skills were weak, and working with Deangelo would strengthen his multiplication and division skills. Marissa helped Becca, Becca helped Detamara, Nathan helped Matt, and Ian helped Delonzo. Marissa who never had homework was capable of double duty. She tutored Shay first and then moved on to Becca when she arrived home from school.

We accomplished the task of getting homework done, but books and papers were lost and completed homework never delivered back to the teachers. Delonzo never brought anything in the house. His homework showed up in the mailboxes of our neighbors on the four-block walk home from school. Finally after dozens of neighbors returned Delonzo Yurcek's homework, we asked for Deangelo or Matt to pick up the backpack from Delonzo's teacher to ensure its safe arrival home and they carried his backpack back to the teacher on the way to their classroom each morning. The system worked and Delonzo's grades came up.

We soon discovered our kids had many deficits. Things didn't add up. They appeared bright, yet what we taught one day, disappeared the next, only to pop back up on another day after tests were taken and failed. We started the first school year with no school records. Shay needed an Individualized Education Plan (IEP) which is the special education document kids with special needs are entitled to under special ed law. This is a transferable document and needs to follow the child to any new school. We couldn't get a copy of Shay's paperwork. The requests for their records went ignored or were lost.

How could we plan for what she needed when we had nothing to work with? Her verbal skills were very deceiving, and according to the social worker in Minnesota, Shay's full scale IQ was only 58. It wasn't long before I realized she didn't understand what they were teaching her. When I told that to the school, they did not believe me. They said she her IQ score was in the 70's and it did not make sense. We were forced to retest everything, and she qualified for services. She was enrolled in a middle school sixth grade classroom with special education for both math and reading.

▼

Many of the things Shay would do didn't make sense. She loved to help me set the table. Yet we lost many glasses as they tumbled to the floor when she set them on the table and missed. Finally I realized Shay had no depth perception. I taught her to place her hand at the edge of the table, and put the glass or plate over the top of her hand so she could do it successfully. No matter how many times we practiced left and right for the silverware, we never got it the same way twice. One day it was her turn to clear the table. I was just flushing the toilet when I heard a terrible crunch. Instead of placing the dishes in the dishwasher, Shay placed them in the trash compactor. All thirteen place settings of my cherished new dishes and silverware were now a mangled mess. I resorted to plastic silverware and Tupperware plates. She had been in a foul mood that night, and I wondered if she did it on purpose or was it an accident?

Discipline was a constant problem, and we needed to come up with an idea that we could use for every child. I sentenced the children to writing as the consequence. I gave sentences for the infractions that needed to be addressed. They wrote what they did, why it was wrong and what they were supposed to do. They wrote apology letters to wronged persons or siblings. I placed all their infraction papers in a binder for the future and the binder filled in a hurry. The papers helped reinforce the rules.

After I caught my children trying to reuse their apology letters and sentences I changed the protocol. Once the sentences were finished, I inspected them, complimented the child on its completion, and while the child was standing there, I ripped them down the middle. I told them the consequence was over, it was forgotten and forgiven, just as God does for us.

I was learning to parent by the seat of my pants, like medical crises for Becca when she was small I now had to be prepared for the unexpected parenting crisis. I had to be one step ahead of everything. I had to have answers for problems I had never faced, for there is no book for parenting in the trenches.

Everyday was a new challenge.

- 32 -

Puzzle Pieces

With moving to Michigan we found much more than training for Jim's career. We found a new home and a new start for our new family. An unexpected blessing was that Becca had to change doctors. The doctors in Michigan had no experience with Noonan syndrome, they did not know her complete history, and they had a fresh new outlook to take care of her. In Minnesota some problems had been discounted because they needed to look at the bigger problems. The bigger problems overshadowed the little ones and they did not look for other causes. They blamed her heart, or her immune problems. She was doing much better with the changes in feeding, but feedings still hurt.

As we left Minnesota the endocrinologist had started her on growth hormone injections. She needed the shots everyday to grow and even with the tiniest needles she had huge bruises. Soon bruises covered her thighs and there were no more sites to give her the next injection. I worried going to the beach, as prying eyes noticed her intense bruising. I began to explain to strangers that my child had a bleeding disorder to avoid abuse allegations and carried documentation in my wallet along with her medical card.

When we arrived in town, I needed to find a new pediatrician. I called every clinic in the town and found that no pediatrician would take a new Medicaid client. Even the clinic where Jim was in residency denied my daughter a doctor.

How could this be? In Minnesota I had never heard of doctors refusing to take Medicaid clients. We had always gotten what we needed for Becca, the kids and myself. We all had been on and off Medicaid since Becca's birth and had not been refused help anywhere.

I called back, frustrated and explained I was a resident's wife, that we had recently moved here for residency and we needed care for my daughter.

The clinic manager asked me why didn't I tell them this the first time I called?

I was saddened. I hadn't always been a resident's wife. It shouldn't matter whether my husband was a part of their clinic or not, I was simply a parent of a child with special needs. Quality medical care shouldn't matter if I was poor or on the way to becoming a surgeon's wife. Once upon a time I was also very poor and the wife of an unemployed carpet salesman whose family was receiving food stamps.

I decided to look elsewhere to find a pediatrician who had experience with children with special needs. I asked Jim to talk to the doctors he was training under and ask who was well-versed treating kids like Becca. I talked to other resident wives at the residency gatherings and I finally got a name.

I called the doctors' office I had called once before and been turned down. This time I told them that doctors and other resident's wives had referred me to them. I still had trouble. Jim's attending doctors came to our rescue and made a phone call on our behalf, so Becca had a pediatrician.

Dr. Page listened and understood that I knew my daughter. He trusted my intuition and wrote orders after consulting with me about what works and what doesn't. He helped me set up all Becca's new specialists in Kalamazoo . . . cardiologist, endocrinologist, gastro-intestinal doctor, ophthalmologist, neurologist, orthopedist, ear nose and throat specialist, and hematologist. We had found ourselves in a town with a small children's hospital and all the doctors Becca needed were in our community. All the worry about who was going to manage Becca's care had been answered; Dr. Page would become

Becca's most favorite doctor. According to Becca, he had magical powers to help cure anything.

I was prepared for the new doctors; and I had continued the reporting system when the nursing service left and I had binders of chart notes. The home nurses made sure we had copies of clinic notes, lab slips, and surgery reports and I had anything a new doctor asked for. After reviewing the paperwork, the new doctors added a fresh perspective on the whys and reasons for Becca's problems.

Becca was now beginning to voice her own concerns, but she would only tell me and not tell the doctors. I worried the doctors would think I was an over-concerned parent.

We lived our lives under a microscope, we were examined, and watched, and judged, to make sure we were doing the right things for our children. I learned early that this was part of the job description for a parent of a child with special needs. Now I was in a new place and no one knew me. Veteran parents of children with special needs forewarned me to be careful. If I didn't react early enough, I could be faulted for not helping my daughter. Over concern could warrant accusation of Munchausen's Syndrome by proxy, the parent who gets attention by causing their child's problems. I had heard horror stories of parents being accused and I remained attentive and cautious.

I had to start again to explain my daughter's medical problems to the professionals treating and working with her and prove myself. Over the years, I became versed in medical jargon. I had to learn the lingo if I was going to speak with the professionals who treated Becca. I discovered not all doctors and professionals were comfortable working with parents who may know more about the child's medical problems than they did. I tuned in carefully at our first meetings, watched for miniscule reactions and responses to know when and whom I could work with to entrust my daughter's care. Sometimes I had no choice, and I remained cautious in my statements and answers.

It is a precarious game that parents who are the experts on their children play, to help their children, without alienating the professionals. With some doctors we became partners and with others I learned it was better to set them up with a trail of pieces so they could discover their own answers and treatments for Becca. It took the first year for the new doctors to learn to care for Becca and with each appointment we gained trust. In time, together we uncovered more of the puzzle pieces of Becca's Noonan syndrome. Thankfully, most of the doctors were family friendly.

Having the opportunity of a completely new medical team provided second looks at Becca. We found more puzzle pieces; she was placed on Ritalin to help her be less impulsive and more able to focus. A medically fragile child with attention deficit hyperactivity disorder was something the teachers would not believe until I 'accidentally on purpose forgot' to give her the Ritalin before school one day. After that experience, they no longer questioned the medication. Becca could not remember, could not focus and was completely off task that day. The Ritalin provides Becca the ability for a more healthy school experience, yet when she wanted to try something new, she requested we withhold the medication. Becca had learned that if she is very anxious about trying something new and she doesn't take her Ritalin, then she can try something new without anxiety.

Because of the severe bruising from the growth hormone shots we visited the hematologist, which led us to more blood testing. We knew that they felt Becca had Von Wildebrands disease, a bleeding disorder, but that did not explain the severe bruising. Dr. Mattano listened and sent us off to the lab at the Cancer Center at the University of Michigan where a well-known platelet researcher finally came up with the answer – Becca's platelets did not clot appropriately. This meant she would need special planning for surgery, using medications or platelet transfusions to prevent or stop her bleeding. Having this knowledge gave us a tool to help us keep Becca safe.

Becca's ankles have always been weak and when we are out and about she uses her wheelchair. She cannot walk from the car in the handicap space to the front door of the store without tiring. Many times it is easier to put her in the shopping cart seat since even as a teen she fits. The orthopedist sent her off to physical therapy and her weak ankles and tight heal cords were strengthened using foot braces that fit inside her shoes and went past her ankles. Becca was much more stable with the supports and she began slowly to walk further and further.

But what one doctor prescribed another one argued.

Poor Becca ending up paying the ultimate price while I tried to balance out the professionals' differences. In a new city with new professionals, I was viewed as 'just' a mom.

The Michigan GI doctors faulted me for having my child still on a feeding tube. They stopped her feedings, made me feed her gluten and her severe immune deficits returned. Becca was now eating more by her mouth and losing weight. Eventually, she fell apart and finally proved to them why she was on a feeding tube. The problem was real, it wasn't Mom being overprotective.

One day after Becca had been placed on a new medication to help control her migraine headaches by the neurologist, she demanded she would not leave the clinic until I made an appointment with her heart doctor. She told me that there was something wrong with her heart. She had told me before, but therapists felt it was anxiety and panic attacks and she was making it up to avoid going to school. I knew Becca always has a reason for the things she does so I needed to listen, despite the professionals' best judgment.

The trick was to figure it out how and what.

Becca was not going anywhere, and she was about to make a scene. I did not want my ten-year-old daughter throwing a temper tantrum in the corridor of the medical office building. She was a stuck mule and had dug her little heels into the floor, and would not budge. Luckily most doctors, who treat Becca, know that I understand Becca, and more importantly know that Becca knows herself and we got an appointment for the heart specialist, six weeks down the road.

Dr. Loker told Becca that her EKG was clear.

Becca told Dr. Loker he didn't find it yet. We all learn lessons from Becca; she has a reason for everything she does. She may look small, but my wise little one knows her body.

We left the clinic to run errands and Jim, in the operating

room, got a page from Dr. Loker to find me and get Becca back to the hospital at once. Her heart was in third degree heart block. He had just taken a quick glance at the EKG when we were in the office, and once he had time to look further he found that parts of Becca's heart were not communicating with each other. Her teeny tiny heart was once again in trouble and she had been walking around for weeks with her heart out of sync. The doctor hoped that by taking her off the calcium channel blocker, her heart would began functioning normally, but for the near future, she needed to be closely monitored.

Looking back Becca has protected herself from many disastrous outcomes. She has proven to the doctors who listen, that she is the one who knows her body and when she tells us something we better listen. She does not complain, unless there is a 'real' problem. Even as a teeny baby, she didn't eat to protect her lungs. She keeps her body in balance with limiting her precarious fluid balances by drinking just enough. She knows the difference between the yeast ear infections that plague her tiny ears and the bacterial infections that pop up in between. Before culturing, Dr. Prophit always asks Becca what it is and her diagnosis is proven right time and again. She is now telling us her medical issues and it is our job to figure out the reason.

Right before we left Minnesota I found a mom of a daughter with Noonan syndrome who was forming a support group. The group grew and they were now holding the second annual Noonan Syndrome Support Group Conference in Baltimore, Maryland. Becca was on a state funded program for Children with Special Health Care Needs and sometimes they provided scholarships for parents and kids to go to special conferences to see the national specialists. I wrote my proposal and we were accepted. Jim's parents came to watch some of the kids. We did not want to subject Granny and Grandpa to them all at once, so we took Detamara, Becca, Ian and DJ with us to Baltimore.

At the conference Becca finally met other children with Noonan syndrome just like her. She found Darcy, and Jenna, and Brenda, and Taryn all around her own age. She looked up to Darcy who was a couple of years older. She carefully watched the other children, while she held onto my leg. In time, she ventured to hang out with her preteen peers. She was excited to see that some of the other kids had plastic buttons for feeding just like she did. She had been self conscious about letting anyone see her extra plastic belly button. I was astounded to hear Becca telling a tiny lad it was great to have a button because you don't have to taste nasty medication.

In the conference setting, Becca was normal among her peers. Becca had always been included and her life had been mainstreamed as much as her health had permitted. I came face to face with the reality that life is always a balance; it needed to be a balance of inclusion for opportunity and segregation to build strength and cope. We now understood how that inclusion had actually made her feel isolated and different, as she compared herself to those around her. She had never had the opportunity to play and share her truths with peers who faced similar challenges. Doctors dialogue with doctors, persons with similar professions don't think it strange to meet and greet and learn together. It was only right that our children with differences had opportunity to meet with other children with the same or similar differences to get to know each other, share details of their lives and grow strong in each others' supportive friendships.

I watched social walls come down as Becca interacted with her female peers who had Noonan's syndrome. The young ladies giggled and laughed, ditched their parents and sat at "their own" table while Jim and I embraced the idea that Becca had a right to be herself and be free of all the unwritten rules and expectations those of us without her differences put upon her. At the conference we found sup port and Becca got a chance to meet Dr. Noonan and have her picture taken with her. That picture remains in a prominent place in our home. Becca had found friends and Jim and I found a place to get answers and support.

Each year or so Becca looks forward to the conference and we make sure that we get her there. Her 'sisters' with Noonan's syndrome remain in contact and it brings joy to our hearts as we watch the unleashed freedom they have when they are together. We have seen the importance of unity in difference. Together, they are simply themselves, as they chase boys and stay up late to talk about boys. The together moments these young women share build strength and health and commitment to life and each other. The unity Becca feels with her friends empowers her, shattering my earlier belief in complete inclusion.

My tears fall as I watch them tearfully say goodbye at the end of each conference. I realize that together, these young men and women need each other and through them we will find more of the missing pieces of Noonan syndrome.

- 33 -

CHEAPER BY THE DOZEN?

Feeding my tribe took careful strategic planning and though residency pay is enough to get by on, it is not designed for a family with a dozen children. Thirty plus thousand dollars a year seemed like we had won the lottery compared to when we lived on less than a thousand dollars a month, but when we doubled our family, it still left us living just below the poverty line. The new kids had never had anything to care for and were just learning how, plus they had faced starvation and had bottomless stomachs. They received an adoption subsidy, but that barely covered their therapy and the repair work for constant breakage, let alone food.

My grocery bill, even with careful planning, was nearly as big as our house payment, and not only had our grocery billed soared, but our garbage bill doubled. Each week we used two trash toters and our recycling overflowed.

▼

Remember the scene in *Yours, Mine, and Ours* where the cashier in the PX had to call for reinforcements to fill the large order to feed the family of eighteen? Jim and I felt like Henry Fonda and Lucille Ball every time we went to the grocery store. We were now feeding fourteen plus the all extras young men my boys brought home for dinner.

Jim was at work much of the time so I left Nathan in charge and took a couple of the kids with me to push the carts. Cashiers cringed when they saw us coming with our three full carts. I'd scan aisles looking for one who seemed competent to handle my orders plus all the coupons that went with it. People stared at the line of carts while my children worked together putting up the groceries. Store managers and security staffs were especially vigilant when my children came shopping. I kept a keen eye on a couple of the kids who were known to pocket irresistible packages from the checkout displays. I was thankful they still had grocery baggers and even the manager offered help to bag the huge grocery order and get the line moving.

While they bagged my groceries, I matched the coupons from my coupon envelope with the things crossed off my list. The large wad of coupons only increased the interest of the store patrons. By this time we had gathered a crowd, and when the final tally rang up, gasps from the onlookers broke the silence.

To my delight, I had discovered they doubled coupons in Michigan and twenty minutes away there was a store that doubled coupons worth up to a dollar instead of just fifty cents. I missed the days of putting papers together and gathering up all the extra loose coupon sections so now my extended family sent me their unused coupons by mail, and soon my new neighbors gave me their extra coupons too. I also bought two or three Sunday newspapers if the coupons were good figuring the Detroit Free Press and Chicago Tribune articles would come in handy for current event homework assignments that my children proudly handed since theirs were different from their friends.

The kids joked that I could teach the Coupon Queen a thing or two, and mom had even one 'upped her! Many times I was able to purchase four hundred dollars in groceries for fewer than two hundred by buying on sale, in quantity and using doubled coupons for the week. I used every trick I had read in women's magazines about how to save hundreds of dollars on your grocery bills.

Only seven gallons of milk would fit in the refrigerator and disappeared in three days so I always seemed to need more gallons! Three giant tubs of oatmeal and fourteen boxes of cereal quickly disappeared. I bought gallon size cans of spaghetti sauce, tomatoes, vegetables, and baked beans at Sam's Club. I bought jumbo-size bags of frozen broccoli, corn, and mixed vegetables. I needed eight-pound bags of French fries, chicken nuggets and hash browns. Most times, it was much less expensive to buy in bulk than to open five cans of the same items. But, bigger was not necessarily cheaper, I compared costs, and sometimes with coupon I could get more for less than buying bulk. Each shopping session filled my garage sale purchased freezer and I added a second garage sale refrigerator freezer to our garage! Sometimes it was hard to find the space for our weekly treat of a five-gallon pail of ice cream, but after one night of milk shakes the entire pail was gone.

The savings did not end at the store. I saved all my UPC codes and box tops, and filled out every rebate. Our mailbox was filled with unusual prizes, and much needed rebate checks.

I found bakery thrift shops, and for twenty-nine cents a loaf I bought day-old bread and reduced price bagels, cinnamon rolls, and donuts. I didn't mind letting the boys eat an entire bag of donuts and drink a half-gallon of milk as an after school snack.

The only place I could not save is at the health food stores, as nothing ever is on sale. It was a real treat for Nathan, Marissa, Matt, Becca and myself when I could afford store bought gluten free cookies or treats. Since I had little time to bake, Marissa and Nathan baked cookies and muffins once a week using Grandma's favorite recipes and rice flour at over a dollar and a half a pound.

In summer we shopped for vegetables at the farmer's markets and visited local fruit growers to pick blueberries, strawberries, peaches, cherries, and apples. We made do by eating more fruits and vegetables instead of snack foods.

Cooking for my new army was a challenge. I was used to cooking for eight, and when I had my daycare kids, up to a dozen. But these kids were different, and five of them were teenagers. Meals with meat required at least six pounds. To stretch the budget casseroles, chili, or sandwiches were our staples. My kitchen became a tiny mess hall. If anyone was in the kitchen with me, we could not open the refrigerator or dishwasher door. The kitchen was small when we bought the house and it seemed to shrink when we added a dozen children with its single short counter. I turned my laundry room into a pantry and ran downstairs whenever I needed something. I learned very quickly that my newest children had no limits on what they could eat. They were never full; in fact, they didn't seem to have any sense of having their hunger satisfied. Thank God, for bulk buying and my two huge canning pots.

Chili was a family favorite, and it took six pounds of hamburger, three pounds of onions, a gallon can of stewed tomatoes, a gallon can of tomato sauce and cupfuls of spices. I topped their bowls with a three-cup bag of shredded cheese and served with two boxes of soda crackers. At the dinner table, the kids raced to see who could get to the second helpings first. Trying to get them to use manners when they were racing for the leftovers became futile. The loser was destined to peanut butter sandwiches if they were too slow.

Two loaves of bread, one of rice bread, two packages of different sandwich meat, two packages of cheese, a half a jar of salad dressing made thirty sandwiches. When that was gone and anyone was still hungry, they made additional peanut butter sandwiches.

Each lunch I'd serve all those sandwiches, plus two bags of potato chips, a five-pound bag of apples, a gallon of milk and an entire bag of cookies. On cold days my five bottomless kids ate two gallons of soup, while my five gluten free children ate another gallon.

Four of the kids were eating gluten free and had to pack school lunches. A loaf of rice bread cost nearly four dollars a day or almost $90.00 a month for bread alone! There was no way I could cut back on that expense, and I ended up making two versions of everything since we could not afford to feed everyone wheat free. I adapted recipes and made two similar but different dishes, one smaller rice based casserole and a huge wheat based casserole.

The boys were especially bottomless and after three hamburgers each they were still hungry. While the six boys ate me out of house and home, the girls were picky and wouldn't try much out of their comfort zone.

Nathan and Marissa helped me in the kitchen, and I was thankful that Nathan often took charge. I could not see around the corner and watch the kids and cook or clean at the same time. Dinner dishes completely filled the dishwasher with the plates, silverware, and cups. The sink overflowed with the pots and pans and my massive pots had to be washed in the laundry tub to fit under the faucet. We had to clean the kitchen carefully to not get cross contamination on the surfaces and the dishes so Becca, Marissa, Nathan, Matthew and I did not get sick.

Thankfully the kids were eligible for the free lunches, and that offset our school year grocery bill. But the receipt grew a foot longer in the summer, the bill hundreds of dollars higher and the number of shopping carts doubled when school was out.

When we chose to adopt the children, I hadn't thought through the challenge of outfitting them. The older boys grew taller by the day. I made friends with Old Navy's markdown person who filled me in on when they marked down and it was close enough that I could stop by once a week during clearance season. Old Navy's Markdown Madness became my major shopping time. For the boys, I bought size 8, 10, 12, 14, and 16 slims and for the young men, I filled my shopping cart with selections from sizes 28, 30, 31 by 30 or 32. Eventually everything I bought would fit somebody. As the older boys grew they passed their clothes down to their little brothers. Poor Delonzo was the last in line and had replaced Matt as the receiver of all the hand-me-downs so I made sure to always buy a few new things just for him. Anything worth purchasing needed to last and I bought the best quality I could get at the lowest price. I bought our winter jackets in January. Jackets and pajamas were passed down the line until they were worn out. I learned that buying clearance name brand with guaranteed replacement was money well spent. For the cost of postage, a broken zipper on a jacket or a damaged new backpack was replaced or repaired by the manufacturer free of charge.

Shoes were purchased when they marked them down fifty percent off the clearance price. I always made sure I was first in line for the fifty percent off summer tennis shoe clearance. I could get Reebok or Nike shoes for less than twenty dollars a pair instead of the usual sixty to eighty dollars each. The little girls got name brand new dress shoes or sneakers for seven to eight dollars. The clerks shook their heads as they bagged my dozen to two dozen pairs of shoes for under three hundred dollars. My boys were thrilled with the name brands and fought 'the war of the shoes' to see who got which pairs when they sometimes wore the same sizes.

I bought plain shirts and sweatshirts and used my embroidery sewing machine to sew swooshes in place to go with their embroidered swoosh basketball shorts and sweatpants. No one ever knew they weren't the real thing and I probably shouldn't have shared my secret, for fear I get in trouble for creating one of a kind knockoffs for my army of quickly growing boys. Overall, the boys were easier to outfit than the girls. Jeans, pants, basketball shorts, jerseys and sweatshirts were their staples and one dress outfit for each.

But the girls! I found keeping two rapidly changing adolescent females outfitted more challenging than the boys. The girls wanted to fit into their schools. Marissa and Shay were different shapes and sizes. Marissa was skinny and tried not to ask for much, but I knew better. She and I enjoyed special times bargain hunting on mother-daughter dates and while we were driving we sang to the radio.

Shay wore regulars and was expanding to plus sizes as her body changed. We solved the problem with overalls and character sweatshirts. Shay hated shopping. Shopping was overwhelming, the movement of many shoppers, the multiple smells, the bright flickering lights and colors, not to many wanting to buy everything and the disappointment because she couldn't. She preferred staying home to play basketball with the boys.

Becca and Detamara began at the same size, and they got upset unless they each got something. To solve the problem I started buying two of everything and they liked wearing twin outfits. When Detamara grew, and Becca didn't I ended up buying one size for

Becca and the next for Detamara, that soon meant Becca wore the same style twice as long and by the time Becca outgrew things, they were no longer in style or much too babyish for a tiny budding adolescent. I began recycling the girls' too small clothing for new outfits in resale shops.

In time I became just as thrifty with my clothing budget as I was with groceries. I learned my way around Kalamazoo finding the areas with the best garage sales. I found last years name brand clothes, toys, skates, sleds, and boots that filled in the needs for the entire family. Every once in a while somebody got hand-me-downs from a friend, and we were incredibly thankful for the gifts.

- 34 -
DREAMS COME TRUE

It was the positives in blending our families that kept us going. The miracles sustained us through the times when our circumstances seemed hopeless. The uplifting moments were a welcome relief from the day-to-day chore of surviving children with attachment issue.

I had not truly believed Jim when he told me of his residency program that provided easy financing of our home. I argued with him that it couldn't be that simple. But it had been true. We found the house, we closed by mail, and when we arrived in Michigan, the keys were waiting for us. It was that easy. No other residency program had this kind of unique set up. It was the miracle we needed.

Before leaving Minnesota, I planned that the Medicaid that paid for Becca's formula and feeding equipment costing over $3,000 a month would take a couple of months to get the casefile opened. The months of red tape I expected never appeared. I had made sure we arrived in Michigan with an extra two months of formula to be sure we had it until we had Becca enrolled in programs to help with her catastrophic medical costs. The Social Security Administration made sure that the connection with Medicaid in Michigan was seamless. The day we arrived, Becca's new Medicaid card was waiting in our new mailbox with our keys.

I had been worried that Jim would be the only resident with a family, but the surgery residency program had a couple of other families with children and the family practice group even had more. I worried about making friends, but the residency program had get togethers and our children were treated to picnics, and parties, and boat rides. What fun to see all my children trying new things and playing in the soft white sand of the Michigan beaches.

It was always a challenge to keep our newest charges from eating too much at the smorgasbord picnics and I had to check pockets for sodas and goodies collected from coolers to bring home. I used these teachable moments to make the children return the 'free' goodies to the owners and teach them social etiquette.

We took advantage of the climate and we picked bushels of peaches, and apples, and cherries at the orchards near the lake. Once we almost got kicked out of a blueberry farm, and it was not my children causing the commotion. The naughty child belonged to another resident family!

The kids and I froze bags and containers of fruit and tried to figure out how to make jam and preserves. Working together to build memories we could eat was a time of bonding that was therapeutic for all of us.

But, the battles continued.

DJ was not learning. Something was amiss. The school resisted giving him an assessment for special needs. Why would I possibly want special ed for a high schooler? He was fifteen, and a sophomore. What was I thinking? I pushed, and they appeased me with a screen for achievement. An hour later after the school psychologist started the test, she called asking for my permission to give DJ the full battery of testing. She had discovered what I already knew; DJ had severe learning disabilities, and was way behind in school.

His early life skills of providing for his siblings had established efficient street smarts, which compensated and hid his deficits. No one ever got close enough to understand his 'real' needs. My heart hurt for him. He had been left behind while he worked double time as a small child to keep his siblings safe and together. He needed success and at fifteen he finally had a chance. DJ had spent the early years with his mom transferring from school to school and in one year alone he had attended eight to eleven different schools. It left him years behind his peers and he was unable to catch up without assistance. He needed help and finally he qualified for supports in his major areas of missing knowledge in reading, writing, and arithmetic.

For the first time in his life, DJ would get services that fit his 'true' needs.

▼

I love spring, but the change in seasons brought additional deterioration for my children. Detamara and Shay's behaviors worsened while Becca struggled with the school transition and became ill. She was over-stressed with all the changes in addition to being tested by her newest siblings. We needed another miracle to unite us.

Jim's parents gave us their old computer and it opened the world of the Internet to me and provided access to other families of exceptional children.

One day on the newly formed Noonan Syndrome Support listserve, a parent wrote of an organization that granted wishes for children with catastrophic or chronic life-threatening disorders. The wish criteria for kids such as Becca was narrow. She had already exceeded her life expectancy, and only God knew how much time was left for her. I knew many kids' who had wishes granted after they became too sick to enjoy them and I had seen other children die waiting for their wish to come true.

This organization took into account that these kids live an unfair life, and uplift them while they can still enjoy it. They work to build family memories of the good times instead of heartbreak. I e-mailed them and silently asked God for something good to happen.

The answer came less than two days later when they called to ask me what Becca wished for. They wanted three wishes!

The first was the easiest. Becca wished for whales and Disney. She had loved Free Willy and Shamu for the past two years and Disney movies and music had been constant companions to help her cope thru the sleepless nights of sickness. A second wish was for a computer. She told me she needed one because her hands won't work. Her third wish was an above ground swimming pool for the whole family to play in. The Children's Wish Foundation sent the paperwork, and the pediatrician immediately completed it.

Just as summer vacation was to begin a white envelope arrived, and inside it declared that one of Becca's wishes would come true!

▼

We were to go off to Florida.

Becca's wish granted our whole family two days in the Keys in Marathon, and five days at DisneyWorld with 'all' expenses paid.

Can you imagine the expense?

Two adults and ten children needed airline tickets. We needed multiple hotel rooms to hold us all and we needed two rental cars so we could get from place to place. Not to mention the shuttles, and admission tickets, and food! To my surprise the program also bought Kristy a ticket and Brian, her boyfriend purchased his own ticket to join us.

As soon as school let out, the entire Yurcek family was off on an incredible adventure. It was Becca's wish that hopefully would give our family a welcome break and most of all I hoped it would unite us. That would be a dream come true for all of us.

The logistics of packing for thirteen was overwhelming. Since we had not yet adopted the children, I needed permission from the social workers in both states to transport the children across state lines. I needed the notarized documents to prove they were supposed to be with us. I had to figure out how to protect Becca from Detamara who was night wandering. We had taught Detamara about how to behave appropriately but she was also a victim at the hands of DeShawn and two older foster siblings in her last placement. She was learning boundaries and when she was awake I could keep both girls safe, but she had experienced traumas and I could not take another chance in having Becca hurt. I could not trust her completely and I didn't know at that time how secretly bonded the two girls were, that Detamara had already saved Becca's life and the two girls watched out for each other.

My children seemed to be nocturnal and were afraid of the terrors that haunted them in the depths of their sleep. Somehow I had to sleep to enjoy and care for the children and I asked for support for an extra room to separate more children from each other. Detamara prowled, Shay couldn't sleep and she rattled in her room, self-talking, singing, and constantly interrupting the rest of the family's sleep. The foster care system refused helping with additional accommodations so I felt I had no choice but to ask for Detamara to remain behind in respite. They refused access to respite care and said she would feel rejected and abandoned.

I called child protection to explain that I was being asked to take a child on vacation that I could not possibly protect another from. The child protection authorities told me that I was protected as long as I made an attempt and had documentation of Minnesota's refusal.

But I still had to protect Becca. Her near fatal encounter with DeShawn's sexual assault and beating left her traumatized and fragile. I spent many a sleepless night thinking about how to make this work. Finally the answer emerged out of a deep sleep. Detamara was small enough to fit in a crib and I would bring my toddler Port-A-Crib. I could make a covered bed like I had seen used in my *Exceptional Parent Magazine* for autistic children to keep them safe during the night. I used my talents as a seamstress to design the perfect answer for my unusual problem. Detamara could easily get out, but she was a compliant child.

I met with the therapist and the Michigan social worker and promised to remain in the room with her to protect her from fire or disaster. The professionals gave me the approval I hoped for, and we were all off to Florida.

The baggage handlers took our luggage for fourteen and the port-a-crib. We watched over the feeding pump, wheelchair, and nebulizer and each child carried their own backpack of necessities to alleviate boredom.

Would we arrive in Florida with everything intact?

We flew from Kalamazoo to Chicago, Chicago to Miami, and

then took a puddle jumper to Marathon — three flights, and a parade of fourteen Yurceks. We assigned each kid a buddy, and miraculously we made the trek without losing anyone, though we almost left Deangelo in the Miami Air Terminal rest room.

The head count Jim said was unnecessary proved to be Deangelo's salvation.

In the Florida Keys, we found two matching white mini vans waiting for us at the airport. Jim took the boys, and I took the girls, and we were off to the hotel. The hotel reception watched as our multitude of children continued to come out of the vans. We would use the same strategy in the hotel, the girls got one room with me and the boys got two more, one with Jim and one with Brian.

Ian found that the outside walls were crawling with tiny green geckos and he was in heaven. Ian loves creepy crawling things, and as a precocious two-year-old he was going to be an entomologist, then by age three he decided to change professions to paleontologist. Soon Ian and DJ ganged up on chasing the girls, especially Marissa with the new-found creatures. Screaming and squealing, the girls ran from their teenage brothers. I worried that Ian would try to sneak one of his pets home, as he had always wanted one and I later confiscated a potato chip container filled with a dozen green geckos out of his suitcase and made him release them back to the wild.

The following day we were off to explore the islands going across the Florida Keys Seven Mile Bridge – the bridge that would live on in Yurcek infamy. I took the girls in one van and Jim took the boys. He placed the cooler of twelve sodas in the back seat next to Delonzo. Soon Delonzo was begging to use the restroom and Jim was at the 3.5-mile point of the bridge. He told Delonzo he had to wait since there was no place to pull off.

Jim quickly pulled off as soon as he reached the end point and Delonzo raced off to the bathroom. He was a bit too late; the back seat was already flooded. It was hot outside and Ian and DJ were ready to pummel him when they discovered their little brother had drunk the entire 12 pack of family sodas.

In fact, it was 105 degrees outside and Jim and I were hot, yet

DJ wore his black wind pants, a long sleeve sweatshirt, and his hat and refused to take them off. He was not sweating and was complaining about being cold.

Cold at 105°? I checked him to see if he was running a fever. He wasn't, and it made no sense that he was freezing while the rest of us waded to cool off in the ocean where we captured family photos on the Florida Keys beaches. I pinched myself. Were we really here? Was this happening? I was afraid I would wake up and find myself back in my bed at home.

Becca swam with the dolphins at the Dolphin Research Center. Kristy and I chickened out, but Jim and Nathan were up to the challenge. DJ recorded the event on our new $20.00 reconditioned garage sale camcorder. The kids and I watched as the dolphin and Becca did tricks. AJ the dolphin became Becca's new best friend and as we left the center, we let her buy a stuffed dolphin. She happily picked one nearly as big as she was. It was her day and her wish, but how were we going to get the dolphin home on the planes with everything else?

Our time in the Keys was short and soon we moved on to the next secret. We stuffed children, luggage, medical equipment and the huge dolphin into a puddle jumper airplane, then unstuffed them and restuffed them onto another plane to Orlando and finally packed everyone and everything into the shuttle to DisneyWorld.

We were surprised as we drove up to two beautiful villas that were our new temporary home. Our villas were on the grounds of the Disney Institute and we were staying in the lap of luxury with room to spare. We were in heaven.

Jim claimed one villa as his and the boys home. I claimed the other villa 'just for girls.' Everyone had a place to sleep! We had two, two bedroom villas with queen size beds and a great room with a pull out sofa bed. The villas had full kitchens, and I was able to stretch our money by cooking breakfast and dinner in our rooms. I surprised Jim and Brian with a round of golf at the Disney Institute.

The temptation of alligator hunting in Florida was too much for my explorer Ian. He rallied the younger boys for the prowling adventure and they found a 'gator. Luckily Jim was nearby to stop them from exploring him closer and redirected them to a game of gecko catching and tormenting the girls.

The midday sun was too much for Becca to handle because her body still cannot cool itself so we waited off the midday heat at the pool. My kids loved being in the hotel, and a swimming pool was a real treat for everyone except Detamara who wouldn't get wet. She screamed at the thought of going into the water and patient Kristy soothed and coaxed my scared little daughter, who by the last day clung to her big sister like a leach in the water. On the other hand, Becca pretended to be Shamu or Free Willy and never wanted to leave the pool. She rode on Shay who patiently pretended to be AJ the dolphin. The boys dove off the diving board and chased each other. Jim and Brian joined in the dunking, squirting, and playing. If Shay wasn't playing with Becca she quietly sat alone.

DisneyWorld was our next big day. The older kids separated from us with Kristy and Brian in charge. They tried working with Shay, but she kept wandering off and getting lost. After an hour Shay was returned to us to hang out with the younger kids and she was not happy about it.

Jim and I, along with Delonzo, Becca, Detamara and Shay set off to enjoy the parks. Shay pouted. She was thirteen and she was not a little kid! It wasn't fair. She did not appreciate tagging along with Mom and Dad, while her little brother Deangelo who was only nine got to stay with Kristy and Brian. Every picture we took showed a sullen and very sad young lady. We couldn't understand it since we were in heaven, on a once in the lifetime opportunity. But Shay would not be happy.

We ate dinner at the 50's Diner at Disney World. Our waiter assigned each member in our party a nickname, Brian became Skippy, Kristy became Muffy. The laughter from our mammoth crew still echoes in my dreams. The dinner tab was nearly $400.00. That was a car payment. I had found a Disney discount gold card on the Internet before our trip and that $60.00 investment saved $40.00 on that dinner alone. It was the best money I had extravagantly spent. It saved

10% at any Disney Venue, so I even used it when I bought milk. Even on our wish trip, I still had to bargain hunt. I felt responsible to stretch the budget for the Wish Foundation. I couldn't even waste somebody else's money.

Time flew by. The next day Becca got to meet and pet Shamu at Sea World. Shamu splashed and completely soaked DJ, and everyone laughed. Shay and Detamara, overstimulated and mesmerized by their surroundings, followed whatever caught their interest, and even with Jim and me watching closely, we still lost them. We worried because if silent Detamara got really lost she would have kept wandering because the only person she dared talk to was me. We worried if Shay got lost she would have talked to everyone and probably gone home with someone she didn't know. At thirteen she couldn't remember her phone number. She had absolutely no understanding of stranger danger.

I bought a Velcro hand holder and a clip key ring. I velcroed each end to a girl and took the middle of the cording and clipped the key clip to my belt loop. We were quite a sight. I pushed a tiny girl in her hot pink Zippy Quicky wheelchair and had two other young ladies hanging off my waist with five-foot leashes. Jim and I could finally relax and stop the worry about losing kids.

We had fun, and everyone "stuck" together.

I prepared ahead by shopping for Disney gear at Target, and I surprised the kids with Disney shirts and memorabilia. Delonzo, Deangelo, Detamara, Becca and Shay each had dollar store Minnie and Mickey Mouse canteens of various colors that we kept filled with water. Each child had his or her own autograph book with Disney characters. I passed out disposable cameras, and each morning at breakfast the child named his or her favorite character and set out on their adventure to get the coveted autograph and picture. It became 'Mission Possible' to see how many characters they could collect and Becca always found Snow White who made her feel like a princess.

The Wish foundation had set up free passes to all of the parks. The kids played at Epcot, Universal Studios, and the newly-opened Animal Kingdom until they dropped. We sat through the production of Beauty and the Beast, and bought a magical snow globe to remember our family dream vacation.

After seven days of dreams come true, we left Florida with exhausted children and parents. We searched and retrieved lost shoes and socks, we had to check under all the beds, under the sofas and in the cushions for lost belongings. We went back for a third pass through the rooms for a forgotten toothbrush or wallet. We searched a fourth time and counted heads before turning in the keys.

It was a true miracle. In eight flights for fourteen people the airlines didn't lose one piece of luggage and we arrived home tired and happy with a lifetime of happy and exciting family memories we had created together. The opportunity to have fun together as a family away from our normal everyday life, mixed and matched and blended the Yurceks into one.

My wish had come true!

▼

A month later when our family returned to Minnesota we were already one family in our hearts, now it was time to become one family on paper. On July 31, 1998, our adoption of the children was complete and they were officially ours. Delano (DJ), Shay, Deangelo, Delonzo, and Detamara were now legally Yurceks. We belonged with and to each other. We made Susan, the guardian ad litem, an unofficial extended member of our family. The more the merrier. We snapped courthouse pictures and then rushed off to the church for a very special wedding.

We expanded the celebration into the whole day with the wed ding of my sister Martha, who had survived her battle with ovarian cancer and found love. Her special wedding became part of our very first new Yurcek family celebration.

I stood in the church where I grew up, the place that surrounded us during our families' hard times. I remembered back to the day of Becca's dedication when we had brought her home to die. Becca survived and now the Yurcek family spanned two church pews.

I remembered the words of Pastor Rick telling me my tiny dying baby had a calling. Becca had been instrumental in strengthening faith and hope for Martha as she dealt with her cancer.

Our Tiny Titan had changed us, and we had changed the persons we now called family. Because of Becca's birth and sicknesses we had a new family, a new career, and new perspective on life.

Most people go through life never taking risks, but we had learned through Becca that each day of living was a risk. Jim took a risk to begin Medical School so late in life. We took a risk to move six hundred miles and begin a new adventure. Jim and I took a risk to adopt our new family.

We learned that life is not fair and life is not easy.

We learned to work hard and that dreams do come true if you're willing to step out. We learned that blessings come from adversity and everyday is a gift.

- 35 -

Activities, Schedules & Logistics

With ten children at home, it required scheduling, planning and logistics to get everyone to where they needed to be at the right time. I feared I'd forget someone someplace. I remembered reading about a newly adoptive family who forgot one of their twelve children at a rest area on a trip to their grandma's. The kids laughed at me when I stopped to conduct roll call to make sure everyone was accounted for.

I had always been able to count on remembering my schedule, but when life became too much and I could no longer count on my memory I began to carry a day planner. I found weekly planners did not have space enough to handle the logistics of my tribe. I plotted everyday hour-by-hour, figuring out how to sometimes be in two places at once. We had games for the younger boys on Tuesday and Thursday evenings, and games for Matt and Shay on Monday and Wednesday. I charted the strategic plans to get everyone where they needed to be and when and how to pick them up. I charted Nathan's work schedule at Menards, DJ's work schedule at Burger King, and Ian's hours at Hot and Now, commonly referred to by my kids as Rotten Cow.

Settling in meant finding activities to keep each kid busy for little or no money? We could not afford fancy basketball and soccer leagues or private music lessons. The kids needed to make do with elementary and secondary school activities. Matt played Rocket football, Delonzo, Deangelo and Matt played boys Bantam Basketball and Shay played on a girl's Bantam Basketball team. Ian and DJ joined the church basketball team the year after he broke Ian's nose and DJ's success came on the court. They gave it their all.

We filled our evenings attending games and cheering for our team players. The driveway was our practice court, and someone was always dunking hoops or willing to join in a game of HORSE. Becca and Detamara dropped basketballs into their Little Tykes basketball hoop, copying the game the older kids played. Mom held her own when I challenged my kids, and they were shocked to discover that I actually beat them once in awhile. When the family played ball at the park, we picked teams and Becca played on Dad's shoulders. Happy times evened out the emotions when things were at their worst.

Marissa joined our community theater. She soon auditioned for a small professional theater and was cast as one of the members of the Crachit family in a Christmas Carol. From October through Thanksgiving Marissa practiced every weeknight after dinner to be prepared for her over thirty holiday performances. I was thankful Nathan had his driver's license and he shared the driving with me when he was not working. He also volunteered at the theater, but his shyness prevented him from acting when they needed young men for the many Dickens characters.

We seemed to live in our van with three boys working, all the sports practices, Marissa's rehearsal and performance schedules, the little girls weekly dance classes or craft activities, conferences, school activities, Becca's doctor appointments and the kids therapy sessions. We sang and talked. We played games as we passed our time on the road. My time in the van with the children reminded me of our old paper route moments and our discussions drew us closer and away from the chaos of the world while the activities cemented two families further into one. Looking back, it was the perfect bonding time we needed as a family. We had time to chat about school, sports, or anything anyone needed to say. The time on the road was a welcome sanctuary, no one could get into trouble – they were all buckled in and the doors were locked. I knew their whereabouts and nothing could turn up missing or create a near disaster by accident or on purpose. We were working together, playing together, sharing together, and cheering each other on. Brothers and sisters watched each other on stage, on the basketball court, and at dance recitals.

Becca loved animals and needed something to do to get out of the house. After DeShawn abused her, she had shut down, was afraid of strangers and had become very dependent on me. Reading the newspaper I discovered a therapeutic horse-riding program for children with disabilities. Her pediatrician agreed it may be good for her and signed the thick pile of intake papers.

Hippotherapy and riding lessons were expensive, but they had scholarships to help defray the costs and Becca was off to her first horseback-riding lesson. I forewarned the instructors that she did not like to be touched and the staff seemed to understand and listened.

As I walked up to the entrance of the Cheff Center holding my tiny daughter's hand I saw a statue with a poem and a horse and I knew immediately Becca would belong. The poem was by John Anthony Davies, England's foremost authority and practitioner in the field of riding for the handicapped. It was entitled *I Saw A Child* and in it's words I saw Becca. My daughter would be welcome just for who she was and over time gain skill and self-confidence.

Becca cowered behind me and held onto my leg for dear life, yet she was smitten by the horses. She peeked from behind my jacket and watched every movement. Eventually, her inquisitiveness helped her venture from my side to reach out to pet a pony. Soon she walked around Kissy who became her cute shaggy irresistible pony.

Kissy had thick black fur and his patient demeanor won Becca's heart. She watched as they put on the tiny saddle. The instructor held Becca's hand gently, guiding her to brush and groom Kissy before riding. As Becca brushed Kissy, the pony turned and nudged Becca's cheek causing her to giggle. I held Becca's hand as we led her new pony friend to the arena. I was shocked when Becca let someone besides Mom lift her, and set her upon Kissy.

Becca looked so tiny on the little pony, but there she was sitting tall and proud. At seven, she wore toddler size-four clothing and weighed barely thirty pounds, but on Kissy she was a 'just a little girl' who loved her pony.

She was proud, 'just like other girls' she loved horses. She had something she was good at, all by herself. Now, she had something to talk about. Horseback riding opened up a whole new world for Becca. Her newfound independence migrated from the barn to the riding arena and into other areas of her life. She talked with other young ladies about dogs, and horses, and horseback riding. She had something she could be successful at, and learn about. She spent hours cruising the library shelves to find books about the horses, and their care.

Becca had found a whole barn of pony and horse friends and real girlfriends. As time went by Becca needed me less and less and she soon was walking in alone, putting on her helmet and waving "Bye Mom."

I wasn't needed!

On the way home from her lesson, Becca told me when that Dad is a doctor, Dad is going to buy her a pony of her own. A week later she wanted two ponies when Dad was done with residency, because she didn't want the first pony to get lonely.

By the end of the school year, Becca rode solo for the very first time. She had learned to trust the staff and her new confidence was apparent. She eagerly anticipated each day she was scheduled to ride and she endured the price of pain and exhaustion on the following day because she had pushed her little body too hard.

Becca had become a horse expert, when we were at a park where they were offering pony rides; the owner was astounded that a person so tiny knew what kind each horse was. She correctly identified the breed of each pony and flabbergasted the owner when she declared the last pony was a flea bitten grey Arabian.

The two little girls signed up for Girl Scouts, Becca in a Junior

Troop and Detamara became a Brownies. The boys participated in the youth groups at two local churches. In the summer, we took advantage of local park and recreation programs where we qualified for community scholarships to lessen our programming costs. The kids rode horses, went on field trips, and played summer sports. Becca even ventured out to the elementary school summer programs with Deangelo, Delonzo and Detamara on cooler days. On hot days, she stayed home in the air conditioning and had alone time with Mom.

Everyday I washed five to six loads of clothing and I finally broke down and purchased a used second washer and dryer. I sandwiched them into my laundry room and it didn't take long before I'd worn them out. Since the laundry room fire, I never left the washer or dryer unattended. If I had to leave to run an errand I shut everything down and fell further behind as I could seldom stay home.

The summer programs gave me a breather to get the house cleaning done undisturbed from the constant monitoring it took to keep my children on track. Keeping up on the house while eyeballing kids was nearly impossible. Each small household chore had to be carefully taught and then taught again, and surprisingly taught even more times. Our five new family members took ten times the training and instruction than my first six had. Often the time teaching and the attempt to help created more of a disaster than we started and it was easier to do it myself.

At therapy, Colleen questioned me about how I kept so much straight. How did I know who was where, when, and doing what at all times? My brain filled in the logistics. I had it all memorized. Before going to bed, I planned my day the best I could. I figured out who needed to be where, when and once it was thought through, I fell asleep.

If a kid needed a ride they had to ask the night before or they walked or got a ride from someone else. The schedule was too busy for unplanned excursions. The family policies were enforced and Mom did not give rides to kids who got themselves in trouble. One of the school counselors thought this unfair, but I did not want to reward bad behavior by making it too easy. The poor downtrodden child usually got 'lucky' because one of my errands passed by the path home.

Our new family celebrated firsts in a new community away from everybody and everything we were used to. I believe the first is always the most special. All the together firsts, the first Christmas, the first thanksgiving, the first dates, the first conferences, the first dances, the first game, the first everything was a time remembered by someone, and cherished by me with happy tears. My two handsome sons, now brothers' double dated and invited dates to the winter formal. We shopped for their dress clothes and the young ladies' corsages. Since neither boy had their driver's license Dad chauffeured in the mini van, cramping their style and I confused my children with my tears of thanksgiving.

Our children belonged to each other and were finding their places. They were developing friendships with peers in the community, relationships with each other, and at long last for our new children, much needed permanency and security.

- 36 -

FALLING FAST

The first year was a challenge and we hoped after finalization we would be over the hump with our kids. There were a million adjustments, but somehow we made it through. We couldn't help DeShawn and the loss left a legacy of trust issues for the remaining children. Up until now we had little say about anything for our new kids. Sometimes, I had to go against my gut intuition to please the half dozen therapists who were working with each of them. Even the therapists did not agree with one another, and at times contradicted each other in multiple ways. I needed to be able to find the help that made sense, and quit trying to please them all at the same time. Hopefully with finalization of the adoption, Jim and I would have a say in accessing and choosing help for our children and we looked forward to having a voice in our children's care.

As the summer came to a close, the kids headed back to school and it was obvious that Shay needed more help. The celebration of adoption opened the years of struggle and dealing with grief and loss of her mother. Even she was asking for one-on-one support and an IEP meeting was set up. At school Shay tried to fit in and this added to her depression.

I was told the prior year to give her independence and don't stigmatize her by having someone shadow her every move. They were the experts and had done things like this before, I needed to trust them and her social worker agreed. I had let it be, but now I had spent more time with my daughter and I had watched her push away her friends. I noticed she didn't know what to do with other kids.

Marissa was exasperated with Shay and reported she was threatening students and talking to herself in the hallways. Behind Shay's back the middle school students chided and teased her and told Marissa that she had a crazy sister. Shay had picked the girl with the worst reputation as her friend and now Shay's reputation was even worse than that. Yet the reports, early on from teachers and the office staff conflicted, they adored her.

I knew to believe Marissa because she doesn't lie. I figured it must be just like at home, when you are there they were fine, when you turn your back - watch out!

Shay wanted friends so bad and according to Shay everyone was her friend, yet she had no idea about friendships. Shay had no idea how to make social connections. One moment she acted silly and the next moment she acted disgusting. Her moods fluctuated all over the place. She no longer cared how she looked or smelled. She refused to change her clothes and left her hair uncombed. She rejected offers of support and her offensiveness turned many of the other teens away including her siblings. Her behavior was quickly deteriorating and to top it off she never seemed to sleep. I knew I needed to get her help.

Marissa was a high achiever and she worked hard to have friends and become popular in her new school. Her friends were now the eighth grade class leaders; Shay was in seventh grade, followed by Matt in sixth. It was no fun to have people call your sister 'crazy.' One of Marissa's friend's was the top student in her class and Shay reported that this young lady was smoking pot in the girl's bathroom.

Why?

Shay was mad at Marissa. She wanted to alienate Marissa from her friends and fun she didn't have and didn't know how to get.

The girls were called into the office and luckily the administration saw through Shay's gollywog. Shay got detention for false reporting. Shay's behavior continued to escalate and now teacher's brought issues to Marissa's attention, telling her in front of peers they would be contacting her mother and they hoped she would be home for the phone call. Before she had only gotten negative information about Shay's behavior from peers who snickered and laughed, now angry teachers and administrators cornered her to loudly discuss her new sibling, while teens in the hall struggled to eavesdrop and then asked her all about it later. It was embarrassing.

I was seeing more signs of depression in Shay and Detamara's therapist gave me the name of a psychiatrist to work with Shay. The psychiatrist immediately placed Shay on an antidepressant.

I was relieved; finally someone saw what I was seeing. Poor Shay was so unhappy and she had reasons to be sad and depressed. The finalization of the adoption meant closure from her birth mother and history. Their feelings conflicted. No matter what the kids went through, they still loved their mother. She was their mom! And they hated her for not taking the help offered for her substance abuse problems.

Even after finalization, Minnesota would not give us any of the children's records; but luckily, we came across some paperwork through unconventional channels. In Minnesota, Shay had had two psychological assessments and these documents helped fill in the blanks. Shay's behaviors at home and school were beginning to make more sense to me. Like our diagnosis with Becca, this information gave us a starting point for further research and knowledge.

Shay had been diagnosed with Reactive Attachment Disorder (RAD), along with her mild retardation. Reactive Attachment disorder meant Shay was unattached and we could expect her to push away anyone trying to make a connection. She was a complex child. She could not let anyone get too close because if any attachment or caring began, it threatened her perception for survival. Any close moment triggered a negative reaction and sometimes crises.

Push them away!

Make them leave!

Stop the feelings of comfort! All five new children jumped on the push-pull roller coaster ride of attachment disorder.

Finally the stealing, hoarding, and crazy behavior began to make sense. The love of a family pushed her away and infuriated her. The need to be loved pulled her back. Shay was lovable one moment, and self destructive and acting out the next. The swings from defiance to compliance and back again were consistent. She required supervision twenty-four hours a day, seven days a week and without the supervision we had disasters. We were on a roller coaster ride of good and bad days and we never knew what to expect.

Shay could be helpful, controlled and happy one moment, and violent, uncontrolled and angry the next. The other kids also had their bad moments, and thankfully took turns.

Was I doing something wrong, or was it the school? Shay seemed to be able to start a task, but couldn't follow through unless she was guided. How could school expect Shay to succeed if she failed at home when we provided careful supports and structure? I was in new territory with my new children and I returned to my 'just' a mom role and followed what the professionals told me to do.

One day, after Shay left for school the smoke alarms sounded. I found a smoldering sheet placed over the lamp in her bedroom. It ignited before my eyes. I grabbed the sheet and stomped out the small flames. Shay's decision to block out the light could have burned down our home. I was shaking. What if I had not come home after taking Detamara to school? What if I had gone to the pharmacy like I had planned to do?

We would have lost everything!

Another day Shay chased a wayward paper airplane into the bus lane oblivious to the oncoming bus. It seemed she never paid attention to where she was going and I constantly reminded her to look before crossing the street. My words floated on the wind and she repeatedly darted out in traffic.

The therapist we found to work with DeShawn was now our family therapist. I enlisted the help of Colleen to accompany me to Shay's IEP. She was now counseling Shay, Detamara, and our family in family therapy. The school team of teachers told me Shay was doing well and did not need a paraprofessional.

Was I off base?

Yet, Colleen saw what I saw. The psychotropic the psychiatrist placed Shay on worried me even more and we were both concerned. She was flying high and her mood swings were worsening. Each day, her defiance mounted. Shay had been so helpful and this behavior was out of character. I asked the doctor if perhaps the meds were causing this behavior change and he told me to bring her to his office.

I complied and he upped the medication disagreeing with me. I still believed it was the medication that was changing her demeanor, but I followed the doctor's orders, I still viewed myself as 'just' a mom in the mental health world.

In a couple of days life for Shay worsened even further. During the day she bounced off the walls, and my walls were actually shaking. She talked constantly to herself and was now carrying on both sides of a conversation along with the incessant animal noises she was making. She was unable to sleep. Her behavior was alienating her further from her siblings. She was jumping in her bed and she had the top bunk! Her hygiene remained abysmal. Anything we asked her to do was met with negativity.

The psychiatrist advised me to leave school issues at school. I had enough to worry about at home.

Then the school called. Her mid-quarter grades were poor and the school alerted me that Shay's behavior was now causing problems. She had many lunch detentions and she was not showing up to take care of them. The list of infractions now had her in school suspensions for the day. She needed to stay after school to slowly make up her consequences.

Shay walked in the door from school in a foul mood.

We had to talk about the phone call and she erupted.

She slammed things. She screamed.

Thank God for small miracles. Jim walked into the house after an all-night hospital shift. Shay settled down and grabbed an after school snack.

Jim gave her an assignment choice of sentence writing. She could write about what she did or she could write about what she should have done differently. He handed her a blank piece of paper and told her to sit at the table until she completed the letter.

Shay seemed settled at the table with her snack and assigned task, so Jim took Matt, Ian, DJ and Nathan to the YMCA to play basketball. With winter coming, I was grateful for the membership. It was the perfect place for energetic teens to run off excess steam and hormones. Our house was too small for a single cooped up teen, much less a half a dozen of them.

I was alone with the rest of the children. My two younger boys and little girls had buried themselves in after school cartoons in the living room and Marissa was downstairs.

Shay sat seething at the table and within minutes of Jim's departure she bolted from the table.I instructed her to return to her work. I was standing near the stairs and I didn't see her coming behind me. She captured me at the top of the stairs.

Half way through the sentence, she grabbed me by the shoulders and I felt myself being lifted off the ground. The metal railing gave way as I went head first over it toward the floor below. My belly hit the railing and my thighs tried to grab it as I was hurled over. My left arm was pinned below me, so I reached out with my right arm. I pulled my lips in hoping to protect my teeth.

As I was falling, I felt as if someone or something was underneath me shielding me from the full force of my fall, everything felt slow motion. My head struck something. A piercing pain shot up my arm. My hand hit the wall. I was lying atop the metal stair rail and something else cushioned me.

For a moment I laid stunned, crumpled in a heap. As I regained my consciousness, I realized my kids were screaming. Marissa had run up the stairs mid-fall. I landed by the front door. Deangelo ran to Jeannie's across the street to get help. By the time he returned with Jeannie, Marissa had helped me to my feet and I had called the YMCA. I left a message for Jim to meet us at the hospital.

I was in shock, my adrenaline allowed me to keep moving. I knew I had to keep moving. If I stopped I could not get back up.

Jeannie and Deangelo were stunned by what they found. My

lips were torn off. There was not anything left but a small piece of bottom lip about 1/2 inch. By pulling in my lips to save my teeth, my teeth had torn them away. I was covered in blood. I should have been dead or paralyzed, but something saved me.

I looked at the stairs, at the blood, and at the stair railing. Then I realized that the hooded cat box I had yelled at Marissa for not putting away earlier in the day was still where it was not supposed to be. The hood was dented the diameter of my head. The cat box probably saved my life. Marissa, under five-feet, tiny and petite, ran up the stairs and pushed Shay, seventy pounds heavier and much stronger into the wall with all the energy she could muster and ordered her not to move.

Jeannie called her husband Scott. He rushed across the street and took Shay to their home. She did not even react to what had just happened. She watched TV, while Jeannie drove me to the hospital.

▼

Marissa stayed behind with her little brothers and sisters looking at the mess. She had come up from the lower level as I lay in a crumpled heap where she was busy pouting because I had yelled at her about the cat box. The bloody cat box she forgot had probably saved my life. Marissa took charge of the homefront. She put the dented cat box away and cleaned up all the blood. Then she played with the kids to keep them busy. Shay's behavior at school and the phone call home had almost cost her mother her life.

▼

I realized that my arm was twisted and contorted and it was undoubtedly broken in multiple places. The shock was subsiding and pain began to overtake my body. I couldn't move my neck. My lips were bleeding uncontrollably. The triage nurse immediately placed me in for treatment and x-rays. The orthopedist said he needed to reset my arm. Another doctor began stitching back my lips.

Jim arrived at the hospital with Shay who stood sobbing, saying she didn't mean to do it. He wanted her to witness the aftermath of her tantrum.

They numbed my arm.

The x-rays revealed I had multiple fractures.

Both bones were broken clean through and the bones in my wrist were completely out of place. They placed my hand in metal mesh gloves that looked like they had been designed in the middle ages and then they yanked it all into place. Then with my arm immobilized they released me to go home.

The security guards asked what had happened. I knew if I told them the whole story Shay could be arrested for assault. I told the guard she accidentally pushed me down the stairs, but behind the doors of the emergency room the doctors who Jim worked with day in and day out soon knew the truth.

This was the second time almost a year apart; we found ourselves in the emergency room with a family member due to the anger of our newest children. The domestic abuse they knew so well now roosted in our caring home.

I am not sure what hurt more, my neck, lips, arm, and hand; or my heart. I had to face our kids.

The pain pills hardly dulled the severity of my discomfort. When we took on the kids, we were trying to do something good. We hoped to take them out of an abusive home. We would provide stability, love and structure. Now our home felt like it was no better than the home they came from. The kids worked hard to make sure peace and tranquility never existed.

It seemed as though they thrived on chaos.

Within a week the swelling was down enough to have surgery on my hand. I awoke post op with six steel pins protruding out of my skin and black metal bars called a fixator stabilizing and holding everything tightly back together.

My right hand was out of commission. I am right handed. The level of parenting and housekeeping from my new tribe was immense. Learning to function one handed was nearly impossible and everything I tried to do caused pain or frustration. I now understood Becca's frustration of hands that don't work. I relied on Nathan and Marissa's help for household tasks as I took on the role of chief operations officer of chores and chaos.

The other kids were angry and traumatized from their past and now it was compounded by this last experience with Shay. Shay would not look at me. I triggered something she did not want to face. I tried to not blame her. Perhaps I had to experience that level of trauma and posttraumatic stress to help my new children deal with their histories of abuse.

In therapy we addressed these issues.

Shay shut down. She refused to do anything. She was very agitated. Her psychiatrist felt she needed to be on her medication for longer to even out.

Colleen upped her therapy sessions to twice a week and Shay deteriorated further. She was self abusing. She tore up the carpet in her room. She banged her head on the concrete floor. How did she tolerate the pain? She would not shower, bathe, and change her clothes. Her appetite was gone. She fluctuated between distancing herself from us or being disrespectful and angry in our face.

If we told her to do something, she threatened us. One time she grabbed the fixator on my arm and yanked until one of the boys stepped in to free me. From that moment on, it became a weapon to threaten to grab my arm. We found knives hidden in her room. I had locked them up, but she somehow stealthfully stole them.

Shay was a very disturbed thirteen-year-old. She gained weight as her body matured. Her hormones raged. She acted up. She stole. She hoarded. She made fifty-five long distance phone calls to friends from camp. Even when presented with the two hundred dollar phone bill, she lied and said she did not place the calls. She wrapped an extension cord around her neck and the boys had to help me remove it. She prowled at night and we placed an alarm on her door. I locked my bedroom door, yet one morning there was a large sharp knife on my dresser.

Her violent temper tantrums increased. She threw anything she grabbed. She said things to bait Ian and DJ and seemed to enjoy making them get angry. She erupted when the boys told her to stay in her room because she was not acting appropriate. Soon all hell broke lose. The boys, not wanting to fight, would hold her door closed, while Shay screamed obscenities at the top of her lungs and pounded the door with her fists. Then she banged the door with her head and threatened to put her fingers in the light socket. I called Colleen and she agreed that after therapy on Wednesday we would place Shay in the hospital. It was unsafe to keep her at home.

Jim and I would take Shay to the hospital together.

Shay pulled herself together enough to put herself in the car. She knew she needed help. I got the brunt of her behaviors and her hatred. I was her new mom. I was not her mom. Ever since finalization, she was trying to get us to give up on her as we had given up on DeShawn. She wanted someone to help her and she could not control herself. She had been in a downward spiral for months.

The therapists said she was testing us and with Reactive Attachment Disorder her behavior was to be expected. It was normal for children with this diagnosis to not let anyone get close or control them, but this was more than just attachment issue. Something was wrong and at last she was in a place to get help. Our insurance company did the right thing and from the emergency room she was admitted to the adolescent psychiatric ward. Jim had worked in both emergency rooms and we were not strangers in the hospital.

If not for those coincidences our road could have been far different as Shay and our family tumbled fast to the bottom.

- 37 -
HANGING ON

I juggled hospital and social service meetings with managing my tribe. My life seemed a repeat of the scrambling from when Becca was so sick. My neighbor, Jeannie had serious mental and physical health problems and she shared a special connection with Becca very few other people had ever been able to. With Jeannie's help I could drop everything when the hospital called.

The psychologist wrote that Shay was impulsive. I still believed her medication was making her worse. The new testing results echoed what had been discovered and hidden from us before. The results repeated what we already knew. I needed help and we were not getting anywhere. Regardless of how hard it was sometimes, I loved each of these kids and I wanted our family as a whole to make it. I didn't want my children taken away, so I tried to please everyone despite knowing I was going against what was right for my children and our family.

Colleen assured me it was all right to fire a doctor, but I wanted to maintain peace with social services and medical personnel. She helped empower me to trust my intuition and began to move off my 'just' a mom position with my new children. Colleen helped us find Shay a new psychiatrist who immediately changed her medications.

Shay's new psychiatrist talked to me about the possibility of my daughter having bipolar disorder.

Shay's moods switched so quickly from glee to despair, joy to fury. I wondered if she was right.

She then shared she thought Shay might have some special kind of syndrome. She asked me about the substance abuse history of Shay's biological mother.

I told her we knew DeShawn and Detamara were born with cocaine in their systems and that there was suspicion from the foster mom that Detamara may have Fetal Alcohol Syndrome. I also told her DJ had confirmed his mother struggled with alcoholism and he'd seen her drink when she was pregnant with the younger children.

The psychiatrist thought Shay and a number of my other new children may also have been prenatally exposed to alcohol and incurred permanent brain damage because of it. This would explain many of their puzzling behaviors. Prenatal exposure to alcohol and street drugs could cause structural brain damage, which manifested as learning disabilities and unusual behaviors.

I was surprised to learn of all the street drugs, alcohol has the greatest impact on the developing embryo, and results in the most permanent damage. I was glad I had a new psychiatrist who listened, explained and took an interest in my daughter and me.

▼

When I placed Shay in the hospital I was shocked when the attending psychiatrist was the same doctor who wouldn't listen to me regarding Shay's worsening symptoms from the antidepressants. He simply would not believe that the medication could cause this. I had just fired this doctor and now I had to work with him as he again worked with my daughter. It was an awkward situation and I made sure staff had him communicate with the new treating doctor, leaving me out of the discussion. I made sure the hospital knew upon discharged, Shay was to be followed up by her new psychiatrist.

The Federal Drug Administration has since issued black box warnings on the use of antidepressants in children and adolescents. I was right. Other children placed on antidepressants had also become 'manic' or suicidal.

In the hospital, Shay acted as though everything was all right. Only when I received the discharge records did I fully understand her needs. She was sad, had self-esteem problems, and anxiety. The hospital records stated that "she did not have any explosive episodes but it was clear each day her behavior became more stabilized as the meds were exiting her system."

A chart note stated, "Shay tends to be rather impulsive and enjoys becoming involved in activities that are inappropriate. She likes to join in with other children who are being disruptive." She had moments when she became very angry, but she could now talk about it and calm down. As time passed it became easier to redirect her from inappropriate behavior.

The testing showed much of what I read about a child with Fetal Alcohol Spectrum Disorder. Was this what we were dealing with Shay? Was Dr. Bui right?

After thirteen days in the hospital Shay was discharged to home and a partial day treatment program. She had settled down. Little was said about her explosive behavior, what do you do when the child wants to hurt herself and there is nothing to do to stop her? How do you handle head-banging, which she did to settle herself down?

The testing and the doctors told me she needed clear and consistent boundaries. Shay's life needed to be structured in order to make progress. There were huge differences in her intellectual and her performance IQs. The testing confirmed what Minnesota had told me – Shay had mild retardation. She would need help in many areas and I felt better.

After only a few days of outpatient day treatment, Shay was discharged to spend Christmas with our family. I had only three days till Christmas and I spent late nights getting ready for the holiday.

Day times were busy; I could not take my eyes off of Shay, Detamara, Delonzo, and Becca.

I had to protect Becca from her new siblings in addition to attend to her medical needs.

I had to keep Delonzo from getting himself into something and stealing.

I had to keep Detamara on task and make sure her acting out behaviors did not reoccur. She was beginning to trust and always needed someone to be present.

If I left the room, chaos ensued.

Jim was buried in his residency work.

Home life fell onto my shoulders and I planned a low-key Christmas. I had learned we didn't wire anyone up. I had learned my lesson last year. Everything in our lives had become consistent and highly structured. We kept everything simple to avoid adding chaos and keep things from being too good for the kids to handle.

▼

In January, the worker from the Kalamazoo Community Mental Health Services arrived to discuss the problems leading Shay to the psychiatric hospital. It had been part of the discharge report that a referral would be made to get me some help to help Shay remain in the community. I told her about Shay and the other children's problems and gave her our Medicaid cards.

She told me I couldn't use my therapist with their program or our new doctor. I had to switch to their professionals who didn't take our health insurance, which had to be used first before Medicaid paid. We were stuck in the 'no man's land' of mental health. The budget was two million dollars in the hole and there was no respite funding available. The worker didn't offer any help and I didn't know to press further.

What I didn't know hurt me, I learned later that this was the door to get the kids services through Medicaid. All five adopted kids had Medicaid as part of their adoption subsidy and Becca was eligible because of her disability through Social Security.

I continued watching, referring, and trying to keep things from falling apart. Shay met with her new psychiatrist. She was off the antidepressant and the new mood stabilizer seemed to be helping. We had weekly therapy for Shay and Detamara with Colleen and Becca had numerous medical appointments. I seemed to always be on the run and there was rarely a day where I got to spend the day home. The only break I got from the running was when one of the kids was home from school sick and I got to cancel the appointments. We paid for their therapies ourselves and used our private insurance whenever and wherever possible. The bills mounted.

Each child was allowed twelve post adoptive therapy sessions paid for by Minnesota using the adoption agency therapist. Delonzo and Deangelo had therapy with the therapist twice a month. I fired an agency therapist for going behind our backs and allowing the boys to call DeShawn in his foster home, which violated the recommendation of Detamara and Becca's therapist.

Just before finalization Jim told the therapists and social workers there would be no more contact with DeShawn as the acting out behaviors by the kids showed us this was not in their best interests. We had been advised to save the ones we could and trust the system to take care of DeShawn's intense needs. He had little chance of having a good outcome and was too sick.

The boys were told not to tell us that they were making phone calls to their brother and exchanging letters. It was their secret. Deangelo revealed the truth when he shared a secret about DeShawn's inappropriate behavior on the overnight visit to the foster home prior to finalization.

Colleen worked with us in family therapy to bring issues out in the open. All twelve of us sat in the same room and talked about what was expected. We talked about how we felt about things to help us cope. But, this only made things worse. The kids acted up further. Now they knew which buttons to push. We had provisioned them in therapy with all the ammunition they needed to push us further away. Children from abusive and neglectful histories recreate the chaos with which they are comfortable.

There were no books on parenting children this disturbed. I parented from the seat of my pants and decisions were made on a moment-by-moment basis. I placed the offending child in 'boot camp.' Boot camp was located in the hallway off the living room. It was quiet and away from the commotion and I could see every movement while they stood facing the wall. They could watch TV from their positioning and it allowed them a secluded place to gain control so they could rejoin the family activities. They thought they were sneaking a peek watching TV, but I just wanted them to calm down and get themselves back under control. Most times everyone was out of boot camp in less than five minutes. Shay, however was often too stubborn to apologize or admit that she did anything wrong, as was Deangelo. Deangelo would declare a war of wills and choose to leave himself there until bedtime.

"I don't care. I won't apologize. I don't have to say sorry. I will stay here all day," either child would say. Unlike our birth children who accommodated us with a slight verbal correction, Shay and Deangelo gave into no one.

Jeannie, from across the street, helped me understand living with bipolar disorder. She had become a dear friend and support person and had a diagnosis of bipolar disorder. She listened as I poured my heart out with frustration and helped me help my tribe.

Shay had been matched with a mentor, and with Colleen and her psychiatrist's help we hung on. Shay's mentor, Edna, was the African American grandmother Shay needed. Edna shared her grandmother stories and black history with the children. Shay and Edna spent days and weekends together. Shay went to Edna's to watch TV, or just hang out. Edna took Shay to church and on outings and family gatherings. Shay had one-on-one time with someone who shared her ethnicity. Edna was the angel Shay, and I, and our family needed.

Summer was nearing and I worried about how to keep Shay busy as she did not know how to entertain herself and she was faring poorly with her siblings. In the middle of May, I spied an article in the newspaper that Mental Health had some money available for respite. I called the intake number and Shay was hooked up with Monday thru Thursday summer programming activities. Every other weekend she spent with Edna. She was busy and I hoped the extra attention lessened her crazed behavior at home. Sometimes it was good to have her out, yet other times it distanced her further from the family.

Shay spent the summer attending activities and doing things we could not afford for the other children. She taunted them with where she was going and what she got to do. Shay stole, threw tantrums and kept her huge privileges while the other kids were disciplined for their bad behaviors and they grew angry at the unfairness.

She picked fights over sibling shoe theft, only to discover later they were where she left them. She didn't need to do anything to put everyone else on edge. We never knew who did what, now her siblings were setting her up as the fall guy.

At least, when Shay was at her activities and out of the house her siblings had moments of sanity. We began to have times we felt like a 'normal' family and I overheard more than one sibling wish out loud that Shay never came home. I could hardly blame them because from the moment Shay came in the door, the air thickened with tension. The more Shay was given one day, the worse her behavior was the next. A bad day followed a good day. I came to understand the push and pull of attachment in all my newest children.

I spent countless hours transporting Shay between her therapies and programs. The summer flew by revolving around Shay's schedule. Any distraction or change of plans sent her into a tizzy.

One day my mind wandered while I waited in traffic and we were caught in the middle of a five-car pileup. I rear-ended the car ahead of me. Luckily the garbage truck behind our fifteen-passenger van avoided hitting the back of our van and only skinned the entire left side. I did not cause the accident, but if I had not been reliving the tension of the morning's battle with Shay I could have avoided participating in the pile up and gotten safely to the side. It cost seven thousand dollars to fix our van's damage and we also had to pay for the car ahead of us. For the next month we survived on one vehicle. I had to get up at 5:00 A.M. to get Jim to the hospital and then pick him up at the end of his day. This only compounded my stress level and soon I was exhausted from lack of sleep.

Because of Shay's schedule, summer activities for the other children were limited, but I did find a week of adoption camp for Shay, Deangelo, and Delonzo that was free to the adoptive family. For a whole week the Yurceks had no stealing, no fighting and no bickering. We rested, and relaxed, and worked to get our house back under control. It had been two years since I could leave my children alone in a room. It felt good to have everything cleaned and clutter free, but chaos returned as soon as Shay, Deangelo and Delonzo came home. I was looking forward to summer ending so I could do my housework and sleep again.

▼

I had learned if I did not take time for me, I could not do my job. On the days that Becca was well enough to attend school, I had peace and tranquility and some mornings I simply crawled back to bed. Once rested I filled my days with appointments, therapies, cooking, cleaning, watching, and trying to find time for something for myself.

Jim's residency kept him away from home for over 120 hours a week. Sometimes we did not see him for days and it was common for him to work thirty-six hours without sleep. By the time he came home, he was in no mood to deal with the kids' misdoings. In essence I was again in charge of the kids single handedly. Jim ate and talked with them for a few minutes and collapsed into bed. He caught up with fathering on his days off and then spent entire days learning about what was going on. He threw footballs, instigated family basketball tournaments, or curled up on Friday nights to watch a Disney movie with buckets of popcorn.

Each child needed a quiet space to share day-to-day school events and I christened the half bathroom as my office. Every moment revolved around our kids. I savored small moments of special time with each child and I held private therapy sessions in the half bath off the living room. Each child needed private time to talk about memories that haunted their dreams. I frequented the library and checked out books written on adopting hurt children, children with attachment problems, and explosive children. I used the techniques in the books to help restore order in my home and begin to teach my children to control their anger.

My children were beginning to process their grief and verbalize their losses. Finally, they were beginning to connect with their siblings and me.

Life continued on, and the craziness of our kids began to feel normal. At least, as normal as one could expect with eleven children, six of them with a variety of special needs.

Nathan was incredibly helpful. He helped me with my cooking, cleaning, watching the kids and manned the home front to give me a break as I ferried Marissa to rehearsals for the Christmas Carol. Other times, he offered to drive her and pick up Ian and DJ from basketball practice or any errand that needed running.

DJ and Ian were now inseparable. They laughed, and joked like brothers while the little boys shadowed them. With the boys bonding, our home once again had times of joy. Becca and Detamara were becoming friends. Becca and Detamara trusted each other and played together as the best of sisters. Nathan was working and Marissa was busy with school and acting. Shay liked spending time with Matt, even though Matt wasn't thrilled at the thought.

We were establishing a routine. Our homework buddies system kept homework in check. The chores were delegated and done without too much grumbling. Laundry still was a problem. Mount St. Yurcek kept erupting and most days my asthma prevented me from getting into the laundry room. I didn't have time to visit the doctors to get my inhalers refilled. The little boys decided instead of putting their laundry away, they would dump it in with the in dirty stinky socks and return it to the laundry room mountain of clothes. My pet peeve became rewashing and turning clothes right side out.

Shay continued to have problems and without sleep she was too impulsive, and could not focus. The doctor added more medications to help her sleep. After they had her moods stabilized they added another antidepressant, but she became unstable, this time with paranoia. She saw things we couldn't see. She heard things we couldn't hear. Somebody was going to steal her. She covered her window and blocked the lights during the night. Shay scared Detamara as she talked about ghosts and devils.

Detamara was now afraid to go to bed and she screamed at bedtime. Shay tried to protect Detamara by placing all her teddy bears and dolls around her to scare away the bad dreams. Shay used Mom's bad dream spray of a calming scent and water and sprayed the perimeter of her bed.

The ups and downs of Shay's nights disrupted Detamara's sleep and without sleep Detamara raged and melted down. I played another round of musical bedrooms and moved Detamara into the family room and she hauled out her portable crib with the cover we had used when we traveled to Florida. She refused to sleep in any bed without her cover for protection. Ian agreed to sleep on the couch in the family room to help Detamara feel safe. Ian became Detamara's protector and best brother.

Then one night, Ian awoke with a knife through his comforter and the backside of his t-shirt.

The evening before he and Shay had gotten into an argument over something trivial. Shay had been removing the batteries from her alarm so we could not hear her night prowling. This was the third alarm system she had outsmarted. We were running out of options. Shay stayed up all night in her room with the lights on. She swears she had not gotten out, but someone had bothered Ian.

We tried to find answers for Shay's behaviors and her psychiatrist ordered an MRI to rule out problems. The MRI discovered a pituitary adenoma. (A small tumor on her pituitary gland). That knowledge increased Shay's anxiety. In therapy, Shay revealed being abused by a boy at the Boys and Girls Club in Minneapolis when she was in foster care. In time she accused her foster brother of abusing her too, yet DJ denies it and his job was always to protect Shay.

Colleen, as a mandated reporter, had to report that information to the authorities. Shay got edgy and refused to talk about it with the police. She revealed that one of the girls in respite care was also making unwelcome advances.

We were now beginning to wonder if the stories she told were true. The more we questioned the more violent and angry Shay became. The doctor prescribed an antipsychotic. Each day we lost ground with Shay and it felt like we were hanging onto her with only the tips of our fingers.

- 38 -

IN A SHOE

After my flight down the stairs, I had found myself in the scenario of the woman who lived in a shoe. I had so many children that I didn't know what to do. I had moved Detamara from her room with Shay into the family room and placed a door alarm on the door between the two rooms. Ian guarded her by sleeping on the couch while she returned to sleeping in her covered bed where she felt safe. We were now out of compliance. The other two bedrooms held three boys each. I had no place to put Detamara. We needed an extra bedroom. The house was not big enough to handle my tribe of children.

One day I was talking to an organization that offered parent support, and I told them of my dilemma. I had to figure out how to keep everyone safely in his or her rooms and the only place we could expand was to put a room above our garage.

I knew we could not get a loan to cover the cost with eleven children and residency so I approached the Minnesota Adoption Subsidy program. They would do home modifications for children with physical disorders, but not with mental health problems. I was in a quandary about what to do.

If child protective services came in they would see we were not providing a bedroom for Detamara. I figured with making the family room her bedroom, and having Ian there, I had a good argument since it was her own space and Detamara was protected. The family room was small, and it now contained all of Detamara's girl stuff – her dolls, and dollhouse, and a highchair for her babies. It felt like the space appropriate for a little girl, but this was also where the boys hung out with their friends, and they let everyone know that 'all pink' was not cool.

The parent support group had an idea. A barn raising of sorts for the addition and a fundraising campaign. The newspaper did an article and it was launched before Christmas.

Our prayers had been answered.

The builder asked for volunteers and materials, and he set up a trust fund for anyone who wanted to help with the addition. The article quoted him to say "I'm hoping to do it in a Christmas spirit barn raising. I would like to have a large crew build it in a weekend." I trusted they knew what they were doing on a snowy January day; a crew took off the roof of our garage exposing the main part of the house and open wires. The trusses and lumber lay in the front yard ready and waiting. The next day a couple of carpenters begin to start the second story, but the weather did not cooperate. It shut down the work with 20 inches of snow.

The project was at a stand still and the roof remained off our garage. Without being there it was hard to understand our predicament and we heard comments like a doctor can afford it, take out a loan, or if they couldn't afford the kids, why did they take them in the first place?

The words hurt. We had been blindsided. We told Minnesota that we would not adopt children that put our other children at risk. We just wanted to keep them together. Colleen said the red flags were there, but no one exposed them to us and we never got complete files. When we adopted the children we were promised there were no problems to prevent the children from sharing rooms.

Spring turned the weather from ice and snow to rain.

The rafters were in, but the roof and walls were not up. Nathan tacked up plastic to help shield the rain from coming into the house. Earlier in the day we came home to a flooded dining room and two inches of water on our wood floors.

Now the water was seeping into the downstairs' family room ceiling and it was the middle of the night! I gave Nathan my cash card and he hit the all night superstore to pick up another roll of plastic sheeting, and buy a wet and dry vac.

When it rains it pours for the Yurceks, from all angles. Water was filling my house. Shay was in the hospital. Jim was working a hundred twenty hours a week. My injuries still hurt. The other kids were causing their own chaos. And now the house project went from bad to worse. The mold was triggering my asthma and I wondered if I should have built an ark instead of trying for an addition.

I needed a life preserver.

Nathan, Matt and I struggled with the plastic and I thought it was under control, but as we climbed back to bed we realized the wiring to the house was soaked and now our power was flickering and creating a fire hazard. I hit the breaker for the electricity and turned off all power to our home.

The next morning I called an electrician for advice, and was told it needed to dry out. For the next two days, we limited our electricity by only turning on breakers far from the side of the house that was wet. We ate from the freezer as quickly as we could. The kids were happy and they had never been told to 'eat anything and as much as they wanted.' The freezer in the garage remained off for several weeks and we lost hundreds of dollars of food. My children polished off dozens of boxes of frozen snacks, but even my bottomless eaters weren't up to the task of eating that much food.

The unfinished addition sat motionless and the wiring was now obsolete. I tried to figure out what to tackle first. I blew our tax refund to update the wiring, and found a contractor, but that soon fell into disaster too.

Now our entire house was flickering.

I made a panic stricken call to my father and he confirmed my thoughts that we had an overload of circuits. Once again, the power was turned off and I called for help. The new electrician explained he could not work on another's work unless I had the city electrical inspector's approval. I learned the first contractor had not taken out the electrical permit as he told us he had.

It was Friday night. I had ten children in the home and I called for emergency response to get the inspector out. That meant the fire department had to come out to the house and make a report, and then the electrical inspector could be paged for a crisis. It didn't seem like an emergency to me, but little did I know the electrical inspector would reveal that it was an unsafe situation for all of us. It was not wired properly and we were now required to leave the house.

Twelve of us would need at least two motel rooms.

The electrical contractor who answered my panicked phone call came to meet with the electrical inspector. When he heard what the power was doing in our house, he knew that he had to intervene. We were lucky the house had not already caught on fire, and my quick thinking and calls had prevented disaster. He heard the voices of the children in the background and offered his help. He worked through the night so that we could remain in our home.

The arrival of the fire fighters triggered a panic reaction in Deangelo. He was afraid of anyone in a uniform and he was old enough to remember the old family drill for authorities. His job was to get out of the home with DJ for fear of the threat of removal from their birth parents. They had been taught never to talk to anyone in uniform and never to talk to anyone from social services, schools, or mandated reporters. Uniforms and people in authority were not to be trusted.

Since we had no power, the firefighters spent time with Deangelo and they talked of sports and football reassuring my scared little nine-year-old. The firefighters watched the five younger children while I was occupied with contractors and inspectors. As the uniformed authorities left, each little kid now proudly showed off their junior firefighter badge.

The next day the electric contractor returned and I wrote a five hundred dollar check for repairs. The next month's menu would include a lot of macaroni and cheese for wheat eaters and rice and hamburger for myself and the kids who had to eat gluten free. When we moved to Michigan I hoped we never had to return to a time of not having money for food. I was mistaken. With a now empty freezer we would be out of money for groceries. I was used to cutting costs, but this addition was making it virtually impossible to pay for anything on time and there was nothing left to cut.

Spring was in bloom and the volunteer contractor returned to put up the walls and the roof. The OSB sheathing on the garage floor was now moldy and mildewed and sitting in standing water. They salvaged what they could and I was relieved when it was cleaned up and I could get my wheezing under control.

Hopefully I would no longer have to run across the street with Becca for air. I would miss the tender ridiculous moments of watching television with my neighbor Jeannie who had an oxygen tank. What a pathetic sight we were with both of us sharing oxygen and Becca attached to her feeding pump. The motley three musketeers would then spend the afternoon sharing a movie and oxygen while Becca played with the dog and the cat on the floor and eating out of her feeding tube. It wasn't exactly the old neighborly cup of tea I used to share with my neighbors in Minnesota before Becca was born. We were now sharing medical equipment.

The news channel had been alerted that the project was being resurrected in June. They talked about our family, showed workers working, and our kids playing in the backyard. The story shared the generosity of the community and the builder. We had been roofless for six months, and I finally had some hope.

My boys and Jim helped the contractor with his two person volunteer crew. A single volunteer returned to shingle the roof and my older boys made me proud though petrified as they worked twenty-five feet in the air shingling.

After a time of committed hard work, the contractor had to leave. Months later the shell of our promised bedrooms remained abandoned and my phone calls were not be returned.

Shay deteriorated as fall moved into winter.

She had a hard time facing me. I couldn't reach out to her as she enclosed herself in a shell of depression.

▼

The unfinished house was a constant reminder of the chaos of Shay's illness. The roadblocks to try to fix the addition frustrated me. I was too busy with all my children to work on it myself. Even when I tried to work, my hand could no longer grasp a hammer and my neck, still frozen in place, would not allow me to look down. Anyway, my children still needed too much supervision to allow them to do anything without Jim or another skilled adult in attendance.

My hand and arm was a continual reminder of the wrath that Shay could bring. My hand was in constant pain and each ten minutes I was required to stretch my fingers and hands to prevent them from becoming permanently fisted. My wrist no longer rotated. I felt its stiffness with each use. My vision was blurred and my lips reminded me that my face would never be the same. My neck was locked in a forward position causing headaches, and needle-like sensations to run to my fingertips. There was nothing medically available to repair the nerve damage. Medications that worked came with the added risk of addiction and limited my mental function to parent my tribe.

My health worsened as I tried to parent all the children. My energy was drained and my friend Jeannie often helped me.

Mandated therapy with Colleen to deal with my 'inappropriate' fear of Shay was a welcome respite. My biweekly therapy visits were forty dollars a month, a family therapy session added another twenty, and the ongoing therapy sessions for Delonzo and Detamara pushed our therapy costs to over a hundred dollars a month. This was all supposed to have been covered by Medicaid, but our Medicaid would not cover anything until my children were severe enough to qualify. Fires, floods, perping, rages, stealing, death threats . . . I questioned when severe was severe? Jim's insurance had limits on mental health coverage of twenty visits per year with a co-pay of twenty dollars a visit.

At Thanksgiving, Kristy and Brian helped Jim and Nathan put in the windows for the winter. They finished sealing up the unfinished walls so at least no more water could get into the house.

Everywhere I turned for help we fell into another hole. I tried to make things work minute-by-minute and hour-by-hour. I had the tenacity to hang in there for the long haul. Living with Becca's catastrophic illnesses groomed me to instant changes and frugality.

We were advised to sue the contractor. How can you sue someone for a volunteer project that was promised out of goodness? Jim and the boys kept plugging away limited resources – one box of nails and one roll of insulation at a time while we waited for spring and a miracle.

I remembered back to the days of thinking about adopting the kids, and Becca's survival. I wondered if this wasn't a test of my patience and how long this test would last. I must be a hard learner. Maybe I needed to be reminded I didn't really have any control in my life. The point was proven - all the balls I had thrown up in the air were still floating and sinking and rising and I couldn't jump high enough to figure out how to catch them. How much patience did God want me to have? I just had to trust God to provide, and remain thankful for what I had. For now, at least, we had a dry place to call home, and it was together enough so we were safe from the authorities condemning our home.

We had managed to find the money to repair the wiring; and find people to fix it, and our family miraculously still ate. If I had known that the contractor did not have all he needed to do the work I never would have let him take off the roof. We would have found another way to provide a room for Detamara, even if Jim and I slept in the living room for the remainder of residency. The contractor had tried to help, he was serious and committed and had set aside the time. We could not blame him for the weather.

We could not blame people for misunderstanding.

We would wait.

This old woman who lived in a shoe, hopefully someday would have a place to put all the children, and hopefully know what to do.

- 39 -

HOLIDAY BLESSINGS & BLUES

Shay spent Thanksgiving in her room. She remained distant and refused any type of family interaction. In early December, Jim's parents joined us and Shay held things together for the witnesses. It was a welcome relief from the day-to-day routine and chaos. She stayed home with her Grandparents while I took Becca, Detamara, Delonzo, and Marissa to see Santa at the mall. Becca had written a special letter to Santa.

Dear Santa,

I'm Becca. I'm nine-years-old. I am special. I have disabilities, because I have Noonan Syndrome. It is very hard and makes me sick a lot. I will go on my pump like I am supposed to, even though it makes me feel bad.

I will go to school even though it is very hard and noisy. Santa please tell the other kids to be nice and quiet. I don't like being called a baby. I am just very little.

It makes me feel bad. I don't want them to call me names. Will you tell them for me?

I want a white Furby very badly. She will be my friend and make me feel good. She will talk to me. I want a Holiday Beanie Bear. I want a computer to do my schoolwork on. My hands don't work.

Your friend forever,
Becca

It was her wish to hand it to him personally.

Becca truly believes in Santa and that anything is possible. There was no way possible for us to fulfill Becca's wish - that would take another Santa miracle.

At the mall, Delonzo refused to sit on Santa's lap because he did not feel well and was afraid Santa could get sick. If he got Santa sick, he figured he'd miss out on his Christmas presents.

Becca waited in her wheelchair for her turn. I placed her in Santa's lap and she handed him her letter. She was quiet when she whispered to him and I did not hear what she had said. But the tears on Santa's face gave me a clue.

He reached into his pocket and handed Becca a special bell. He told her it was only for very special little children, and to remind her that she is Santa's special child. He understood it is neither fair nor easy to be her.

I was tearing up knowing what was going on – a little girl truly believing that Santa could help with anything. My heart was breaking knowing I couldn't fulfill her wishes. When I turned around I saw the tears on the cheeks of the others who had witnessed the exchange.

As I took my daughter from his lap, Becca smiled as she accepted the coloring book. She carefully held her special bell. Becca showed such faith as she told me that Santa would fix everything.

Becca believes in miracles.

How could I tell her that neither of her miracles were going to happen? I did not know how to even fill one of the impossible requests on her list. Jim and I could never fulfill her request for a computer. Our budget was bleak. I didn't have time to find the scarce furby. They were the sold out season rage. I prayed for a miracle – that was my only hope. I knew that Becca needs hope in her life to keep up the fight against her chronic pain.

Becca proudly showed Granny her special bell while we prepared dinner. Just as we were about to sit down, I received a phone call asking for "Becca's Mom."

It was the manager of Santaland saying they wanted to help with Becca's wish. I moved into the privacy of my bathroom office and turned on the water to filter my voice. He had seen the letter and the mall wanted make Becca's Christmas wish come true. He had a lot of questions about my tiny daughter and her needs.

He told me one of the ladies behind Becca in line wanted to know what the letter contained, and she was surprised to read of Becca's request for a Furby. She had just been to Toys'R'Us and picked up two of the impossible to find toys and wanted to give a 'white one' to Becca.

I pinched myself as I got off the phone. Was I dreaming? Over the next couple of weeks, the letter circulated from store to store as they collected funds from all the employees at the mall to build a custom computer for Becca.

▼

Shay was not happy as the weeks before Christmas flew by. Something was changing and her dark dank mood affected everyone.

▼

I had a hard time keeping the secret Christmas wish.

I am the worst when it comes to secrets and Jim makes fun of me insisting that I am no better than a little kid. I had to tell someone and had shared it with Granny and Grandpa and my friend Jeannie. I wanted Becca to be surprised.

On December 23 the manager called saying that they wanted to deliver the computer Christmas Eve. I spent the next day trying to keep the kids busy. Then as dusk fell, a loud knock sent my two little boys scurrying to our front door and there right in front of them was Santa, his Elves and a camera news crew asking for Becca.

Becca jumped off the couch proclaiming she knew Santa would come! She knew it!

Santa gave Becca gifts in boxes as big as she was.

The manager of Santaland played Santa's elf to not miss out on the fun, and my kids remarked that he sure looked a lot like Al from Tool Time. The elf helpers quickly set up Becca's precious computer on the kitchen table. On the computer tower was a gold plaque inscribed "Merry Christmas Becca from the Crew at Crossroads Mall, December 1999."

The Christmas spirit was alive in my living room that evening.

Miracles can happen. This was not the first Christmas miracle in Becca's life. I remembered back to that very first Christmas and all the miracles of the season and how blessed we all have been. There is a Santa in the hearts of those who give and who make wishes and miracles happen. Christmas is the season of miracles and love. Yes, miracles do happen because of some very special Santas and angels who care.

Her Santa letter was read on TV and the reporter asked children not to see her as a baby, but as a small girl who can do anything. No longer was Becca teased for her small stature. The miracle Christmas computer became Becca's door to the world of learning.

The kids and Becca opened the rest of the gifts given by the generous employees of the mall and no one was forgotten. Happy tears and squeals of laughter surrounded us. I will never forget the miracles of that Christmas and Becca hugging her Santa.

But Dad missed out on the fun, he was on call that Christmas Eve. He was preoccupied and missed the newscast while working in the emergency room.

Jim came home shortly before dinner and told me of his Christmas Eve. He had a young black teen that had aged out of the foster care system come into the emergency room by ambulance. He had no home for Christmas; he had lost his family, and no one to call family. He had tried to commit suicide on the freeway and was hit by an oncoming semi and survived. Jim told me he reminded him of DJ, and that is why it is so important for these older kids to have a family forever. We may not have much time with DJ, but we were someone to come home to, to bring his children to, and to share in the good times and the bad. DJ had a connection to his past and a place to call home. Looking at our kind handsome son, Jim and I realized DJ was lucky he was adopted as a teen when so many others sat aging out of the foster care system. We were thankful we had kept most of his family together.

This was our third Christmas together building new holiday traditions. We drove out into the night for a Christmas light after dinner ride and tucked happy and contented children into bed with sweet dreams.

Christmas Day was full of our kids, gifts, and our smorgasbord dinner, while Becca sat for hours playing and learning on her new computer.

Within a couple of days, the holiday blues returned. The kids mourned Christmases of the past. They missed their parents and their brother and Shay was having an exceptionally hard time. The happier we all were, the more she tried to undermine the happiness. I became afraid of too much happiness and we tried to keep things quieted down. At any sign of laughter, Shay erupted. Unless she was happy, we were not allowed to be happy or we paid a secret nasty price. Her stealing increased. She raged and brought her violence and temper tantrums out of her room and into our living areas to get her siblings to react.

One day, Shay announced she smelled smoke coming from the downstairs bathroom. I met a stunned Delonzo coming out of the door. The smoke came from the vanity under the sink. Running to check underneath, I soon discovered a burnt tissue box with smoldering embers. Whoever did it had wet the box to extinguish the fire, but the dry tissues underneath continue to try to ignite from the embers. I threw the whole box in the toilet, grabbed the wastebasket and filled it with water from the tub and doused the remaining flames. Delonzo pointed his finger at Shay and Shay said Delonzo did it. I quizzed them, but never discovered the real culprit.

As the stealing increased I enacted a version of "Peoples Court." The living room became our courtroom. We gathered evidence and marked it as Exhibit A and Exhibit B and so on. The accused offender was assigned a defense attorney. A judge was appointed and we selected the jury. It was definitely a jury of their peers. The bailiff read the offender his rights as they swore on top of the family bibles; *The Bible* and the book *Adopting the Hurt Child* by Gregory Keck.

We drew the name of the defense attorney from a hat; no one wanted to have the job of defending the guilty. By the end of the court session, the child understood that it wasn't mean Mom and Dad handing down the sentence, but a jury of their own peers. The family court episodes seemed to make an impact and slowed the stealing.

'Just the facts,' I felt like Detective Friday on Dragnet. Most evidence pointed at Shay. I knew her siblings could set her up as the fall guy and there were a number of instances I still do not know who did what to whom.

The knives and acting out behaviors escalated. Her tantrums were now bizarre. One day she was screaming in her room saying she was 'shooting squirrels' and seemed to be reenacting the recently watched Patch Adams movie. Another day she broke her door down during a rage and chased me with a three foot piece of door frame she had broken off the wall when she pulled the door down. The piece came to a point, and she came after me with the dagger yelling that she was going to kill the vampire and was going to put the stake through my heart. Ian and DJ grabbed her, tackled her and then carried her to her bed. They held her there until she settled down. Then they let her go and she escalated and came after me once again. This time saying she was going to bite off my ear like Mike Tyson. The boys grabbed her as she came toward my ear.

After most of these episodes she'd fall asleep. Other times she stared off into space unaware of what was going on around her. Most of her tantrums lasted less than an hour and things went quickly from bad to worse. We thought she needed to go to the hospital, but we couldn't get her there safely. Besides, by the time we arrived everything would seem all right.

We scheduled more therapy and another doctor appointment.

Then one day I let Shay out of my sight to go to her room to get a book. Soon Becca was screaming. Shay had grabbed her by the neck because she wanted to change the television channel. Becca was ten-years-old, barely 40 lbs. and the size of a tiny four-year-old. Shay's finger marks were bright red on Becca's neck and turning to dark bruises. I told Shay to get back upstairs when she began throwing whatever she could grab. She began banging her head in extreme anger. Afraid she would hurt herself; Jim had no choice but to restrain her.

Shay seemed to understand that she needed the help. After she settled down, we told her we were taking her to the emergency room. We had no choice but to admit her this time. She was not safe to remain at home. We were met by the social worker who had few options. Shay was now sullen and withdrawn while we filled out admittance paperwork.

After the ER docs reviewed the records, they recommended Shay needed long-term care. It appeared these recommendations were already in place during her previous admission. Her medical records stated that Shay may need an out-of-home placement but our insurance was running out and no one told us of the guarded prognosis. It was the middle of the night just after Christmas and the psychiatric hospital beds were full. The doctors found her a bed in a hospital thirty minutes from our home and transported Shay by ambulance. Jim and I followed the ambulance to meet Shay and we spent the rest of the night filling out mountains of paperwork to admit her to the unit.

The intake disclosed that Shay had thoughts of hurting Jim, myself, and her siblings. She also wanted to hurt herself and she would use anything to make it happen. We could not bring her home.

If Shay's diagnosis of Bi Polar and Fetal Alcohol Syndrome were true, she would need intense help to learn to manage her behavior. Complicated with reactive attachment disorder, she may never attach to the family ever.

Shay told her best friend and staff that we refused to bring her clothes and her stuffed animals. We brought what she asked for but she told us they were now the wrong ones. I received a phone call from Shay's one and only friend who was being raised by her grandparents. The two girls had common histories that had brought them together. Both birth mothers had substance abuse and mental health problems. Shay's friend had been shaken by a phone call she received from Shay and she told me of the changes she had noticed. She was scared Shay was hurting herself at the hospital. I convinced her to write a letter to us to help Shay.

Shay's best friend's letter confirmed the things I was seeing.

She wrote "For the past two months Shay has been hurt and not feeling like she belongs on this earth. She started talking about death. Coming from a person who was suicidal and was very depressed, I strongly feel that Shay has made it to the stage where she will try to kill herself."

Desiree closed her four-page letter with "The girl I knew is not there any more She is really depressed. There is a girl who is really nice and sweet who is my best friend, but that girl I talked to that night at the hospital was a totally different person."

The girl's grandmother asked that we make sure that Shay would not call her again.

Shay's last and only friend had been driven away.

The news that Shay wanted to hurt me again sent shivers up my spine. I became afraid to visit Shay alone and Jim or Edna accompanied me to the hospital. Yet, Shay acted as if nothing was the matter.

We were told that kids like Shay need intense help and it may take two years or more for her to be able to learn to control herself. They warned us to be prepared that it may never happen, Shay may be too disturbed.

What had we gotten ourselves into?

What was Shay's future?

- 40 -

REPEAT, REPEAT, REPEAT

As the kids settled in, I discovered my new children did not learn like my others. They seemed to forget everything. I would send someone out to the garage to bring in a bag of corn, and French fries returned. I learned to go over what I wanted the kids to 'get or do,' and then ask them to repeat back to me what they were to 'do or get.' Even with the repetition more often than not, the mission was never completed.

I'd tell Delonzo to take a shower, and soon he'd be sitting in front of the television watching his favorite cartoons. I'd ask him where he was supposed to be?

He'd reply, "I don't know."

For a long time I thought these responses were excuses, but in time I learned when any of my new children answered, "I don't know" they were telling the truth.

They forgot.

They forgot everything, including something they had told me two minutes earlier. My new kids did not remember what just happened. I was baffled. One day they were able to do something they had practiced, the next it was completely forgotten.

How could my kids do something well one day and completely forget how to do it the next day and then a few days later be able to do it again?

I taught day in and day out.

Repeating the lesson, re-explaining to the children why we do this, re-teaching why we do not do this? They wrote sentences for inappropriate behaviors. Some days my discipline brought on a tirade, other days they were cooperative and finished their sentences or wrote their apology letter in record time.

If only they'd understand my simple routines, life could be much quieter and the house could magically return to order. I kept trying to get them programmed into a rhythm of structure. But if I left the room, chaos followed. It appeared that without a monitor my children were unable to control their behaviors. I soon learned to leave Nathan or Marissa in charge while I went downstairs to start laundry or go to the bathroom. As long as someone was in charge, the room remained calm. What went on when I was out of sight or earshot was another story.

My repetition drove Jim crazy. He found fault in my redundancy over trivial things our other kids picked up by osmosis. I felt like a broken record and I frustrated Marissa who learned everything the first time. She couldn't handle the 'stuckness' of everything. She'd run to her room, or wander around the house with her headphones and CD player turned on to tune out the ever-repeating instructions. She took on performances for three plays at one time to keep busy.

Yet my new children seemed to thrive on the very 'stuckness' that drove Jim, Marissa, Nathan, and Matt crazy, especially if my repeat method washed over into their lives.

Deangelo only took two to five times to get it.

DJ just needed two or three prompts to start.

Detamara started at me with confused eyes, but once everyone else got moving, she watched vigilantly to copy their actions, and soon she was participating in the activity or helping clean up the room. Delonzo seemed glued and it took the boys to physically unstick him. Then once he started he'd sneak off to bed and sleep while everyone else cleaned or got dinner on the table.

It didn't make sense. This was more than attachment issues or trauma experiences or my children growing in up poverty.

With Becca's new computer I discovered an Internet support group and found that other adoptive parents were dealing with the same thing. I had enough history from DJ and Shay to know that their mother struggled with drugs and alcohol. DJ talked about his mother drinking while pregnant with Delonzo, DeShawn and Detamara.

Many years ago I had read the book by Michael Dorris called *The Broken Cord*. Was I dealing with the same thing?

Could it be possible all my new children had Fetal Alcohol Spectrum Disorders (FASDs)?

Naming it, opened the door to knowledge, to solutions and power to get appropriate help so they could be successful. Dr. Bui questioned that Shay had the disorder. In further reading, I realized probably all my new children's brains were injured before they were even born and I couldn't change the damage they had, but I could change me and the environment and learn how to help them.

My mom did an excellent job reprogramming my siblings. She learned techniques to help my wild little sister who was exhausting her and in constant motion. She needed to find something to channel that incredible energy and brightness. With mom's strategies my sister calmed and began reading at age two! My little brother was born in the early 1970's and mom went into labor at five months and they used alcohol IV's to stop it. My brother had been born with Dyslexia and learning difficulties and he didn't really start talking until he was almost three. My mother never drank. Could the alcohol the doctors have given her caused his struggles? My mom had worked hard to help him gain skills and thirty years later my brother is an engineer, a fine father and caring husband. Becca had coded twice and she was now learning and growing and a very much alive little girl. I knew the brain could change. I listened and learned from seasoned foster and adoptive parents whose strategies seemed to help my children become more successful.

They challenged me to change my paradigm from trying harder to trying different and it worked. The ideas weren't at all like I had parented my birth children, but as I tried them my frustrations lessened. The more I learned about FASDs, the more I realized that the dreams I held for my children to achieve were bleak . . .unemployment for persons with disabilities was at seventy-five percent . . . sixty percent of people in our prisons are thought to have fetal alcohol . . . ninety percent need mental health services.

I wanted to cry, and stomp, and meltdown myself. I vowed to not have my children become those lost souls in the statistics. I had to get help for them!

I told Colleen about what I had discovered. I learned that dealing with FASDs the early years makes the biggest difference. I dug through Detamara's file at the school and found a note from the early intervention specialist that the foster parent asked if Detamara had Fetal Alcohol Syndrome when she was barely two. Now at nine, we were finally getting the long awaited diagnosis.

Detamara was struggling so hard in school and she wanted to learn! In kindergarten she threw temper tantrums because she did not have homework like the bigger kids. I had to assign her 'homework' each night and the tantrums ceased.

Now she hated school. Detamara forgot her memorized addition problems when the class moved on to subtraction and lost both addition and subtraction memorization when the class moved into multiplication. Division soon replaced multiplication, addition and subtraction. Detamara cannot understand much of what is said to her and she couldn't keep up.

I had learned to speak slowly, carefully, and check for level of understanding each time I talked with her. When I did, she understood and complied.

Repeat, repeat, and repeat! Marissa kept on her headset!

Flash cards, manipulatives, and letting my children "cheat" with a calculator saved their math facts. Repeat, repeat and repeat, Detamara finally gained basic math skills. DJ rarely got them so he used the 'assistive technology' of a calculator and Delonzo could do algebra and forgets his multiplication tables.

We used our insurance and got a referral for a neuropsychological exam to learn understand Detamara's strengths and weaknesses and know how she learns.

We discovered Detamara had an Auditory Processing Disorder (ADP), common to many children with FASDs. Even though she could hear fine, she had trouble understanding what others told her. Now it made sense. That was why she was carefully watching what everyone else was doing. She told us that is 'how come' she watches the other students to see what page they turn to, and which problems they do. That's why she is so quiet when the teacher calls on her to answer a question.

I changed my frame of reference to discover tools to help my children. I wear glasses – they assist me to see better and if I were totally blind I wouldn't need such silly contraptions. If I were blind, electric lights could be considered assistive technology for the sighted. Becca needed a computer because her hands didn't work. She had needed oxygen as a baby to breath and a feeding pump in her stomach to eat. Little Kim from my old daycare with Spina Bifida needed a wheelchair to walk. So what if Delonzo needed a calculator because a certain part of his brain worked differently!

I was not afraid of assistive technology.

The next thing I discovered was that what they knew one moment evaporated the next. If I taught my child in her slippers, at the kitchen table, when my child moved into the classroom, and left her slippers in her bedroom, she also left her spelling knowledge there too. My kids had perfect recall in one area and not the next. I learned I had to repeat the teaching in multiple environments; in the car, in my home and in the schoolroom were all different places.

My new children did well when they were surrounded by firm structure, loving support and a safety net. They seemed to live in the present and have little knowledge of time, money, or sequencing. I learned when the routine or plans changed; I could expect not just one meltdown, but five! I began preparing them for transitions – we are doing 'this' today. Then a fifteen-minute warning . . . ten-minute warning . . . then a five-minute warning, and finally verbal prompts to coax them on to the next thing.

It drove Marissa crazy and she wished I'd just say it once and leave well enough alone.

I learned when I backed off they failed.

Jim enjoyed roughhousing with 'his boys' and soon learned that if he wired up his new set of kids he couldn't settle them down. He learned that if he bumped someone, the next day the child told another 'Dad, hit me.' We learned that if a kid tripped over a shoe I left on the floor, 'Mom, tripped me', even though I had been in the next room when the child fell over. What happened and what they said happened were two very different things.

It didn't matter that they ate us out of house and home, if the dinner served wasn't what they hoped for, they forgot they had eaten and told a friend, "I didn't get dinner tonight."

I had to do much of my parenting very differently for my new children and it exasperated my first set of kids who thought I was too easy on the 'misbehaving' ones.

When something was missing and someone had 'stolen' it they denied it and said they only 'found' it. We made a rule that anything you 'find' cannot come in our house. I sewed pants pockets shut to ground them from putting anything in them. I instigated 'Ground Zero' which meant the offending child didn't have the right to do anything without me until they worked their way back to privileges.

Delonzo asked us why we didn't keep our promises. The social worker had told him "we were going to be his forever family and he was going to have fun."

We tried to explain that it's not always fun in a family and being in a family took work. Work and fun were very different in his understanding. The world my children lived in was crystal clear - yes and no, black and white, on and off - and the middle ground of communication confused them.

I learned from other foster and adoptive parents that children with FASDs can succeed, but as expectations increase they begin to fall. I determined not to let that happen to my children. I am on guard 24 hours a day, seven days a week, for Becca's medical condition so I learned I to be on guard 24 hours a day, seven days a week to intervene and supervise my five children with FASDs to keep them safe from their behaviors.

I allow them to do things by themselves, but I realized due to their brain injuries they couldn't monitor themselves all the time. They have off days and off hours and I must be ever present to prompt, encourage and provide a safety net.

I worry that something bad will happen when one of my children melts down. My children pay the price and fall backwards when educational, judicial and mental health systems do not understand their brain damage and exceptional needs. I pick up the pieces after lack of understanding or support causes my kids to lose it. I worry about my children's first words after getting caught. The initial reaction is to take the focus off them and when they are fearful or angry, they can easily make untrue allegations that ripple through communities and families. They seemed to have no understanding of cause and effect.

I had been threatened early on when asking for help for one of the kids, that if I pushed too hard, they would just take them all back as I was not equipped to handle them. So I persevered without files or paperwork on the children.

I began 'really' knowing and understanding their severe needs and finding ways to help them myself. Detamara's assessment opened our eyes. Further research into FASDs and years of living and parenting my children made me believe we were dealing with organic issues built into the minds of my children.

To help my children I had to learn to do what was in their best interest, despite being labeled, branded, sanctioned for being overprotective, not allowing my children freedom, or whatever the behavior they faulted me for. I was warned that professionals often construe this as overprotective and since I had always worried about what people thought about me, this was a big lesson.

I learned it was okay to have thick skin, but I also had a healthy fear of child protection.

- 41 -
PINBALL

It was fourteen months since my accident down the staircase and we could not protect Shay from herself. The hospital recommended a long-term placement. When we adopted the kids, we were promised that Medicaid would cover medical and mental health costs for whatever our insurance would not pay. This was spelled out in our adoption contract. Little did I know that we were now on our way to a long and drawn out arcade game with our family as the pinball. Shay bounced from here to there and back again to find help. We were in a new game we had never played and didn't have a rulebook

Somehow we had gotten thrown into a fiscal tournament and we were out of our league to help Shay. Shay had talked about wanting to hurt herself and the family, especially me. If we brought her home, and something happened, we could be charged with failing to protect the other children in the home. I had been warned the next time something bad happened, we might not be so lucky. Shay, at 170 lbs., was strong and muscular. When enraged, she was too strong for any one of us to handle, including my husband and he was rarely home. Jim and I met with Colleen to discuss the close call with Becca and we all agreed, medically fragile Becca was at risk and the other kids did not need the chaos of Shay's deteriorating condition. We couldn't let anyone else be hurt. I already had been disabled by the wrath of her illness.

Shay was discharged from the hospital to a crisis respite placement about an hour from home. It was a crisis residential setting with an onsite school. Each placement forced me to relive the sordid story again to new professionals in Shay's life. I should have recorded it or had it transcribed. Each retelling opened emotional wounds and left me shell-shocked. Jeannie joined me and stayed with Shay while I filled out the mountain of intake paperwork for the residential treatment center (RTC).

I was shocked as I walked through the unit to the office. It seemed chaotic and disorganized. The hallways were cluttered with kids' belongings everywhere. I tried not to gag from the stench of body odor, urine, deodorant and cologne. The childcare office was locked, as were all the other doors on the way. Teen girls screamed and overreacted. The young ladies looked lost and abandoned.

I wondered how could you have control without structure?

The RTC psychologist confirmed what I had already been told at the hospital in Battle Creek. Shay's road to recovery would be long. He warned me that I would have to fight hard to get what Shay needed. He knew of only two others who had won the battle we were destined to fight.

It seemed a curious statement and I had no idea what he meant. Shay hung close to the staff, Jeannie told me Shay seemed afraid of this place and the other girls. Yet I knew I could not bring her home, as we could not stop her from hurting herself or the others. After the paperwork was done, I got the contact phone numbers. Shay gave me a stiff hug and walked away.

While Shay was at the crisis RTC I met with the head of the Mental Health's Children's services manager. I had been advised to not meet with her alone so I invited a friend who sat on the community mental health board to join our meeting.

The services manager said they could authorize six to eight months of care for Shay. Then we would have to bring her home and work through her issues. She also told me that with her diagnosis of

Reactive Attachment Disorder (RAD) when she came home, her behavior might be rougher before it ever got better. We should expect her to test us. This time the ante would be higher. Shay knew how to escape from our home and she would be mad at us for "locking her up."

I asked for another meeting to discuss residential care and present recommendations from Colleen and Shay's psychologist and psychiatrist. The services manager sent one of her behavior therapists to sit in for her. The behavior therapist told Jim and I that many parents in similar circumstances choose to disrupt the adoption to get help for their children.

We told her of the recommendations of six to eight months of care did not match the differing second, third and fourth opinions of long-term placement with a connection to her family.

She told us we were asking for something that did not exist. They do not pay for residential placement, they only pay for home and community based services.

Luckily Shay acted out in RTC and they realized it was dangerous for her to return her home. They had to find another placement until we could figure out what to do. The only placement they could find was to have Shay return to Kalamazoo and be placed in a shelter for runaway teens.

Once again I rehashed the story, reliving the pain and trauma of the recent past. The more I told the story, the more I felt like a failure. We were judged wherever we went. We were good enough to adopt, but now that things were falling apart, fingers pointed and heads shook that we jumped in way over our heads.

Jim and I were confused.

What more could we do?

We had pinballed from hero to scapegoat.

The runaway shelter was close to home, but the teens were street-smart. It was not the place I wanted my mentally challenged and severely disturbed daughter. Shay for the most part functioned at a young elementary age child. I had learned from my research that kids with FASDs need to be protected from negative influences. Shay mimicked others behaviors, both good and bad. For two weeks, her new housemates, a mixture of males and females, introduced her to a whole new spectrum of challenges. She was learning behaviors that made it increasingly impossible to return home.

I met with the program to discuss what to do about Shay. Jim fervently studied for his Absite exams, the measurement for surgery residents. His schedule was exhausting and mental health was making demands we thought incredulous. Jim snapped at me as I relayed more bad news from the program. As the bearer of bad news, I got the brunt of his venting.

My hands were filled with my children's needs; Becca required watching, and medical cares while Detamara and Delonzo acted like three-year-olds, constantly getting into trouble and creating disasters. Ian and DJ needed guidance, homework reminders and grounding. Nathan was in his first year of college and working full time so I lost my taxi driver and chief cook.

Colleen and the psychiatrists convinced Community Mental Health we could not bring Shay home until we knew what she needed, the exact diagnosis of disorders and her treatments stabilized. Somehow they made arrangements for her to be sent to the only state run children's psychiatric hospital in Michigan. Hawthorne Center was about two and a half hours away in a Detroit suburb, but currently had no open beds. We needed a powerful angel to help us open the doors.

On February 16, 2000, a month and ten days after Shay blew out of our home, she moved into Hawthorne.

▼

The hospital looked like a large brick college building, with several wings. A desolate basketball court with dead weeds that popped through the melting snow was the only sign that children may live there. It was off by itself and the trees surrounding it projected a park-like appearance in the glistening snow. From the road, no one would know it was a hospital.

Jim and I, and Becca and Shay entered the building. This time there was even more paperwork. Shay appeared unaffected by this sudden move. She seemed to enjoy the trip and eating fast food. It was hard to understand her blasé attitude. Perhaps because she had moved so many times, this felt comfortable or maybe she had to dis-associate to protect herself from feeling pain and rejection.

I retold my story of my flight down the stairs. My body quivered and I tried not to become too emotional. I held back my tears and tried to quiet my trauma as a victim of secondary trauma. In time I learned I was not alone and that parents and families who adopt these severely disturbed children may become victims of the same trauma that was present in the adopted child's birth home.

We met her new therapist and a new doctor. The doctor told us that we had a long journey ahead. They asked where we thought she should go after discharge?

Jim and I checked the box indicating recommendations for long-term care and a placement with 24/7 supports. Most families check the box home, fearing they will be nailed for abandonment. That one tiny checkmark saved us from hanging when Community Mental Health refused to pay for Shay's treatment later. On the other hand it could have sent us down the very real path of being nailed for abandonment for not wanting her to come home.

He told us long-term care and 24/7 supports was incredibly hard to get and we may have to go to huge lengths to make it happen. I asked if this was achievable? He told me only a person or two had ever won the battle I had to face. He knew of no one winning the battle in the past few years, since closing psychiatric hospitals was the current trend, and support in the community is considered the least restrictive placement.

What was I to do?

We toured the unit with Shay; the place was much cleaner than the crisis residential. The long desolate hallways were empty of children. The only sign of kids was on the unit. The children were orderly; the noise was not chaotic. There were locks, locks and more locks. Every door had to have someone let us in.

Were we in a hospital or a jail? The two seemed the same.

After the tour it was time for us to leave and I hugged Shay goodbye. She turned away and skipped off with her new staff. She did not look back and appeared happy to be going to dinner.

I spent the drive time home wondering why and how we had gotten to here?

Our lives felt as though they had fallen apart, the dream of the family we had tried to help was shattering.

DeShawn.
Now Shay.
Both had to leave our home.
I wondered what I could have done differently?
What didn't I understand?

I was glad Jim was driving back to Kalamazoo. My head was spinning, and my heart was heavy. There was little hope for my new daughter. Every place Shay had pinballed to have the same bleak prognosis – she may not get better and she could not attach. Now, someone had pulled the plunger on the pinball machine and we were in a new game.

Shay needed to get help and no one knew how to help her.
She needed a guardian angel.

My dream of a forever family grew dimmer.

- 42 -

SURVIVING

Shay had now been at Hawthorne for almost a year and I had trekked five hours each month to visit her. Sometimes just Becca and myself visited, other times Jim joined us. As time went on I brought the other children, all except DJ who refused to come. DJ, Shay's older biological brother had been alongside her through foster care, but he abandoned her in the state hospital. All month Shay waited excited about our visit, then when it arrived, she bounced all over the fast food restaurant and sat at a table off by herself. The other kids were confused by her behavior and it didn't make sense that she wanted to see them, but not sit with them? Was it possible to build back unity? How do you parent and run your family when you have a child in a psychiatric hospital? Where is the normalcy in that?

I worked with Shay's therapist to help Shay see how her behavior affected others. After months of rehearsals Shay begin to sit with the family and act more appropriately. She also began to carry on short conversations and ask the other kids questions about their interests. We journeyed as a family for her birthday and celebrated together by splurging at a sit down Mexican restaurant. Shay beamed with happiness we had not seen for a long time.

Each visit was costly as we resupplied Shay's lost clothing and personal care products. Her clothing ripped, or was lost, or became too small. She lost her shoes. She lost her winter coat. The laundry lost many of her tagged clothing and she was constantly short on socks and underwear. When Shay went into placement, we lost much of her already meager subsidy and the difficulty of care expense stopped. What we received was a drop in the bucket to what she cost, even when she was not living under our roof. The damage Shay had done to our home was left unrepaired. We boarded up the broken window, we epoxied the broken toilet tank cover, tore up the carpet, and we filled the holes in the walls. These were only band-aids and everywhere we looked our house screamed at us from the trauma of living with Shay's illness and our other children not knowing how to care for anything.

The unfinished addition was a constant reminder of the wrath of Shay's mental health issues. If Shay returned home, we needed that bedroom to separate Shay from Detamara. Our home sat unfinished. Jim added a few more meager pieces of insulation to the unfinished garage addition.

To follow the ultimatum given to us by Community Mental Health, I contacted attorneys. Estimates ranged from ten to fifty thousand dollars to fight the charges. If we were charged, Jim's medical license would be suspended and our names placed on the national abuse and neglect registry checked nationwide. We could lose another job due to a daughter's need for care. One attorney told me that there was nothing I could do until they charged us with something. Then it would cost us thousands of dollars, to clear our names. We would have to prove ourselves not guilty if we were charged with medical and mental health neglect because we could not keep her safely in our home. Just like with Becca's million dollars in health care bills, Shay's mental health needs could cost us everything.

The only place I could find money to hire a lawyer was to take it from the car payment. I used that van money to search for a lawyer to follow the rules imposed on us by the Mental Health Supervisor. Within months we were in repossession of our broken down minivan and we were down to our fifteen-passenger gas-guzzler.

President Clinton had appealed to the American public to help a child from the foster care system. We had done it six times over and reunited five siblings together into a family. We had added them to our own. We had provided for everything she needed, food, shelter, clothing, and a family. And now we were being charged with not being able to provide the monies or therapies for our daughter's catastrophic mental health care.

We stood in no man's land. We were failed by Minnesota and their promised support for the post placement of the children, and the State of Michigan refusing to honor the post adoption support promised to federally funded foster children.

We were guilty, for being too poor or naive to believe the promises made to us when we adopted the kids.

Jim's residency hours increased from one hundred twenty to one hundred forty hours a week and on this one weekend day we drove to see Shay, the other he slept.

The path Jim and I were on between residency and Shay's illness placed us at a fork in the road. We had little time to talk. The house was in chaos and when I tried trying to explain the demands of mental health on us, he couldn't believe it and got angry.

I listened to him vent, but it made me feel like he was attacking me for bringing him news that he did not want to hear. Sometimes I wondered if he blamed me for our broken dreams.

Jim distanced himself from me. He remained good with the children, and spent each spare minute between books and work, with them. In the medical world Jim was surrounded by rules and regulations, and protocols and procedures that had to be adhered to with utmost care. To him, the world of mental health was absurd and the things I told him seemed ridiculous. In medicine errors this big would cost lives, where was the preventative care? Where was the established triage team? What was the continuum of care in the 'fail first' mentality of mental health?

I felt lonely and responsible. I had no answers.

I was the one who wanted to help children who needed a home.

Isolated, Jeannie was my gift and I came to rely more on my best friend from across the street. She was a mother of three teens and had bipolar disorder, severe asthma and an immune deficiency like Becca. For years she had been buried in her home afraid of the germs of the real world and then she fell in love with Becca.

If Becca could go out and challenge the world, Jeannie would try. Jeannie became my respite care provider for the children. She sat beside me and quietly listened when things got tough. She told me what I needed to hear, even when I didn't want to hear it. Jeannie was there when I needed her and I was there when she needed me. We pulled through together. I had found a best friend in my loneliness.

Jeannie witnessed Mental Health's demands, they later denied. Jeannie explained Shay's bi-polar from the inside out. Jeannie recognized things in Shay early and became my safety net in crisis planning. She spent the summer supporting me and for the first time in years she ventured out making a trip to California to visit extended family. Jeannie knew her asthma could kill her and more than once I transported her to urgent care for a severe asthma attack.

The last time she requested no ambulance because she didn't want to be intubated again and I ran red lights to meet Jim and the emergency room crew. The ER doc had never seen such a bad attack.

My best friend was living on borrowed time and she asked me to be there for her family and help them cope just as she had been there for me.

How could I bury my best friend?

I hoped the time would be long in coming, but it wasn't.

Jeannie's health worsened. I wanted to take her to the doctor, but she said she was all right. We argued and there was nothing I could do to change her mind. She had been wheezing all day.

That evening she called me to say she was doing fine. She had just talked to her daughter Shannon who away at her first year of college and they had talked about their relationship being stronger and mending. Shannon had faulted her mother for her lost years of childhood of managing her sister and brother when her mother could not do it. Everyone noted that Jeannie had changed and was finally happy.

Jeannie believed she came for a purpose and her time was soon ending. She came to be my friend and help me on this journey and in return Becca and I gave her newfound freedom and peace. That evening her breathing sounded relaxed. The next morning, after the children left for school and I was alone with Becca when I called Jeannie at 9:00 A.M. like usual and her husband Scott answered and I sensed something was wrong. Scott told me that Jeannie passed away during the night. She had collapsed after going to the bathroom, and the paramedics could not revive her. She strangled to death by blocked airways.

Gasping for air, my friend died?

I was paralyzed by the news.

I went to check on Becca and without me saying a word; Becca awoke in a panic I have never seen in her before. She told me that Jeannie had died. She was sobbing from grief and big alligator tears rolled down her cheeks as she reached out to hug me. I asked her how she knew and she told me that Jeannie had come to her during the night. Jeannie had told her she was leaving and Becca was to take care of Mom for her and remember the angels!

Two days before her death she reminded me that she needed to get a necklace chain for the Austrian crystal angel I had given her. The chain had broken.

▼

Jeannie was a firm believer that God has a purpose for all of us. She had recently told me that all things happen for a reason and Becca had come to change her life. She was thankful for the life she was given back. Becca, Jeannie and I had spent the last two years together. She told me my mission was being fulfilled each day, and that my mission required much of my guardian angel that often worked overtime to protect me. She laughed as she told me I was so much trouble I really needed two angels and even then they would be pressed to keep me safe. I needed one to protect my front side and the other my backside. Evil had to work overtime to fight the successes or supports I needed to find to help my children heal.

I laughed and told Jeannie I was working moment by moment to steal back from the hurt and evil they knew so well. My weapon was Love. My children did not understand love, and safety, and security. Those felt foreign and uncomfortable to them, so they fought love, and safety, and security; while I fought back for their hearts and souls. I promised Jeannie, I didn't care where or how much I had to fight, or how badly I'd be beaten down. I would keep on fighting. Jeannie had held me up in that fight like Aaron held up Moses even if it meant fighting at the state hospital. Now my best friend was gone and I fought alone.

▼

Scott asked me to help him find clothes for Jeannie to take to the funeral home. Walking into her room waves of memories flooded back. I walked up to her now empty bed and looked at the empty oxygen canula on her pillow. The sunlight caught a reflection that glistened a little rainbow on the wall.

The crystal angel I had bought Jeannie danced in glorious colors on her wall. Jeannie had brought the miracle of an angel to let me know that I was not alone. She was there, right behind me, my much-needed guardian angel to protect my backside.

I took the angel from the bed stand table and placed it alongside my identical crystal angel on my necklace. Now two angels hung on my chain, reminding me of the two angels guarding me on whatever mission I was called.

I made a promise to Jeannie to take care of things.

Scott got her large family here for the funeral. I had to support her siblings and answer their questions of the changed Jeannie. I told them of how much they all meant to her. I cried with Shannon and tried to help thirteen-year-old Shellie cope, she was too young to lose her mother and my heart broke for her.

The funeral at the Catholic Church was packed with the friends, family, and kids who knew Jeannie and I knew I was to speak. I stood and talked of my friend and companion. I spoke of her kind heart to comfort friends and family. I said a prayer and asked God to help me. The perfect words came without thinking. I thought of the words on the plaque that Jeannie had given me, the footprints story.

God wasn't walking beside me; he carried me through burying my Jeannie, my best friend. I had overcome my fear of public speaking. I looked down at my two crystal angels.

Jeanne Marie Sheldon died November 17, 2000.

▼

Somehow things were magically being taken care, and I wondered if Jeannie had anything to do with it.

Thanksgiving introduced the holiday season and the beginning of the new Yurcek traditions. On Christmas Deangelo announced that the US Marines were at our door.

One of the kids remarked that the authorities were there to take Delonzo to boot camp for stealing. They had come with a mission to deliver my children's Christmas toys. The older boys laughed at their off humor. The local church provided brand new bicycles to replace the now broken ones for children in need of a miracle. Jim had told our first set of children that we would pay for their first wheels and from then on it was their job to keep them in good condition. Matt rearranged and rebuilt everything he owned and his bike never staying looking the same way for very long, but was just the way he liked it. The others kids kept theirs carefully the same.

We were able to borrow money to finish the addition, and I worked with the city planner to cut costs and our house was now out of code compliance. We were no longer 'new' construction so we qualified for help. Our county commissioner joined forces, along with a small advocacy organization for persons with handicaps. Habitat for Humanity sent a couple volunteers, we found a furnace for half-price and a donated central air conditioner for Becca. Every contractor cut the cost of their services when they heard about the dilemma of our family with our new children and we snuck under the loan ceiling.

We were on our way to finishing our long abandoned addition. If we had to bring Shay home, we would have room enough for everyone. The woman in the 'shoe' would soon have three more bedrooms, space to spread out and storage to boot to keep everyone safe.

- 43 -
QUESTIONS

Home was a different place with Shay at Hawthorne. She was getting help. With a heavy sigh of relief I calculated the emotional toll one child had cost her family. We didn't realize how insane our lives had become. Shay was safe and the tension evaporated. I had been hypervigilent to avert crisis. The energy I expended had paid off with moments of calm I thought were normal, but my watchfulness couldn't ward off everything and with a flip of an invisible switch Shay could twist her siblings into tornados and smile as they spun out. Everyone could now put his or her PTSD (Post Traumatic Stress Disorder) radar systems on the low idle. Finally, I did not need to worry about Shay hurting herself or her family.

But I had a new parenting challenge. There was no book to tell me how to parent a child in residential treatment.

- How do I parent a child long distance in a psychiatric hospital?
- How should I act at her meetings?
- How do I explain and cope with everyone's judgments?
- What responsibilities do I have and how much authority did I have in the treatment-planning meeting?
- What about the IEP at the hospital school?

Jim and I had asked Hawthorne at Shay's entrance for workups to understand what we were dealing with. Her psychiatrist wanted her to see a neurologist and have a genetic workup to rule in or out some syndrome and look into prenatal exposure to alcohol like her younger siblings. I had learned with Becca's medical issues that the more I was included the better I could monitor and help them help my daughter. When Hawthorne invited me for a treatment-planning meeting they shared her medication changes and behavioral incidences. It appeared I had no rights of inclusion in decision-making for Shay; they did not want Jim or my perspective on anything.

Like communication lines down after a thunderstorm, we were forced to wait for repair work until we regained contact. Nothing was disclosed to Jim and I for the first few months. Finally it was arranged for Shay to have telephone therapy once a week because of the distance and needs of the kids still at home. We were excluded from much of what was going on. I felt disconnected and judged as being a major piece of Shay's problems. My million questions found answers and support through the Internet group and my sessions with Colleen.

Nightmares hounded me of kids putting their foster or adoptive parents through investigations. It was common for her to make things up as she went along and lie to get out of responsibility. I began to fear Shay's irresponsible reporting due reactive attachment disorder and possible Fetal Alcohol Syndrome would get us into trouble. I had read many emails from my Internet support groups of families who faced false reporting or were investigated for misunderstood allegations. I tossed and turned through sleepless nights.

A couple of months later Jim and I and her siblings journeyed to Hawthorne for an apology from Shay. The kids weren't interested in wasting their time. Shay had said sorry many times with no meaning. This time she must prove herself.

I listened to the kids rant about the chaos she had created for them and they were rightfully bitter.

In the family therapy session, Shay seemed to think things would magically be better by a simple sorry.

Detamara shut down.

Becca curled up on my lap.

The boys folded their arms across their chests and rolled their eyes. When the Hawthorne therapist asked them questions, they remained silent.

Matt and Marissa were courageous enough to speak and I worried what Shay might do to get even with them. I worried about the children's behavior when we returned home. I had my own troubles facing Shay; I felt feelings of betrayal, loss, grief, and fear on the entire trip home. I lost track of an entire thirty-mile stretch of highway and I determined never to drive to and from Hawthorne alone.

During the long drive time for the many trips to visit Shay at Hawthorne I slowly relived, put into perspective and learned to cope with what had happened to us.

I knew I needed to learn not to fear Shay and Mental Health wanted me in therapy to get over being 'inappropriately afraid' of her. I was appropriately afraid! I was rightfully afraid! My lips, hand, arm, and neck injuries were permanent but I understood deep down I had to learn to balance those fears.

Into the springtime the agency continued to tell us that they don't pay for residential care and no neurologist or genetics had assessed Shay. We only had the information of mild mental retardation, reactive attachment disorder, and bipolar disorder. They were asking us to bring her home. I knew in my heart of hearts she would not be better and I could not bring her home. She was still using the locked seclusion rooms, and I was still too afraid of her. I could not sacrifice our children's newfound stability to help Shay.

I read enough about FASDs to know that this was permanent brain damage and I did not have enough help to maintain her in the home without full time support.

A home-based worker met with us, and we scheduled a meeting with the hospital liaison and children's mental health manager. I asked Colleen to attend. I had written to my Internet adoption list our family's dilemma and they advised me I take another professional with us. I chose Colleen, the therapist who had been working and treating Shay and our kids since the second week of placement.

Jim, Colleen and I expected we would discuss options for Shay and our family. Instead they talked about us bringing her home or relinquishing her to the system.

Colleen was stunned and worried about the 'helpful role' this manager could play in getting us help with child protective services. She believed it was a set up for abandonment. We could risk losing all our children and Jim could risk losing his hard-earned professional license. Over time I learned we were not alone in this type of face off. Many a family, teacher, doctor, or social worker who adopted one of the kids from the system had lost their license, career and the other children when they could no longer maintain one of their exceptional children in the home. Pre-adoption training didn't tell us adoption might cost us everything.

Our options were limited. Jim told them, he would bring her home, but they needed to staff the home twenty-four hours a day to keep everyone safe.

They offered twenty hours of help per week.

Jim said he would hold them accountable if she did anything to harm anyone. He used strong words as he explained that this was against what three professional placements stated. We had been told she needed more than a home can offer. It was going to be a long road for her to be able to learn to control herself and they were taking on the liability if anyone was hurt or emotionally abused because of Shay's actions.

They said they could not guarantee anything and could not provide staffing. This left only one choice – to disrupt the adoption and abandon Shay.

We walked away from the meeting astounded.

How could doing something so good and trying so hard cause us to lose everything we had worked for? It was unfathomable that we risked losing both our adopted and our biological children!

Who would care for Becca? No one would be able to care for her intense needs with the love and compassion of a family and her mother.

What would happen to Ian, Marissa and Matt? What if DJ, Deangelo, Delonzo and Detamara had to be separated again?

What could I do?

That afternoon was Shay's treatment planning meeting and I didn't have a babysitter so they made arrangements for me to attend the meeting via a conference call. I was surprised that the children's services manager, the home based worker, and the hospital liaison were at the hospital two hours away in person.

We talked of discharge and the need for residential care.

When Shay had been admitted, Jim and I had checked the box for residential care, which had been written into the admitting paperwork.

The children's service manager asked the hospital psychiatrist to change the discharge plan from residential to home, and move up the discharge by two weeks. So Minnesota and Michigan could battle out who was responsible for Shay's catastrophic long-term care costs.

The doctor told them that would set up the Yurceks for abandonment and refused.

The children's services manager argued that he didn't understand the dynamics and that Kalamazoo Community Mental Health was not fiscally responsible. Minnesota Health and Human Services and their adoption program should be her funder.

I remained silent and invisible in my bathroom office while the professionals argued and the meeting at Hawthorne closed failing to agree to anything. They had lied. They had not told us that they were doing this. Just that morning in our meeting, we had been told to contact an attorney and they had given us thirty days to make it happen. I was shaking.

What were we to do?

I stayed quiet and invisible, not believing what my ears heard?

It was June 23, 2000 and no one could help us. No one wanted to pay for Shay and we couldn't afford to pay for her. Four days earlier I had seen Oprah live in Detroit at the Fox Theatre. Nathan and Kristy had given me tickets for *Living Your Best Life* Premiere for my birthday and Mother's Day to see my mentor. It was an incredibly extravagant gift from my children.

Oprah talked about standing for what you believe in, and on her show the next day BeBe Winans premiered his new song *Stand*. The words of the song spoke to my heart.

I needed to "STAND" for Shay, but how?

I journaled as I had in times of crisis with Becca, pouring out the thoughts that were racing in my head. I wrote of our dilemma with Shay. I wrote about having to tell my daughter that she would lose the only family she had left.

Writing helped me clear my mind and make sense of the flooding thoughts. I wrote into the wee hours of the morning, with Oprah's words and BeBe's lyrics replaying in my head. I prayed for answers. I don't even remember where it all came from. I reread my four pages and changed nothing. I could not face my daughter to tell her we were giving her up. I could not let Jim give up his dream and career. I would not lose my children without fighting the good fight. I would not be a member of all the people who abandoned Shay and I be forced to be no better than all the systems that failed her. I would not face her with the devastating news of having to let her go because she was too expensive, at least not until I exhausted all my options.

Then I decided to write a letter . . .

- 44 -

SOS

Having finished my letter I determined to send it to every advocacy organization, high power person and government official I could find on the Internet. I was told that I had to fight with everything I could muster if I stood a chance of getting help for Shay and our family. Shay was stuck and hope was running out to fund her residential care. I started at the top with the White House, the US Congress, and US Senate.

If I was going to fall, I wanted a long distance.

Two hours, forty-seven minutes and thirty-nine seconds after I pressed the key to the White House, Hillary Clinton's secretary called me. She said they were forwarding my letter onto someone who may be able to help. I dropped the phone after the woman hung up. Was this a dream? Could someone as far up as the White House care or was I now delusional like Shay?

I made phone calls to follow up with the emails I sent and discovered that my email was already on the desk of a number of Executive Directors who said they didn't know how to help me. They had not heard about disruption, or relinquishment. They believed adoptions of children with special needs rarely failed.

Again I spoke with the North American Council for Adoptable Children. I discovered my story was not unusual and their representative told me that we might really have to relinquish Shay to help her.

Many other families had done the same, even though they still loved and cared about their child.

My temperature rose.

This was insane.

We made a promise to Shay and we had to keep it. No one knew how to help a child like Shay. How could adoption services place children with families who were not prepared to raise them? How could we be held accountable for helping when no one could help? How could anyone be prepared to raise Shay without support? I sent my letter to my Internet support group. I received over a dozen letters from parents who had been faced with our dilemma.

It was true!

They had lost their children and destroyed their lives.

Some filed bankruptcy. Many faced allegations of neglect. Some were placed in jail or lost all their children while investigations tarried. Some lost their children forever. All of them! Biological and adopted children? How could that be?

The promise of a forever family, the commitment of an existing family with existing children all lost forever because you reach out to help. To help, the words resonated trauma of what these families lived through. They were left with damaged homes, damaged lives, and broken hearts.

Loving their children unconditionally was not enough to keep them. These children were neglected long before they were adopted. Their biological families abused them and for many prenatal exposure to alcohol and drugs set them up to be challenged before they even took their first breath. Many sat in foster care limbo for years while the very system set up to help, save, and support them neglected them as numbers in a file. These were mentally and emotionally fragile children with compounded losses. The grief and trauma these children faced was insurmountable. We were set up to fail when we lacked proactive supports.

The price was too great. They could not afford the $300 or more a day cost for a residential care bed? There were not enough supports in the community early on when just maybe they stood a prayer of helping their children remain in their homes. Many had no choice but to give up their children to get help from the child welfare world. Jim and I were in over our heads.

We now realized that many of these children had undiagnosed permanent brain damage from being prenatally exposed and there was no amount of loving that would put the missing pieces back into their brains. How could new families be blamed for not loving them enough to heal their damaged hearts when no one was willing to admit many had brain injuries?

No one was willing to say that some children may be too damaged to make it in a family. It would take the unity of families and professionals around the world to discover strategies to support these children and help them grow.

Save the ones you can we were told.

Let her go many an answered. Others told me to fight the system to protect our family and its survival. We had no choice but to fight for the survival of our family and Shay.

▼

I had done everything Mental Health asked me to do. I gave them the adoption paperwork to understand what and how Minnesota pays for things. Minnesota could not understand Michigan's rules. Michigan said Minnesota was wrong. In talking with Adoption Subsidy, they said to use our Medicaid first, and then after appeals and denials they may consider paying for Shay's residential placement after exhausting all avenues.

I was asked by Mental Health to file charges on Shay's assaults on both Becca and me. When I went to the police station they told me they would not accept them, since she was already Mental Health's responsibility and was clearly incompetent. The police told me; if and when we brought her home they would note that there was a mentally ill teen living in our residence and flag it. That way the police would know how to respond to a call from our home.

Colleen told me that they had asked me to do this, to get the courts to help pay for the costs of her treatment or to get her adjudicated.

What was I to do?

Jim and I met with Shay's therapist at Hawthorne, and we explained the entire story. He went and got someone from their office of recipient rights department. It was her job to enforce the Michigan rules for the mentally ill. She was helpful, and told us our experience was not how it was supposed to be.

Very little made sense, I had Medicaid, but in Michigan they do not pay for residential care?

Other states do?

I received a call from my Representative in Congress's assistant, who told me about the Family Opportunity Act, addressing custody relinquishment to obtain services. Families would be able to buy into Medicaid to get treatment and hospitalization for their severely mentally ill children. But I had Medicaid, and could not get help!

I received a letter from the United States Government from the Children's Services section, opening as a response to my email to First Lady Hilary Clinton. It listed many organizations to help sort out the responsibilities of who should pay for Shay. The federal government gives its authority to the states to handle this, but because I had two states disagreeing and the letter was no help. I had no one.

Each state pointed its territorial fingers at the other for fiscal responsibility. The letter from the Minnesota Attorney General didn't help. Years later I would hear from a friend who had fought to get a hearing in Lansing. The Michigan adoption program was under scrutiny of the legislature and one of the clarifications made was that the receiving state was responsible to provide support. Michigan's Adoption Subsidy was out of compliance with Federal Law.

One day I received an email from a friend on the adoption list, who was forwarding an email from a mom who waged war on the State of California for her mentally ill daughter and managed to fight custody relinquishment to get her daughter back. I sent her my story hoping she would tell me where to start. She called me and provided a crash course in federal law. She gave me a phone number from someone from a federal agency called HCFA (Health Care Finance Association) now called Centers for Medicaid Services.

The Centers for Medicaid Services oversees how states use their Medicaid funds. There I found someone to help sort out the Medicaid Funding and Shay had an open Michigan Medicaid case since her arrival in Michigan.

That person forwarded my email to someone in Michigan who called me to provide an overview of Michigan mental health rights and I was told to recontact Michigan Protection and Advocacy. MPA is given the charge to represent the rights of the disabled in our state by Federal Law. The director sent me piles of documents to learn how to help myself help Shay, but it could just as well been written in a foreign language.

I understood very little.

We were advised to tape record the next meeting at Hawthorne. When we tried, we were stopped as it was against confidentiality to record what goes on at the hospital. To appease me, the head of the hospital agreed to take minutes and the meeting was hot and heated.

The doctor said that Shay was the responsibility of Kalamazoo Community Mental Health agency and they should pay for her residential care. Now, they disagreed with what Shay needed. The hospital said she needed more treatment.

I was afraid of her, if she had fetal alcohol and could not learn from experience, how could we control her? Many said it was hopeless. It was too dangerous to bring her home. Shay was sweet and kind much of the time, but she snapped when she became frustrated or depressed. Someone had already been hurt and the next person could be killed during one of her rages. For the time being Shay would stay at Hawthorne.

The meeting was adjourned, deadlocked. We walked away with questions and no answers.

The initial requested testing was ordered. The neurologist and the genetics doctor finally saw Shay and the neurologist wrote that Shay's problems were caused by prenatal exposures to drugs, alcohol and toxins, the affects of neglect and childhood trauma, and her genetics from her biological family.

Mental Health now was being pressured to realize that Shay was their responsibility and they begin to disagree about Shay's best interest. They felt home was the best placement and we would have to work through her issues.

We were in trouble.

They gave us thirty days to prepare to bring her home.

How could I bring home a teen that was still being locked in a time out room? I did not have a padded room for her to rage in. In a family home, that would constitute abuse. Protocol allowed in a treatment facility is not allowed in family care. In addition, Shay had learned new behaviors and tricks from the other disturbed kids in the locked psychiatric hospital and she was no longer innocent. No progress had been made on her attachment disorder. How could I have her around little kids? How could I help her not fail?

I wrote the person at Centers for Medicaid Services about the ongoing struggle for Shay's discharge and residential funding. They sent an email stating they were forwarding my letter to their Chicago office. That email was followed up by a phone call telling us of someone who could help at the Michigan Department of Community Health in Lansing. Mental Health wanted to meet us and Colleen advised us not to go. If we disagreed against their clinical opinion we could be charged with medical neglect by failing to provide mental health for Shay. Instead I called the contact person from the state, and we set up a meeting.

Armed with letters of professional recommendations to protect the other siblings, in addition to recommendations from Shay's treating professionals. I felt ready. Community Mental Health sent four people, along with her therapist from Hawthorne. A mysterious man from the Department of Community Health also attended. We talked about Shay's needs and read the half dozen letters I passed around the table. Finally after eleven months, there was agreement that Shay needed residential care, and I was put in charge of finding her an appropriate placement.

I visited all the places Children's Mental Health and the hospital recommended. Colleen warned me about one RTC she believed misused seclusion and restraint. I knew I could expect Shay to ping pong back and forth between running away and getting sent back if she went there. She had already learned the escape routes in her first visit from the other kids who were her friends.

The recipient rights worker at the hospital was now an ally. She told me of a place an hour from home offering services for dually diagnosed children who were both developmentally delayed and severely emotionally disturbed. The Manor Foundation had helped children since 1920. I called for a brochure.

An advocate joined me while I visited the places I had been recommended and the first place was the nightmare Shay had lived in for her first thirteen days and she was afraid. She would be one of the lowest functioning kids and there was a huge risk of victimization.

Next we visited a group home for girls. It looked neglected, garbage overflowed the entry, all the games were broken and the rooms smelled of urine. The first words from the worker's mouth were that the kids had to want to stay if the come there. Many of them ran away, but in winter they often came back fast when they got cold and hungry. The home was next to the boys unit and she disclosed the kids sometimes snuck out for sexual rendezvous.

When interviewing parents I learned of the deficits of both places, and knew these were not the place for my developmentally delayed brain injured daughter. Shay could not control her behavior, but she was not yet a delinquent.

At The Manor, the coordinator met with us and opened a question and answer session. This was impressive. Whenever I asked a question, she seemed to know what she was talking about. She understood the issues I had only read about and she passed my test.

We toured the boys unit that was attached to the office. We toured the Onsite School. Then we toured the girls unit located across from the field and playground. The girls unit was the newest and separated the middle school and high school students. On each end of the building they had practice apartments with two bedrooms, a kitchen and living room providing independent skill building for the older young ladies who were all developmentally delayed.

Shay would fit in. She loved people and helping. She would not have to measure up against peers with unattainable standards. Some of the children there had also fallen into the same gap in the mental health and child welfare system. They did not fit into the developmentally disabled world and they did not belong in the severely emotionally disturbed programs. They only become that way when we fail to meet their needs. They are the victims of abuse and neglect and prenatal exposure to alcohol and drugs.

My daughter has a brain injury that is not my fault nor hers and medication contributed to the aggression that threw me down the stairs. Shay is an amazing person, but her years of neglect put up walls to believe she was worthless.

My daughter was one of many of societies throwaway children and I did not have to throw away my daughter. I had come to understand that my daughter was just a victim. We had found the program for Shay and amazingly it was only an hour from home.

▼

I held my two crystal angels and thought of my best friend Jeannie who would have been so pleased with all this.

Little did I know I already had an earthly angel who had orchestrated a miracle to save my daughter her family.

- 45 -

TABLES ARE TURNED

I created quite a stir when I learned that our family and Shay had rights to care, and I filed grievances and appeals over the fiasco of our community mental health's denial of Shay's care. My early morning email campaign regarding the request for us to relinquish custody of Shay gained attention and the guardian angel I needed was waiting.

Somewhere in the state of Michigan there was a man I was to call, his name was Manfred. Behind the scenes he orchestrated things I didn't understand. To my face, he challenged me to learn and grow. He guided me in to gain the knowledge I needed and nudged me on to open doors I had to look behind. He confirmed when I was heading in the right direction. He was always there to fill in a missing puzzle piece I didn't have without telling me the answer. I will never know the full impact he played in the outcome for Shay.

Manfred acted in the role of ombudsman though that was never his title. Initially he listened to me complain and feed him information and I bet he got bothered by my persistence. He then investigated in a non-partisan and impartial manner. According to my editor years later, he revealed he found my complaint legitimate. From that point he worked to train me to attain the knowledge and moxie to fight, while behind the scenes he engaged others in resolving our dispute. Manfred had years of expert relationships and a reputation of mediation for citizens while improving organization goals and carrying out the rules and responsibilities of the State of Michigan.

I had prayed for a guardian angel, but I didn't know the job description this poor angel had to have. Manfred worked as an investigator, counselor, teacher, analyst, decision maker, mediator, negotiator and advocate for Shay's cause. He understood the technical side of the process. He knew the language I didn't yet understand. He was not afraid to use additional pressures of contract compliance, but preferred to use informal and flexible processes to solve our dilemma. He was a diplomat in the highest sense, while keeping his eye on Shay's best interests and government funding resources.

Manfred is an incredible person who truly cared and was willing to put up with my questions, and persistence, and frustration. Without Manfred, the Yurceks would not have the next chapters of this story that included everyone.

▼

I was excited about The Manor for Shay. We were going to develop a 'person centered plan' and Shay was going to be included in the planning.

We called a meeting and Manfred, from the Department of Community Health that is responsible for Shay's Medicaid, joined with all the persons from our County's Mental Health. This time things would be done correctly. I did not trust anyone.

Shay was now a part of the team and the Hawthorne people transported Shay to attend her meeting. The adults asked Shay what she needed and wanted. Before the meeting Shay and I spent time talking on the phone about her plan and she had me help her make a list of all the things the residential treatment center needed.

First and foremost she wanted her family, and second she requested a time out room. She didn't want to be the highest functioning teen or the lowest. She wanted to have people she could learn from and she wanted to be able to help and mentor others.

Shay had realistic opinions on services she needed. She didn't want it to be like a foster home, she needed more security than that.

The control provided her safety to grow and get healthy. She told them she needed different levels of support and care. There were times she needed more support and there were times when she felt she functioned very normally. She wanted to gain normalcy.

Shay was ready to roll up her sleeves and do it. She had learned while she was in the hospital, that she had to learn self-control to gain her freedom.

I shared what I had found on my site visits and Shay shared her insight on some of these places. She was scared to go where she had already spent two weeks and the high functioning teens terrified her. We discussed strengths and weaknesses of other options and determined the request for Manor Foundation funding was appropriate. It had all of Shay's requests including a small on-site school with opportunities for volunteer work and a seven girl basketball team.

Shay agreed and so did the rest of the team.

We felt we had developed a person-centered plan. Shay would get what she needed, including time with her family.

▼

A week later we received a letter of denial for the funding even though it was enforceable under Medicaid law since it was written into her plan of care.

They were violating her rights to treatment so I asked for their denial in writing.

They claimed it was in the mail.

I emailed Manfred and the state daily, keeping the rights advisor abreast on the lack of the letter coming from our county Community Mental Health agency. I filed a rights complaint on their timeliness of the denial of care.

They told the rights advisor that I was refusing to sign for the letter and they had sent three letters. When asked in later investigations for the certified letter notices we were told that person no longer worked for the agency.

I filled multiple three ring binders with every piece of correspondence for Shay's fight – every email – every letter – every envelope – was placed in the notebook in chronological order. I had filed a complaint about our being asked to give up custody of Shay the preceding June. All my letters were sent certified and the receipts were carefully stapled to cautiously worded correspondence.

The denial of care came at the same time of the rights violation investigations was complete. Many laws had been broken and they had ninety days to investigate. The rights investigator did not follow state timelines. They seemed to think they could do anything they wanted. They predated letters. Letters were delivered three weeks late, validated by the postmark.

In August, three days after I filed the complaint about the relinquishment of Shay, the director of our community mental health agency was ousted. The newspapers questioned why. But, no one knew why. Did Shay's case have something to do with it? The head of Children's Services said she would do what Hawthorne, doctors, or therapists thought in Shay's best interests. Then when push came to shove, she 'clinically' disagreed with the professionals treating Shay.

They had not yet written the true diagnoses into her plan.

They argued about fetal alcohol and the levels of her mental retardation. They diagnosed her with bipolar disorder and reactive attachment disorder. They determined she was more functional than she actually appeared and ignored the severity of Shay's issues. They would not put into writing their denial of care for Shay. Despite the recommendations of the treating team, it seemed the person with the funding and the power of the pen had the last word.

I called someone at the states rights office to help me. The lady was nice and told me I could file an appeal for the denial of care. I read about this in my books from The Bazelon Center for Mental Health Law that had just arrived. I buried myself in the law book and the words that had initially looked foreign began to make sense.

The more I learned the more pieces I had that built upon older understanding. I understood now that under Medicaid Law, there was a clause for children under eighteen years of age and that anything found during a screen (which would include appointments by a physician) was an entitlement. Anything needed to treat or ameliorate any medical, or mental health problems discovered was a covered service. It talked of residential care being a covered service under Medicaid law in certain circumstances and any denial of service had a federally guaranteed rights and appeals processes.

I learned I could appeal the denial of care for Shay's placement at the Manor. I read we had the right to deny anything given to me verbally. We did not need to wait for the written denial Mental Health was not getting me while their story changed daily about where the lost paperwork was.

I filed an appeal asking for an Administrative Law Tribunal Hearing at the State level and wrote the appeal myself. I submitted it to Lansing by certified mail and let Manfred know I filed for the Tribunal. I didn't know enough to fight the Community Mental Health's Lawyers and I needed to find an attorney to represent Shay's interest. With Manfred's help I contacted Michigan Protection and Advocacy Services. I spoke with their head attorney and agreed to meet at the library with his assistant to prepare to appeal the decision for Shay's right to care.

I arrived armed with two three-inch, three ring binders of documentation. One held the papers on the fight for Shay, and the other was filled with her mental health and medical records.

They copied paper after paper as we worked to prepare for the tribunal through April. The attorney asked for an independent second opinion on what Shay needed from our Community Mental Health agency. They went back and forth about whom, what, and when. Finally agreement was reached and the professional visited Shay at Hawthorne, met with the doctors, and did an extensive interview with me.

The date for the Administrative Tribunal was approaching quickly. We asked for a hearing in person instead of by phone and that postponed the trial for another couple of weeks. We received the second opinion the day before the hearing was set. The lawyers asked us to sit down one last time to try and work something out. With the newly released second opinion in hand, we sat down at the table.

This time, Kalamazoo County Community Mental Health finally agreed to the placement at the Manor Foundation for Shay. Shay had been in the state hospital for fifteen months! It was only twenty hours before the fair hearing and we won the placement for Shay

Shay finally had funding for a long-term residential placement.

My prayers had been answered. Shay could keep her family!

We had not backed down. I kept my promise all the way up the ladder to state appeals and I didn't give up no matter what it took. Now I could fulfill my promise to her of a forever family. I hoped The Manor had the skills to help Shay find self-confidence and a place in our family.

I owed Manfred. He talked to Protection and Advocacy and helped find lawyers to represent Shay and our family for pro bono. The state recipient rights workers from both the hospital and the state office looked out for Shay's best interests.

My grievances and complaints weren't over. The rights system that is supposed to protect the Medicaid consumer didn't work on our behalf. The lengthy reports found no fault in anything the agency did to us. Jim and I were faulted for not being able to pay for what Shay needed. No one could afford to pay the high price of her catastrophic needs and depending who you talk to, I later learned that the cost to care for a person with fetal alcohol costs one to two million dollars over the person's lifetime to families, agencies and society

I spent the next year appealing the complaints to the highest levels. All I wanted was someone somewhere to acknowledge me. Shay had been stuck for too long. I wanted an apology.

I had learned an immense amount since the adoption of our new children. Unlike the medical system, in the social service system I could not count on anyone. Yet I found people to help me, and teach me, and support me in finding help for Shay.

There were many things going on in higher places behind the scenes that supported our fight, and those details I may never know. Somehow he was mysteriously brought in by the Feds to help fix our family disaster. Manfred, my mentor and guardian angel may have had a lot to do with it. He checked out the placements for Shay. He found me help with the appeal. He guided me when I needed direction. He had fine judgment and I will never know all that he did to help my family. I have quizzed him for the details and in his professional respect for confidentiality he remains closed to answering. Shay's story reached many people. I had talked to politicians, lawyers, and reporters trying to figure out how to help her. I spoke with a variety of news magazines. I spoke openly about the issue of custody relinquishment. I knew I was not alone in my dilemma. The parents who replied to my email plea a year earlier wrote of the loss of their children and the support failures of the systems. They encouraged me to not give up on Shay.

I repaid their words by sharing our story with our identities hidden, in the fall 2000 issue of *Adopt Talk* published by the North American Council for Adoptable Children. Somehow we hit the tip of the iceberg. The numbers of disrupted adoptions and custody relinquishment hits on the Internet skyrocketed from less than 500 hits to over 30,000. The ripple had turned into waves, *Time*, *Prime Time*, and other news stations commented and wrote of this awful practice. Our family was not alone. The United States General Office of Accounting, the chief investigative arm of the Congress issued a report on the practice of custody relinquishment to garner mental health services. Only seven states reported in 2002 and in those states over fourteen thousand children lost their families due to the catastrophic costs of their mental health care. Later another report wrote about the criminalization of mentally ill children in the jails because of the closures of the state hospitals and residential care.

We had been asked to relinquish Shay and to disclose her abuse to her family. Luckily for Shay, she did not become another statistic. She was still a Yurcek and my daughter forever.

I beat the odds for Shay by sheer fortitude and answered prayers. I spent hundreds of hours fighting and I studied law when no one was able to help me. I had written a legal appeal, and even the lawyer who took the case commented that it was an excellent brief. I learned way too much. Despite the odds against us, we ultimately prevailed for Shay.

The tables had turned. They had to justify their actions. The appeals took the next year and they sided with the Mental Health

Agency. I know there are more than two sides to our story, and I can only write from our perspective. Once again No one had done anything wrong. Mental health did what they believed best without full understanding of the impact of living with a child who had FASD, RAD and was afraid of being loved. Perhaps there was a glitch?

Over time I discovered the holes that prevented me from garnering services for Shay. There was no one to hold accountable for our heartache and trauma. In the end I was much more traumatized by the systems failure to help than by the abuse I had suffered from Shay. Something needs to change.

A hard-earned and well-deserved victory, we are celebrating a new chapter in the fight for Shay, who was moving to the Manor!

- 46 -

HOME AWAY FROM HOME

I had put Shay on the Manor waiting list when I discovered the system was backlogged and by April she had the top slot for a bed. On the day of the hearing there was a bed open for Shay and in an oversight the agency lost her bed. I couldn't believe it! Now Shay had to wait at Hawthorne until someone was discharged from the Manor. We gave up Jim's vacation to Minnesota to see Kristy and Nathan and waited for the phone to ring.

It was the middle of July when the next bed opened and I drove to Hawthorne for the very last time to move Shay to her new home. Hawthorne helped Shay say goodbye to everyone and cope with more losses. In her short life, Shay has had to say goodbye way too many times. We said goodbye to her therapist and Bev the recipient rights worker. Bev cared about what happened to my daughter, and she helped me help Shay. Bev was Shay's mentor for her weight watchers program and hemmed Shay's dress for the Hawthorne formal. I was grateful to all those who helped us along the way.

Jim snapped a picture at the entrance to the hospital of Shay and I in our victory pose, leaning on the Hawthorne Center sign. It had taken nearly nineteen months after leaving our home. Finally, Shay was moving to a residential treatment placement (RTC) for the long road to learn to control her anger. Until her rage and aggression was under control, we could not even consider bringing her home.

Our trip to the Manor was only an hour and five minutes and it meandered through the small towns of middle Michigan, into Amish country and the buggies. The farms fascinated me. Shay slept during most of the trip to the manor, perhaps to keep her mind off the unknown. I reminisced of the battle we had fought to get us to this moment. It was a peaceful trek we could look forward to on Sundays. The ride was a welcome relief from the business of the passed year and a half.

We were welcomed at the Manor and Shay was given a tour. She was quiet and smiling, and seemed to understand that this was now her new home. Jim took another picture of Shay at the Manor, my daughter, in my arms, happily allowing herself to be close. This was not the same young girl who left our home, but a slowly healing now fifteen-year-old daughter.

The Manor had all the things Shay had asked or in a RTC.

- She had asked for a RTC with a quiet room where she could go to regain her composure. The Manor had a safe small room for her to retreat to.
- She wanted a place with a sports team. The Manor had basketball and floor hockey teams competing with schools in the area.
- She wanted to not be the lowest functioning child; she wanted people who were like her and others who needed her to help them. The Manor had a special school with small class sizes where she could learn at her own rate and her own level.
- She wanted to grow in her independence. At the Manor Shay could volunteer and learn cooking and independent living skills. Shay loved to make food. She could work towards the privilege of living in the practice apartments and get ready to be able to live on her own with supports upon discharge. Our favorite times had been cooking and cleaning together.

I wanted to be included in Shay's treatment plan. The Manor asked me questions, filled me in on medication changes, weekly therapy appointments and made our family feel like we were included in her care. The Manor wanted us to work together to help Shay.

Shay and I began talking and I could feel she was healing. I was too. I explained to Shay I could not help her. I could encourage her, but the wanting to change behaviors ultimately was her decision. She had to do the hard work. I let her know I would be there whenever she needed me.

Ten months after placement she surprised me with a Mother's Day poem. Shay had been out of our home for twenty-two months. I had to prove myself worthy to be trusted. I would not leave.

Thank You Mom

Thank you Mom
for being there
Even though
it seemed like I
did not care.
Thank you for
watching over me
like an angel
I know I made it hard to love
but you did not give up.
You kept on going
because you thought
I could change.
I have changed a little
but I still have a ways to go.
Don't give up
I will try not to also.
I want you to know
You mean the world to me.

Love Shay

I had done the right thing for Shay. At Hawthorne, Shay was stuck and not much work was done to help her control her behavior. Now that she was at the Manor, she worked hard to understand cause and effect. Shay said she did not want anyone to control her, when she could control herself. The therapist and I worked on social skills and issues prevented her from being accepted by her siblings.

Over time I understood the complex issues Shay dealt with, and I was no longer be afraid of my daughter. She tested the Manor in learning to control her anger and acting out, but she consistently came up against structure and rules. In the beginning, she landed in the time-out rooms, but her behaviors improved when she realized the staff maintained clear limits.

Shay learned when she finger-painted vomit on the time-out room wall, she had to clean the walls with soap and a sponge. When she put her hand through the plate glass window, she lost her pass to town for the week, and had to pay for the damaged window. If she was aggressive or a danger to herself, she stayed campus. If she wanted to move to higher levels and gain rewards she had to behave.

The Manor ran a step-by-step program with residents moving from a main unit into a practice apartment, out into a group home and finally to a more independent apartment. The established continuum of supportive care provided opportunity to advance along with a healthy safety net that eliminated unnecessary moves from the program for failures. Shay progressed and moved into the practice apartments, but she sabotaged her success so she could sleep in the support and structure of the main unit. For a while she spent her days practicing cooking and being a part of the young women working toward independence and going 'home' to her main unit bed at night.

Shay wanted to participate, and she worked hard to reach the goal of being included when the Manor took the kids into the community to shop, go to parades, the county fair, and ball games.

Shay celebrated her first year in placement by graduating to the large two-story group home in the community that she shared with five other girls. The girls lived together in a home-like setting with staffing and participated in cooking, cleaning, and living together as a family. During the day they attended Manor schooling and participated in many outings with the other homes. In addition, Shay began work-study at the hospital laundry and volunteering at the nursing home. Shay loved playing checkers and talking with the seniors. She spent two quarters working at the humane society and now she and Becca had something to share. Shay told Becca about all the new arrival animals and all the animals that got adopted. Shay was one of the higher functioning teens, and this gave her a sense of pride. She felt better about herself when she helped others. She was definitely my daughter, she garnered the same sense of giving as I mirror as my own mission.

She made friends and some of the younger girls looked up to her. Shay went to church on Sundays. She had her first paying summer job grooming ball fields.

Slowly, the children began to believe Shay was healing. At first they tentatively listened over my shoulder waiting and watching for my reactions to Shay while I talked to her on the phone. We no longer spent our family visit providing her with things she 'needed.' She wanted family-focused visits. On summer days we played basketball at the park, we ate dinner together, went for walks and stopped at the favorite ice cream stand called the Blue Moon. The kids drooled over the ice cream varieties and their favorite was one with candy bug eyes called Road Kill.

I finally believed she felt connected to our family, and wanted to be a part of things. It may have taken her possibly losing everyone, for her to finally trust us that we were in it for the long haul. The "Glue" family, she was stuck with us, no matter what, State Hospital, Residential, she was still my daughter.

The Manor was not just person-centered practice it was a fully family centered practice. The staff shared everything Shay proudly said about her family. They took into account Shay's place in our family and they respected the needs of all her family members. With the help of the Manor, Shay realized she was one of the fortunate kids who still had families involved in her care. Most of these kids had no one but their caseworkers and were wards of the state.

Shay was finally ready, willing, and mature enough to start to make progress. It took time, patience, mistakes and retrying over and over again before she quit sabotaging her achievements. She didn't believe she was worthy of praise or accomplishments. She felt uncomfortable getting compliments from others when she did good things. It took time, but eventually she found pride in herself.

I explained to professional that some of these children were so broken by trauma and attachment issues it took hanging in for the long haul before you finally caught them. I equated it to jumping off the cliff with my daughter, and running to beat her to the bottom, ready to catch her when she was ready to accept help.

Our goals continued to evolve and every ninety days we met to discuss her future. Shay led the meetings; she facilitated her own agenda and listened as we talked about her progress and future goals. This was a miracle in its own. She sat in the chair and got mad, but she stayed put. She wrung her hands, and her face told the story of her feelings. In time she verbalized what she felt. For children such was Shay with histories of trauma and a diagnosis of fetal alcohol syndrome this was a miracle. I had read that most children with FAS because of brain damage could not learn to do this. Shay proved otherwise, she made progress every month.

Shay celebrated her sixteen and seventeenth birthdays in care at the Manor. The Manor tried to create many memories of a "normal" high school career. She was excited about getting ready for her high school prom. People in the community donated prom dresses to the girls in care. The girls primped and had their hair styled. The boys would get rented tuxes and donated suits. A prom would not be missed out on because of the generosity of the staff, community and the expectations of the Manor treatment teams.

Shay lived at the Manor for two Christmases and two Thanksgivings. The second year of holidays she was well enough and we were healed enough for her to come home for the festivities. The Manor staff transported her home.

We celebrated Christmas with Shay home, and we returned her to the Manor Group Home where she hugged all her roommates. I helped her carry her Christmas loot. We were met by girls who had no family to share the joy of showing off their Christmas gifts. I did not have the heart to walk away and I spent the next hour with the girls. They were so excited to share their holiday with someone.

As I walked out, I thought of how lucky Shay was to have kept her family. So many of the Manor kids had lost their families due to their severe mental health problems, and dual diagnosis of developmental delay. To get care their families placed them in foster care, or abandoned them to the courts or were foster children. Now these poor girls had no one to call mom or dad and only a few still had contact with family or former foster family.

Jim waited in the car while I talked. The four little kids had fallen asleep and when they awoke they just rolled their eyes and explained to Dad that 'Mom was probably just talking again.' I explained the girls to Jim when I finally got back to the car and his long wait longer annoyed him. Would her outcome have been the same if Shay lost us?

Shay and I brought cupcakes to share with all the girls after her home visit at her birthday time. She was beaming with joy as she walked in to proudly to share her mom with the girls and I took my time to stay and visit.

We felt included and their actions showed how much they cared about our daughter and celebrate her successes. I got phone calls when Shay went to the time-out rooms and when she needed a doctors appointment. Amazingly they updated us with all the positive things Shay accomplished and kept us connected. Shay advanced through her therapy and skill-building at The Monor and in time she would be ready to return to our community.

The staff at the Manor were helpful, caring, and non-judgmental and became a big part of our lives.

- 47 -
LIFE GOES ON

With Shay safely in her residential placement, I finally had time to do something for myself. The children adapted into their schools and neighborhood and enjoyed their activities.

The hours upon hours of fighting for Shay had helped me find a new career in the midst of the battle. My phone or email brought questions from families who heard of my battle for my daughter. They asked for advice or help to navigate the complex world of children's mental health and child welfare. My days became busy helping families find answers and offer support and I now had time to connect with my friends who I had found via the Internet or support groups from across the country.

When Jeannie died, I wondered if I would ever find a best friend again. But mental health disasters helped me connect with other mothers who understood what it was like to parent children in the trenches, and the toll it took on the families. I found others who understood my very isolated journey and together we brainstormed, shared celebrations and embraced sorrows to stoke the fire of hope.

▼

Kristy was thriving in college and no longer bored. She had waited a long time to be challenged, and the high-level math classes peaked her interest. When she started at school she longed for a computer from the laptop-leasing program, but financial assistance was not available for rental and we could not help Kristy. We urged her to approach the school about options to make it happen. Kristy had been offered work-study hours and from her request arrangements were made to work in the laptop office and she worked extra hours to pay for her own computer. Within months she was offered a full time job working with the computers for the college and as an employee of the college she was entitled to free tuition with benefits.

Kristy was never satisfied with anything for very long and she called me one day and to tell me her boss, the head of computer laptop leasing, was leaving for another job. She wanted the position, and I empowered her to ask for it. She was afraid, she was way too young, but she had proven herself, and what did it hurt to ask? A few days later, she was awarded the position. She was now in charge of the student workers and the entire laptop department. She was thriving and by the age of twenty managed the laptop department, attended school full time majoring in mathematics with a minor in technology. The bigger the challenge, the happier Kristy became. She and Brian were now living together, and purchased their own home, driving new cars and happy.

▼

Nathan inherited Grandpa Yurcek's love for cooking and mastered baking gluten free morsels and was now a fine chef who cooked better than his mother. I thoroughly enjoyed his contributions to our family. He graduated from high school six months early and his employer at the home improvement store jumped at the opportunity to have him work full time. Nathan was my born saver, and he soon had a sizeable down payment to buy his first new car. More than once we had counted on the Bank of Nathan to float us a loan until payday. Jim was jealous that both of our oldest children had new cars and we drove used older vehicles. I reminded him of his dream to not have to work on cars again, and if his kids' cars had warranties he didn't have to fix one for them. He needed patience and I assured him his time would come.

During spring break from college at Western, Nathan took a

road trip to Minnesota in his new car to visit Kristy and was offered a job working in the computer department at the college that Kristy attended. It would be too good of an opportunity for him to turn down, a full time job with benefits and best of all, just like Kristy they would pay for his tuition at one of the five private schools in the Twin Cities. The women's college paid for their employees to attend college and they could not discriminate so they offered the male employees tuition at one of the other private colleges.

I hadn't needed to worry about providing for my oldest children's college education, their years of hard work was now paying off with jobs, careers with benefits, and attending private school for free.

▼

Ian and DJ were brothers in all the right ways. Our house had been a parade of boys coming and going. Kids of all colors and of all kinds came and went with our boys. Ian was always befriending the underdog and whomever he brought in seemed to fit into our home. We always had room for one more at the dinner table.

Ian floundered after high school and left for the offer of free tuition and structure provided in the Marine Corp. Detamara missed her big best brother, and cell phone calls home brightened her days. With Ian's departure DJ lost his brother's leadership and begin a spiral of self-destruction to the streets of the inner city.

▼

DJ had only three years in our family before he graduated from high school and like most young adults dreamed of spreading his wings. He had studied hard, played sports and made friends in his new community. He worked at a daycare center five days a week and saved his money. He responsibly paid all his bills and finally he moved out with friends and was on his own. At times he did well and at others he struggled. He seemed drawn to wrong people who took advantage of him and I worried about where life would take him. I reminded myself, he was now grown and his decisions were beyond my control. He dreamed of being a famous rapper and I worried that his music would lead him to the wrong crowd. All I could do was hope and pray that he kept himself out of trouble and be successful.

▼

Marissa had spent her free time acting throughout the community and was accepted into a world-renowned arts summer camp. The money seemed impossible on residency pay, but with a partial scholarship, much hard work and determination Marissa got herself to the nearly six thousand dollar eight-week summer camp. She had watched our resourcefulness and held an all-family garage sale, did pop can drives, babysat and ferreted out of Dad's change collection. She still came up short. I called the camp to explain her hard work and our family circumstances hoping to find extra help. Shocked at our story, they told me to write a letter to the board of the non-profit arts association. Two weeks later a letter stated that Marissa's scholarship doubled. She had done it.

Marissa thrived at camp and carried leading roles and was asked back for a second season. Marissa dreamed of going to the year round boarding school for acting, but finances prohibited it. She had to settle for staying in town and acting close to home. Marissa won awards for top dramatic and story telling performances at the State Forensics tournaments; while being looked over for lead roles in musical productions at her own high school. She vowed that someday she would make it to a leading college for acting, to prove to the drama coach that she was neither fat or had little talent.

▼

Matt was developing a strong relationship with Deangelo who looked up to his big brother. Our mini bike drove the neighbors crazy while the two boys drove it around the perimeter of our tiny back yard. As Ian left his job at the Italian Pizzeria, Matt stepped in to replace him, knowing he could count on a Yurcek boy.

Matt was growing fast and already taller than Ian and it would not be long before he passed up Nathan. The prediction of the pediatrician was coming true; Matt would be the tallest brother. I began to wonder if Matt would pass up Jim at six foot three, but Jim continued to hold his high stature.

▼

Deangelo settled in with the family and began to remind me of my biological children. The values and demeanor of his siblings were rubbing off on my angelic son and he had overcome his attachment issues. He had always been silently distant, but no longer.

Early on, DJ teased him about talking too smart or acting too white, but Deangelo didn't let it stop him. He was a smart capable young man with a very gentle and caring demeanor. DJ in time encouraged his younger brother and their homework buddy relationship helped DJ understand Deangelo's strengths and ability to learn. DJ told his brother that he was going to college, and that he needed to keep up his grades and both boys had come far in understanding the importance of education for a better future.

▼

Delonzo was gaining a foothold in the family, but remained confused whether to let anyone get close and had little respect for women. I realize I get the full rampage of his anger at his mother, for being his mother. He steals from me and pushes me away, and every time I tell him no, he faults me for not meeting his needs. I understand the dynamics but someday I 'hopefully hope' that he understands that I am in his corner and lets me into his distant world.

▼

Becca has continued to thrive; her transition into elementary school was slow, but by the end of fifth grade, she was fully included in all of her classes. The school environment however, triggered headaches from all the sensory stimuli and we sought help. We discovered not only did she have Noonan syndrome, but she was secondarily diagnosed with Autism Spectrum Disorder. Her sensory problems impacted her health and visa versa. She missed days of school and by middle school she was far behind. All her life she only had enough stamina to make it through a half a day, and without proper supports she was floundering. By the middle of sixth grade I realized for her own good she needed to be taken out of school and homebound with me. I entered a new career as her academic teacher. She learns interactively and the computer became her best teacher. It limited her anxiety as she struggles with her little perfectionist self. The computer was forgiving, it did not judge, it gently corrected her until she was practiced perfect.

In time we discovered she had severe visual perceptual problems that got in the way of her learning. Her brain reversed things, and her eyesight was impaired. She learned by using her near perfect memory on how things looked to her to be able to read and answer questions. That was one reason she could never get her thoughts to paper. Writing required too many motor skills combined with visual processing skills. It was too many steps. In the complicated process her precious thoughts would be lost. Other times her words failed her. She was a very concrete learner for a long time, and then all of a sudden, all the mathematics we had been trying to teach her connected. In record time she memorized her addition, subtraction, multiplication and division facts. From being unable to understand the concepts of math to math becoming one of her best subjects.

▼

In the stability of our home, **Detamara** grew, and grew and soon she was passing her hand-me-downs up to her older sister Becca. Three years difference were blended by their differing social and emotional lags. What was one of the girl's strengths was the other's weakness. They balanced each other out and learned together. What Detamara forgot, Becca remembered. What Becca could not reach, Detamara helped her get. Detamara tied Becca's shoes, while Becca prompted Detamara onto success. They became an inseparable duo. Becca now had a best friend and the girls hung out together. Becca and Detamara became the best of sisters.

When Detamara needs peace and quiet or is angry, Delonzo steps in to be Becca's buddy. Delonzo and Becca have the infamous love hate brother sister relationship. One moment they are the best of siblings, and the next moment they stare daggers at each other.

At only three months apart and in the same grade, what would you expect?

▼

I had become accustomed to the roller coaster ride of my large family. The quiet moments could quickly become an uphill battle or a downhill spiral of one of the kids illness or misdoings. Juggling therapy appointments, school functions, IEP meetings and the coming and goings of the teachers who joined my home became a daily part of Yurcek family life.

Free classes offered by the school district for summer programming and the inexpensive drop-in summer program at the local elementary school gave the younger kids something to keep busy. Through a community fair for children with disabilities I met a respite provider who helped build a program on Saturday nights for Becca. Now all my children had places to go have fun with structured recreation and safe peers. Our lives had settled down, as much as one can with so many differing personalities and abilities living under one roof.

Colleen bugged me that Jim and I needed time without children. The Saturday night respite program was just enough time to take in a movie, grab a bite to eat, or do a little shopping before the sale ads expired. We soon learned we were not the only parents having grocery shopping dates without our children. Jim and I ran into other parents on Saturday night catching up together and tying loose ends while their children attended the Saturday evening program.

We added Sunday morning 'dates' while the kids slept in and Marissa supervised. We went out for a ride and a cup of coffee or my morning Pepsi along with a paper. Jim and I down our drinks while catching up with each other enjoying our ride. We relish our quiet interlude of sharing our dreams and the next step of life. We had blended into one family and now began the task of learning to let go as our oldest children moved into adult lives. They knew we were only a cell phone call away.

The kids attached to one another long before they trusted enough to attach to Jim or I. The teachers and professionals were struck by their loyalty to one another. No one dared pick on a sibling or you faced a whole tribe of trouble.

The Yurceks had become one for all, and all for one.

- 48 -

THE SURGEON

Jim's final year of residency was exhausting for all of us and flew by in a hurry. Jim was the chief resident and his eighty, hundred, hundred and twenty hour weeks expanded further as he was on call for the other residents twenty-four hours a day, seven days a week for the entire year. I no longer heard him getting up in the middle of the night to answer his pager. I slept through all the buzzing and beeping that called him out of bed to go to the hospital to assist with middle of the night emergencies. Multiple days passed without the kids seeing their father.

Being a surgery chief resident is a huge responsibility and with Jim being in his mid-forties, he was not up for night after night of little sleep. When Jim was home he was completely exhausted. He tried to study for boards and presentations but would collapse with the book in his hands. Days without sleep left him looking worn out and aged. For six months he was chief resident at the busiest hospital, and then the second six months he switched to the other hospital. Both hospitals are level one trauma centers and he not only had the responsibility of handling the general surgery cases but also all the traumas. Jim gives everything he has to his job, and this time his job required everything he had. There was nothing left for his family, even though he wanted to help and be there for his children. I figured we only had to make it through a year of this schedule.

I hoped Jim survived it.

▼

Five years had gone by in a hurry and in the blink of an eye, the end of residency approached. The future held so many unanswerable questions and rolling them over in my mind did little good to solve them. There were already many general surgeons in our area, but maybe we would be lucky and find a surgery job in Michigan.

Moving, changing doctors for Becca and schools for my children with their IEP's and special needs seemed overwhelming. My kids were settled. They hated change and so do I, since I had moved so often as a child. It was Marissa's senior year, I had moved my senior year and it was neither easy nor fair. I worried about what would happen when Jim completed his training and Shay was still in residential. We would love to return to Minnesota? But if we did, perhaps I could stay behind until Shay turned eighteen, and then move on. I played out scenarios in my head. I reminded myself I had no control over any of it. I had to trust that everything would work out, and whatever hand I was dealt, we would make it through.

Jim began to look for a position. We kept the Midwest open with Michigan and Minnesota as our first choices. We scoured his medical journals for openings, and one day we received a phone call from a recruiter. The recruiter had an open position near Kalamazoo in a small town twenty minutes from our home. Was this an answer to my prayers? Jim and I went to visit the small hospital on the lake. We felt we found an answer to our predicament even though we pined to return to Minnesota to Kristy, Nathan and our extended.

We turned down jobs that paid more or were near our parents so our children could remain stable. For Shay's sake and the other kids consistency, we needed to stay put in Michigan. There were definitely positives to staying in Michigan. Michigan had been good to Becca and her medical care, and it was a safe place to meet her medical needs. We didn't need to uproot our children from their schools and Marissa could graduate with her friends. We didn't need to sell our home. We could stay put and get back on our feet financially after the devastating years of residency and the kids catastrophic mental health costs combined with medical costs of Becca.

The day we signed the contract for Jim's new position was a day we had long waited for. It had taken eleven years - two years of undergrad classes to add to Jim's Business degree, four years of Medical School, five years of residency - were now done. We had made it! The contract was unbelievable and they even gave him a signing bonus that was more than we made the whole year we delivered newspapers!

Our big red van had survived residency and part of Medical School and now it sat dead in the driveway next to the white minivan. We needed to replace it. Our little gray car did not hold more than five of us at a time. Jim used the signing bonus as a down payment to buy our first new vehicle. The contract made doors open. Unbelievably with the contract in our hands, we did not have to worry about our mediocre credit.

Jim beamed as we drove a brand new SUV off the lot with only four miles on the odometer! His old dream to no longer change a water pump in the driveway during a rainstorm or a freezing cold blizzard had come true. He now had a car with a warranty and he did not have to work on cars anymore unless he wanted to. The eight-passenger SUV with its heated leather seats was Jim's dream come true. He had toiled eleven long years to put his hands on such a steering wheel and sit in a heated seat. We drove in style to visit Shay at the Manor and we did not need to worry about our van breaking down on the way. Now, everyone could visit Shay and we didn't have to leave the older kids at home for lack of room.

Jim's parents, Kristy and Brian, and Nathan all came into town for graduation. As we walked into the Radisson Ballroom, Deangelo remarked that he never dreamed he would ever be in a place such as this. His eyes sparkled in the lights of the huge crystal chandeliers and stared at the formal place settings on white clothed tables. Our kids watched to see what silverware you used when. Detamara watched while guests placed the linen napkins on their laps and she mirrored their every move. The kids made it through dinner without spilling a morsel. After dinner the fancy desserts were left on empty seats and

Delonzo moved from place to place to finish off the extras, not wanting to waste the scrumptious delicacies.

We cheered as Jim received his diploma; our whole family together made it happen together. All of us were here, but Shay.

I sat at the table replaying our journey in my head, remembering back to when Jim used to be uncomfortable in the NICU, to the first day he went back to school. I thought of the hundreds and thousands of newspapers it took to pay the bills and the milestone of the first day of Medical School, and then the celebration of the graduation of Medical School. I remembered as we drove away from our home of twenty years to Michigan in the moving caravan and the day the kids arrived, our fight to find help for our kids and keep Shay. I missed Shay and thought of her at The Manor. She was still our daughter! Becca was thriving! Dad was a surgeon! We had made it!

Jim is a surgeon!

It was an unbelievable journey.

Now we were on to a new and easier chapter.

Financially we should be able to provide for our family, but it would take a few years to get back on our feet and pay off the thousands of dollars in debt for Shay's lawyer bills, the kids' mental health bills, and repair our broken home. The kids had been hard on things, and the house needed a lot of work. The cost of Medical School and living expenses would have to be paid off at the same time the oldest kids were in college and with Jim's new career they no longer qualified for financial aid.

Kristy, Nathan, and DJ were all in post secondary school. Ian had enlisted in the Marine Corp to find a way to someday pay for Medical School. Marissa was a year from college, and Matt would soon follow. Even with Jim's glorious new career, finances for a time would not be easy, but I could begin to pay back our debt.

The tables had now turned and we were now paying nearly half our salary in taxes alone. Jim was in practice for six months when I discovered that we needed to look for a tax write off. We met with a financial planner and were advised that we needed a home with a larger mortgage. Life was so different on the other side of the fence and it took getting used to.

Afraid of any debt, I scoffed at the idea to take such a risk.

For the past eight years, I had carried a house plan in the back of my wallet that Jim and I had found in my mother's house plan books. It was our dream home and we vowed that someday we wanted to build our home. One day as I was paging through the Home Guide and I spied a picture of a home. The two-story home had everything we dreamed of. I did not want to move from our familiar school and uproot the kids from their friends. Becca who was now homebound and getting some education services and I didn't want to start all over again.

I pulled out the crinkled picture from behind my driver's license where it had lived for a very long time and set it next to the picture in the home guide. It was our dream home! Out of thousands of house plans, some builder was building our dream home as a model house.

I read further. The house was in our school district and it was five minutes from our home, plus five minutes closer to Jim's new job! The house was far less than I ever thought it would be listed for because one of the major employers in the community recently announced they were pulling hundreds of professional jobs out of the community and big expensive homes were not selling. Still, I was afraid of buying another house, as I knew we had not had enough time to repair our damaged credit.

Jim and I drove over to look at the house and found it barely studded in. We walked into the open garage and we're astounded. We ventured to explore the new construction and were soon met by the neighbor across the street and we explained our interest. Jim and I disagreed with each other on which of the two floor plans this house was, but it was definitely our house plan.

We began looking at other homes throughout the area. Then one day while we were looking at a home in the development where they were building our dream home we met with the realtor.

We discovered that banks work with new physicians in the area and they understand that new doctors have overcome huge financial challenges in residency. Just like with residency, they had special no down payment plans to get the doctors into new homes. Could we reach our dream?

After two weeks of thinking and dreaming about the home, I made a phone call to the realtor, and we toured the house. It definitely was the house, but it was the larger version with enough bedrooms for all our children still living at home. The bedroom above the garage was L shaped and could be divided into two rooms for both little girls and the girls could share a bathroom. The boys could be on one end of the upstairs and we on the other end. The house had five bedrooms, four bathrooms, and a second-story laundry room. The gigantic kitchen with an attached great room. I could cook and see what the kids were up to at the same time, plus we could all eat together at the same table. There was even a dining room to boot for when everyone was home and a front staircase overlooking the foyer to welcome guests. Another staircase came off the great room.

We took Becca with us, and she announced that there were horses in the back yard. She was right, the house was on the edge of the development, and there were horses in the back yard to provide pony watching out the family room window. Our dream home was being built on one of the last lots in the development in the same school district where the kids were attending, with horses for Becca?

A miracle or coincidence?

The realtor was right; it was easy to buy our home. The bank was supportive, and we signed papers to purchase it. Jim and I picked out the new carpets, tile, and fixtures for our dream home. We had the builder finish the basement and now I had a real office that was not a bathroom. He completed a family room, extra bathroom, extra eating area, and a home schoolroom for Becca. I didn't have to breathe sheetrock dust. Jim didn't have to do the building. We didn't have to call his parents, or my parents, or the church, or the county for help.

Moving day arrived right before Marissa's senior prom. Marissa and her friends dressed in my new master bedroom suite while their dates waited downstairs with their parents. The girls came down the stairs of the foyer and it felt as though we were watching fairytale princess movies. It was a magical moment and it felt good that we could make her senior prom so special after all the years of struggling. It was nice to give Marissa a tiny token back, for all she had given to Becca and all the help she gave us with her new siblings.

Jim loved his new career and the kids were growing up. It was quiet in the new house. We had so much space that we rarely heard the kids, but with so much space we had another problem. We had space to spread out. We had so much space I had to figure out how to keep it up and keep track of all the kids in it. I learned even on the other side of the fence people had problems. I couldn't keep an eye on where the little ones were and stealing went out of control. There were too many places they could sneak.

In time we honed our ears to hear their little footsteps creaking and I came to know which doors squeak and how each sounded. I could tell where everyone was without seeing them. I was no longer the old woman who lived in the shoe. I still had so many children, but I now knew what to do.

I drive into the driveway reminded of all the miracles, adventures and life experiences of how we got here. I cry happy tears thankful for our journey and survival. We were in heaven, this was a magical place.

-49-

NEVER ENDING BACKPACKS

Through my network of adoptive and foster parents I was asked to speak to a group of caregivers on the east side of Michigan. I shared our story and presented about the importance of keeping siblings together. After the presentation they shared the good news that the group had been given five hundred backpacks from Office Depot for the foster children in the inner city. Each of the backpacks contained a couple of pencils, a notebook and erasers; they were not the well-stocked backpacks my children received so long ago in Minneapolis.

On the way home the kids who traveled with me discussed the importance of having a new bag for the first day of school. Marissa shared how she got her precious My Little Pony backpack and her new first day of school outfit. It had made such an impact she still cherishes it to this day. Deangelo shared watching Shay and DJ head to school out of the shelter with just the clothes on their backs. He had been fortunate that Grandma Dorothy had always outfitted him and Delonzo and made sure they had what they needed.

Marissa and the kids talked about what the backpacks needed to contain, and over the nearly three-hour journey they prepared a school supply campaign. They made a pack that together they were going to fill as many backpacks as they could for the kids they had just met. The kids could not waste time; school started in a month, but Marissa had become the queen of fundraising and the kids had helped her raise money to attend her performing arts camp.

The kids decided to buy supplies off the Sunday Back-to-School sale ads and went door-to-door with empty potato chip containers asking for money to help foster kids get new school supplies. The entrepreneurs had an ongoing lemonade stand and raised money by selling their belongings at a kid sponsored garage sale. They dumped their change jars together; dollar-by-dollar their little nest egg grew. Soon they were collecting five and ten-dollar donations. Ten days later they had enough to go shopping.

They poured over the ads and figured out how to get the most for their money. They made lists of which store they could buy what and bought a hundred of each of the supplies on their lists. A hundred packages of markers, crayons, pencils, pens, bottles of glue, glue sticks, scissors, and erasers were placed into individual zipper plastic bags. Cartons of newly purchased notebooks and folders were loaded into the car to head back for the foster care walk to raise money and awareness about the plight of foster children.

My kids presented the foster children with the school supplies and explained why they did it and they vowed that next year they would get backpacks for the children in the Kalamazoo shelters. The families generously gave my kids ninety-one backpacks for children in the Kalamazoo shelters to start school ready to learn this year.

With less than two weeks till school started, my kids took off fundraising again with a vengeance. This time they reached higher, Marissa, Becca and Delonzo went to the stores asking for assistance.

They were surprised when they found K-Mart gave them two boxes of supplies and two more backpacks. Going door-to-door they found our neighbors wanted to shop themselves for the children and they brainstormed about creating an easy-to-find dropsite where people could go drop things off and they could collect them with ease. A trip to the Children's Shoe Store provided the solution. It was now their drop site. The kids stopped at stores and shared their mission. Office Depot in Kalamazoo gave my adventurous children with twenty-six more backpacks. They went door-to-door dropping off flyers they made on Becca's magical Christmas computer. In record time, their ninety-one backpacks doubled and they had enough supplies to stuff the rainbow of backpacks to the brim.

In less than a month the kids managed to fill a hundred bags of supplies for foster children and the ninety-one backpacks had grown to two hundred thirty-seven more here in town. They had collected enough supplies that they replenished the storage cabinet at the mission and the YWCA to make sure kids went to school with new belongings.

The news channel heard about their project and surprised us packing day. My living room was filled with school boxes, backpacks and supplies. The camera crew followed my children on the Sunday afternoon before the start of school as they distributed the backpacks to the kids in the shelter. It felt like Christmas and a new Yurcek tradition was born. We knew we would always have to remember the homeless kids in years to come.

The news media had brought our little family project to their attention of the public and we were surprised to find checks in the mail from generous people in the community who wanted to help. With the start of school, Becca was homebound and left behind with little to do so she and I filled our days scouring the shelves of the stores for back-to-school clearance items we could buy at 75% off. We made friends with the mark down teams, and Becca soon knew when prices were marked down and when she could buy a hundred or more backpacks at a time. The store crew helped my tiny smiling entrepreneurial daughter load up our vehicle to the roof and after school her brothers carried them into the house.

The 'Backpack For Kids' Project continued to grow. The second year we were up to four-drop sites with newspaper and television coverage and we opened up to the non-profit child serving agencies in the community. The support group for kids with emotional problems generously made available their non-profit status to cover the growing project so donations were tax deductible and they helped us get a couple of small grants to assist with the growing costs. The First Presbyterian Church downtown let us use the Sunday school rooms to pack the mountain of backpacks that Becca found and that had been dropped off in the donation boxes. Becca and I discovered art kits at an after Christmas at 75% off and we bought all five hundred plus of them out of my grocery budget. Every child would get school supplies for school and an art kit and pencils for homework.

Word spread about the multiplying school supplies and we included the kids' friends and other families from our support group in our project. Our small army of kids made quick work of getting out the backpacks to needy children throughout the community.

The Disney Channel announced that the Disney Magazine wanted to hear from kids who were making a difference in the community while Becca was watching. She told me we needed to let people know about kids who need help and begged me rush out to buy the magazine. Within two weeks of school being let out, we begin our summer tradition of working on the project.

The magazine article was forgotten until the first of October when Becca reminded us we "needed" to enter. Delonzo and I dug through our mountain of pictures and wrote the backpack story. We put together a tape of two years of news articles about our growing project and with the help of overnight shipping it arrived just under the deadline. Delonzo and Becca were proud of the nearly twenty-page presentation book and we copied it as a thank you to those who helped.

January arrived with a phone call interview that the kids made it to the top ten list of all the entries. Becca announced, "See, my angels told me that we were supposed to do it and they were right!" Disney interviewed the kids and asked for references to make sure they did what they had claimed.

We were not the only volunteer project to achieve the top ten spot, a local girl scout troop was featured in the newspaper for the hundreds of hours of volunteering they did across our community.

The March first deadline for the winner came and went. I reassured the kids that is was an honor to make it to the top ten. But,

Becca continued to claim that it just wasn't here yet, the letter was coming and once again she was right.

A week later the envelope arrived with the news the kids 'Backpack for Kids' project was the Disney All Stars Team project winner.

Becca announced, "I told you so!"

The kids were excited to find out that they won a $1000 check for their project and that would go a long way to buy school supplies for the upcoming season. Now an individual winner and our kids would be off to California to do a volunteer project with Becca's hero Raven and her cast.

The kids, Jim and I spent a couple of days at the Disneyland hotel where each child found individual gigantic gift baskets waiting them. The baskets were nearly as big as Becca, and the boys and Detamara tore into them to find countless movies, CD's and all sorts of Disney paraphernalia.

The Disney trip came just before Ian was to ship out for Iraq. God must have known that the kids needed to say goodbye to Ian. He took leave, and Marissa joined us at Disneyland.

We shared our story of the backpacks at the volunteer outing. The corporate Disney people marveled at the miracles of Becca and our family's journey while we planted flowers and spent time visiting a Burbank nursing home. The kids got to visit the taping of the *That's So Raven* show and were shy to meet Raven and her cast, but it was Becca who spoke up and broke the silence.

The dream did not stop with Disney.

Backpack for Kids continued to grow, word spread and by the third year of the project it was easier to do the work since now many retailers were on board. Gift certificates arrived from Target. Old Navy called to let us know then the backpacks went on clearance. The two Old Navy stores in our part of the state had a friendly competition to see which store brought in the most school supplies by their employees. Office Depot stood behind the kids, and our drop sites continued to help us. The third year we filled nearly seven hundred backpacks and caseworkers began to help us assemble them and the juvenile court workers had kids do community service hours by helping with the project. Our old house still had not sold and was standing empty so we filled it with supplies and backpacks.

Our children were growing older and the project was now running out of steam. The non-profit group who had sheltered the project was now changing hands, and we had no place to help us with non-profit status. Other community organizations were duplicating our idea. I questioned if we were to continue, but Becca needed the project, and was even getting work-study credit for her participation. My kids would not quit and we decided to go it alone. I was six months into writing *Tiny Titan* and facing writer's doubt. I prayed for a Backpack-for-Kids miracle and people to help us with the project and *Tiny Titan*.

We filled up the newly created storage room at our new house with backpacks. We actually designed two rooms, one for our storage and the other for the Backpack-for-Kids project. We had witnessed miracles of the never-ending coffee can of change; it just seemed to never get to the bottom. Just when it seemed too impossible a miracle donation or something helped the kids through.

Then came the phone call that put back the spark. I was sitting with Becca in June, when the phone rang. I had prayed for 'people' to help me with the book and the Backpack Project and I doubted my prayers value as no one showed up.

The call was from a writer from *People Magazine*, I guess I hadn't specified lower case or uppercase 'p' in my prayer. In my wildest dreams, I never thought of *People Magazine* that wanted to do an article about small angels and had heard about the kids work.

Amy made an appointment and drove to Kalamazoo and she not only found the 'Backpack for Kids' project, she found a bigger story called *Tiny Titan*. For over three hours Jim and I talked of our journey. She told me in her years as a writer she had not heard a story such as ours.

I offered her the first chapter of the book and asked for her impression. She told me she is tough critic and did I really want the truth?

"Just read," I said.

After she finished she told me I had to finish it and it was really good. Several phone calls from Amy came and went. They were supposed to send a photographer and when the phone call never came, the kids and I settled for the fact we were not chosen to be in the story.

We worked on the project for weeks and all of our backpacks were spoken for through caseworkers and non-profit agencies. At the last moment the media decided to come out and share our children's hard work of packing almost nine hundred backpacks. The Department of Health kindly allowed us to use an empty conference room. The noon news reported our story and the phones of the Department of Health started ringing. They received so many phone calls that their phone lines crashed. The supervisor came downstairs and told us what happened and I called the news channel to make sure they announced the backpacks were already gone. It was clear, nine hundred backpacks were not enough to meet the needs of our community.

On the way home, I questioned myself if all this media attention was worth it. Every time, they got involved my life changed. Upon my return home I learn that *People Magazine* had resurrected the story. They wanted to send the photographer to town to for an upcoming issue. We had already given out and backed the backpacks and I didn't have one left and the kids had used up all their money. *People Magazine* is sending their people and we had nothing.

The children did one more fundraiser and we made arrange ments for the kids in the shelter to be in the photo shoot. It was a special day, as *The People* photographer gave my kids and the kids in the mission a lesson in photography and modeling. Each week my kids looked for their story, but it never came. The kids understood that Hurricane Katrina needed exposure and our story was less important with so many people no needing help.

Then on November 14, Becca and I stumbled on the long awaited story while waiting in the checkout line at Target. At the top of her little lungs Becca yelled for Delonzo and Detamara announcing to the store we are in *People Magazine*.

The People article exposed our project to generous people who sent letters of encouragement and small checks. Soon boxes began entering our doors. We had to borrow Matt's truck to retrieve a pallet donation of 585 pounds of school supplies from a wholesaler in Chicago who donated to our project. Our storage room filled with supplies and has overflowed into the triple car garage. We no longer can park any cars in it. We will do one more year of the backpack project and leave it as a legacy to the community.

The community welcomes our project, and others are participating. We are taking on the challenge to move the backpack project to a new level and are adopting all of the children in the two needi-est elementary schools in the inner city. The Kalamazoo Kings baseball team has offered to help us and we are already planning a school supply drive at the ball field. Corporations are jumping on board and the Kalamazoo community and school organization are collaborating to make this a reality.

Our children opened the door to the national attention of Disney and People Magazine. Their project idea this year is to write to corporations to not only get backpacks and school supplies, but new socks, underwear, hair bobbles and bead and clothing so that these children can go to school and have the opportunity to reach for the Kalamazoo Promise. Needy kids need tools to learn to achieve their dreams.

Sixteen years ago, Kristy, Nathan, Ian and Marissa started school with donated backpacks and school supplies and I vowed that someday we would repay their kindness. Our new children understood the realities of not having supplies to begin school. The Yurceks had not forgotten, we multiplied it hundreds of times with nearly three thousand backpacks and counting these past four years.

Becca was right, her angels helped us and did find the "people" to help us along the way.

- 50 -
IRAQ

Our son Ian had no idea what he wanted to do with his life after high school and he wasted his scholarship money from the state by not waking up to go to class. Ian's brightness was not challenged in high school and he had learned to slack off. He had never needed to study, so he never learned 'how' to study. The work in school was much too easy and like Kristy, he didn't see any point in doing it. Both kids aced tests without opening a book and no amount of lecturing by parents or teachers made a difference. Ian was now paying the price for his lack of study skills and initiative.

Ian had been tested for placement in the gifted program, and both times the scores did not show the high levels of uniqueness that I saw in his early years. He was a bright kid and because of Kristy's giftedness, the school district in Minnesota kept an eye on the siblings of those students. As sixth grade approached, he was assessed once again, and with no warning they tested him in a different format. They caught him off guard, and his scores looked much different. He scored in the top two percent.

When we asked Ian why the difference, he finally confessed that he had blown the other two tests because he didn't want to be identified as a 'nerd.'

That is my Ian.

One day he approached his father and I about his need to discipline his life saying he needed a quick kick in the shorts to help him get where he needed to go in life. He was going to join the Marines!

Jim and I knew he may be right, but we didn't want our son put in harms way. We could see that the world stability was getting more complicated and things were not heading in the right direction. His father and I tried to convince him otherwise, we told him Kristy and Nathan had figured out ways to pay for college. There was no changing Ian's bright and stubborn mind once he sets it. We knew we could not hold him back and all we could do was provide advice. Each of our children would have to learn life on their own and make their own decisions.

Ian took the placement tests for the military and was pestered (recruited) often. Ian wanted to be a doctor and with the other kid's medical and mental health bills, Jim's student loans, and the costs of a large family we could not help with tuition. He met with recruiting officers in Portage and they made promises that looked good to a kid – education reimbursement for his time served. Ian saw the military as a way to get the structure and boot in the shorts to grow up.

The Marine Corp now knew they had a candidate that they rarely see and he signed the paperwork. Ian was off to the Marines to develop discipline and provide a way to pay for college, and begin the long road to Medical School. Ian was smart and enlisted with a career goal in mind. He would learn to run computers for the Marine Corp.

Meanwhile the US was talking about Iraq, my heart ached. My heart had to trust that if this is what he wants to do, then we needed smart people to serve our country and God would be there with him. I trusted so many times with Becca. I knew full well that we really have no control over our lives and anything can happen at any moment. Why would it be different for Ian?

I asked God to protect Ian, and I told my son that I was proud that he knew he needed discipline and he had a plan for his future. But from the earliest moments with Ian in the Marines, we found ourselves in messed up paperwork – there were lost orders and dropped urine screenings. He took his physical in Lansing. Jim drove him to the station to ship off to boot camp with orders ready to go. After arriving, he was delayed from his training because of the dropped urine screen, and they lost his place in the computer-training program. Two months later, Jim took Ian to the bus to Camp Pendleton. Saying goodbye to our son was not easy. All the kids were in tears – even my tough guys. Ian challenged them to do things that I couldn't. He is their brother and they now looked up to him. DJ became lost without Ian's guidance and struggled.

My heart ached quietly as I prayed that God would make a way and protect both my sons – Ian heading to military duty and DJ off to make his way on urban streets.

Ian finished boot camp shining;he was a young man with speed and agility. He breezed through boot camp; the challenge sparked the competitive side that he was strong at. He was one of the fastest on the courses and he ran for miles with ease. I remembered my little asthmatic toddler who trained his stamina by running miles with heavy newspapers.

Just as Ian was again shipping off for his training, the Marine Corp changed his contract from being a computer specialist to a Hummer driver. They threatened they would throw him in the brig if he refused to go. It didn't matter that he had lost his slot because of the mistake of the dropped urine screen.

I was angry, they had made a promise to my son, and they were breaking a promise over their mistake. Something was not right. Over the years, my children had taught me I was 'not' just a mom. I called the recruiting office and they said they would look into it. I had heard that before in both the medical and social welfare settings where someone inevitably dropped the ball. It didn't surprise me the military gave me the same line. Not letting it go, I called all the way to Lansing and I threatened to get my congressmen's office involved. I cited law and breach of contract and after a couple of days of haggling, Ian was sent on with everything 'supposedly' fixed.

The officers in charge asked Ian if his mom is a lawyer and he told them that no one messes with us. My mom took on the state of Michigan for his sister and won for her needed care.

Thinking the order mess was cleaned up, he once again found himself with lost orders at the next base. As he stepped in line at the base he heard the Sergeant call for anyone with MOS problems to step in the other line. Ian stepped in the other line.

The first Sergeant argued with him saying there was nothing they could do but go back to the second set of orders and send him off to Hummer training and deployment. A higher up officer overheard Ian's conversation with me on the cell phone and the argument with the Sergeant and pulled him aside.

After the examination of the orders, they told him that he had breach of contract with the Marine Corp and if he wanted he could go home and be out of the Marines. The officer looked thoroughly at his paperwork and remarked that he was too bright to be wasted driving truck. Little did he realize that one of Ian's biggest weaknesses is his ability to get lost. Of all my kids, Ian is directionally challenged. This wise move probably saved my son from driving the wrong way on the wrong road right into enemy hands. *Thank you God.*

Ian saw this as a failure and said he wanted to stay, but do computers. They rewrote the orders back to the original contract and he went off to a base to wait for the opening in the computer training. For a couple of months he swept the dessert, swam, played basketball and did virtually nothing.

Ian excelled in computer training, but his patience was thoroughly tested by the Marine Corp. I always tell my children that the easier road usually ends up being the long hard road back with detours that take them to places they did not want to go.

Ian now understood and would face wherever his new road would take him. He knew for the next four years he had to stand by his commitment and live with his consequence. He enjoyed a brief couple weeks at home after his training and it seemed all too short, especially for him.

On leave he wrestled with his brothers and inspired them with his weightlifting ability. Becca beamed and enjoyed the ride as Ian used her for his dumbbell. The moment was a precious memory to keep in my heart when he returned to base.

Upon returning to the base, Ian called me in a panic. He had orders to ship out to Iraq the following week. He understood that he had to go.

I prayed for a miracle.

About an hour and a half later, he called again. He had been standing in line, when the gunny in the front of the room announced she needed two computer techs to stay behind to run the computers at the base. She called two other young Marines and then she changed her mind and shouted – "Yurcek and Rodriguez, you're coming with me." Ian couldn't believe his ears.

He stepped forward puzzled. He told me he could not believe it. Over the course of the weekend Ian felt like an emotional yo yo as the decision wavered back and forth. Ultimately, Monday arrived, and the determined female gunny prevailed. She took Rodriguez and Yurcek and moved them from the barracks and into a dorm room apartment. Once again, Ian was protected from deployment.

God had miraculously listened to me and answered my prayer.

Both Detamara and Becca would not understand Ian having to go to Iraq. Detamara viewed the world as an unsafe place, especially if her favorite brother Ian, who had protected her from Shay and the ghosts that haunted her, was not safe. Perhaps nothing in the whole world could ever be safe ever again and her progress was in jeopardy.

I prayed that she did not fall apart after she had come so far.

Many more times Ian was protected from deployment. Once he was scheduled to leave and he broke his hand while playing basketball. Then his hand had trouble healing and he sat on the base for more months. When it looked like he was to leave once again, the gunny made him non-deployable by giving him a job on the base fueling jets for six months. Finally, Ian got the call that he 'really' had to go and he was upset when he could not come home to visit.

It was heartbreaking. I so wanted to hug my son before he left for his tour of duty, but Becca, always the believer, assured us we hadn't yet gotten her letter about our trip for the kids Backpack for Kids Project.

Becca was right, just prior to his deployment the kids' tickets arrived from Disney and we headed to California where I had a chance to be with my son who joined us in LA for the weekend. The hard work Ian's little brothers and sisters did in creating the Backpack's for Kids Project provided our whole family the gift of hugging Ian goodbye. All of us hung out at Disneyland. I savored the moments and captured the memories in my mind in case I never saw Ian again.

It didn't matter what we did. It mattered that we were together and we had a good time. It was a perfect answer for all of us to say goodbye and tell Ian we loved him. I watched my military son play with his little brothers and sisters. Ian coaxed Detamara onto a Dance Revolution machine. I recorded it and while Ian was in Iraq the little girls watched those videos over, and over, and over again.

Jim had a very hard time letting him leave and saying goodbye was difficult. Jim's heart sank; worry lines were deeply etched in his face. I noticed how much older and greyer he looked, going through Medical School, especially residency had been hard on him He loves his job so much, I seldom saw the sadness anymore, but having Ian in Iraq took its toll.

Jim traveled to San Diego the week of Ian departure and he promised Ian he would be there when Ian returned. I stayed home with my hands full of the siblings left behind and we said goodbye to Ian via cell phone. After Detamara had her turn she put herself to bed and asked for her medication to sleep away the goodbye. Becca broke my heart, she kept sobbing saying over and over she did not want him to go. She was not one to cry over things, and with her strong determined will and her spirit she didn't allow herself to feel sorry for what life handed her. But today her heart was breaking and silently mine was too. She cried tears bigger than I had ever seen her cry.

That first evening Becca cried herself to sleep on the brown leather couch with Ian's picture held tightly in her tiny thin arms. Marissa grabbed her camera and the black and white picture was a reminder of the price families' pay when sons and daughter go to war far from home. Marissa was home from college in California for the summer; it would be lonely for her when she returned without her brother who had been stationed nearby. At least for the time being she was home with her family to shelter the blow.

I could not break down in front of the kids. I silently squelched the pain I was feeling, and reassured my children trying to convince myself everything would be all right. For the next three weeks, Becca carried her llxl4 mahogany framed portrait of her brother in his Marine Corp dress blues. People stopped in their tracks to watch my tiny Becca carrying her beloved brother's portrait.

The girls' nightly prayers include their brother and every night as I heard Becca's prayers, I said my own. Becca told me that Ian has his own angel to watch over him and not to worry. I have heard Becca talk of her angels and I do not doubt their existence as she's proven they exist to me with all the miracles I've seen.

Our family had mixed feelings on the war; Marissa placed a yellow ribbon on the front column on our new home. I found a single electric lighted candle that remains lit in the window until Ian is safely home.

Ian has shared with Becca that he believe he really has angels too. One night on base in Iraq he was suppose go to the mess hall and something didn't feel right. He decided not to go. An incoming missile hit the pathway he would have been on at the time.

We sent off boxes of things from home. Kristy set up an email list with many of our family and friends to give him a needed boost. With the email, many people remembered Ian in Iraq; he received letters, emails and care packages to buffer his loneliness.

Jim's face lit up every time he got a call from his son. As a computer geek, Ian had access to the email and often the phone so we did not wonder about him. We heard his voice often. This was reassuring to the girls and Jim. Ian and I talked from our hearts, he shared when he returns to Michigan, he never wanted be far away again. This was a change as Ian always said he wanted to travel the world and go far away to school.

He began counting the days to come home. Luckily, with his decision to enlist in a specialized branch, his deployment was not as unpredictable as many other Marines and those in the Army. He received orders to return sometime in late winter of 2006.

Thanksgiving and Christmas were lonely for all of us. His empty place setting and chair reminded us where he was and our normally chattering crew was a bit somber. Then as we were just sitting down to dinner, Ian called from the opposite ends of the earth to share the miracle of Christmas conversations. Even separated half an earth away, the Yurceks celebrated the holiday together as we passed the phone to one another.

February arrived, and I will never forget the phone call that Ian's replacement had arrived on the base for training. He was coming home in a couple of weeks. He gave us cryptic messages about when and he would only say his age plus four when he would land in San Diego.

The tax return had arrived just in time. Jim bought his ticket immediately. Ian used the Internet to purchase tickets for his best friend Kitty, his sidekick and best friend Ethan, and Matt. Matt had crashed the car and was indebted to Mom and Dad for the deductible and he was now broke. Jim and Ethan drove a car to Chicago, while Matt and Kitty headed out a day later. Kristy flew back from Spain to meet her brother. The two determined sisters battled Marine Corp bureaucracy to move heaven and earth to find out the transport plane arrival time.

As Ian stepped out of the plane, he spied his family who were jumping up and down with signs. Matt's sign said, "Sorry I crashed your truck," and Ian was a little worried until he found out that his little brother had played another Yurcek practical joke. Ian definitely had family. He had the biggest contingency at the airbase with Marissa, Kristy, Matt, Ethan, Kitty, and Jim. Jim had promised to be there when he landed and he called from his cell phone to tell me when Ian was safely on the ground in the United States.

God had protected Ian.

I cried, big tears of thanksgiving. I yelled downstairs to the kids and their cheers of happiness echoed through the walls of the new huge house. Even the dogs barked in the celebration. The next call was from Ian.

My therapist asked how come Jim gets to travel so often with Ian, and I stay home. I told her Jim needs to be there for Ian, more than I do and Ian needs Jim, besides we can't afford to fly everyone and the children can't miss too much school.

Jim and the kids spent the week with Ian in San Diego, Jim's sister Carol, her husband Allyn, six-year-old daughter Kyra, and three-year-old Ryan joined them, along with Jim's grown niece Bobbi. With thousands of miles between us, the Yurceks celebrated Ian's homecoming. Not to be left out of the festivities, I participated via the cell phone while they ate out, walked the beaches, and picnicked in the park. I shared picnicking and playing basketball with them in the sunshine while I drove on the ice and newly fallen snow of our Michigan February. Their ten days in San Diego flew by and the kids and I once again drove the two-hour trek to Chicago to bring them home.

All I could do while Ian was in Iraq was to believe he was safe and doing well. I had stayed tough for the kids and kept telling them everything was going to be okay while silently praying. On the other hand, I could not make the children a promise I could not keep. The reality was Ian may have lost his life or gotten badly hurt. It was that secret I kept locked in my heart and Jim and I and the children never discussed. We couldn't dwell on something we couldn't control.

Looking though the pictures of my son's safe arrival home freed my tears. Tears of thanksgiving. Detamara and Becca assured Jim that it's okay Mom's crying, she cries when she's happy. The kids were too hyped to go to sleep, and my day began sleepless. That night I crawled into bed, safely falling into the deep nights sleep that had evaded me since Ian's departure. I didn't need to count sheep; I was counting down the days until he returns home.

- 51 -

COMING HOME

A few weeks after Shay returned to Kalamazoo she turned eighteen. She now had all the rights of adulthood, and with her developmental disability questions rose regarding guardianship. How do you parent an adult daughter with a disability? What were our roles and how could we play them out? I wanted to help her develop her independence, but give her supports to prevent failure. This next year would be a hard road discovering what worked and what didn't.

The group home idea turned into an ultimate disaster. The girls living there were too unstable for Shay to handle. They were higher functioning and she was easily used and manipulated by them because she wanted to be accepted. As Shay was the oldest and now eighteen, they asked her to buy cigarettes or other over the counter medications that were restricted to be purchase by minors. She bought them things to buy their friendship. When the girls in the house had meltdowns that brought the police, we started looking for other options for Shay's placement.

We worked together to find how we fit into each other's lives. I attended her person centered planning meetings. Shay learned from experience and she came to me for guidance when she needed Mom's advice. Shay asked me for help to manage her finances and included me in her medical care. It was a rocky beginning while we all learned what support systems were truly needed. When she is not quite on, she allows staff to help her get back on track. She has moments of depression and ups and downs of her bipolar disorder, but for the most part she is stable.

With the caseworkers help, we finally found a young woman who needed a roommate and a nice two-bedroom apartment with a pool. It is on the bus line convenient for Shay to learn to ride the transit system and stores are just around the corner. Staff helps Shay get to the Y to play basketball. She joins the family for Friday night dinners, and we now have Mom and Shay phone calls. The kids slowly came to trust that Shay was really doing well.

▼

Shay had come along way, and so had I.

I had moved from being 'just' a mom, to someone who knew way too much to do nothing. During these past years, I started volunteering in the advocacy world. I flew to Washington DC, and worked on a grant to help develop protocols to reduce the use of seclusion and restraint in residential settings. My mission was to help garner family involvement for children in residential settings and try to make residential care settings more family friendly.

I testified in Lansing, our state capital, for the Senate Hearings on the failures of Mental Health Services in Michigan. Governor Granholm announced the appointment of a mental health commission. I received a letter to apply. The commission was made up of mostly legislators and professionals.

But word never came. I rallied friends and other advocates and we told our stories in front of the commission. I carried a friend's testimony of her having to give up on her eight-year-old son, for the lack of services and the severity of his illness, all the way to a Lansing Senate hearing. The professionals were now talking about custody relinquishment to get services. Two years previously many told me it did not happen in Michigan, my struggles and truth was finally validated. A reporter for the Detroit Free Press opened the door to a series about the lack of Michigan children's services.

The US Surgeon General reported on the failure of mental health for children. It was true. We had lived it. Not only would I be validated by the knowledge that I was right, but it was not me who failed my daughter. We were set up to fail by a fragmented, under funded, and broken mental health care system. We were not alone. I knew there were others. I learned the numbers of others was too numerous to fathom.

Manfred set up a meeting with the new director of our community mental health agency. The director had moved from being the Michigan Deputy Interim Director of Mental Health to our community. He came to my 'new home' and sat in my 'new' living room. I showed him the five binders containing fifty pounds of paper filled with information on our fight for Shay. He saw what he did not know. He saw the person centered plan that asked us to give up custody of Shay three years earlier ordering us to find a lawyer in sixty days. He asked for copies of the documentation he had seen as somehow they were "missing from the files."

He told me that we had been wronged. He apologized.

I had received my long awaited apology.

Manfred said since we could not go back in time, we needed to move on. I had decided not to pursue a lawsuit for all that had happened. Money would not repair the damage. It would only make the lawyers rich, and take money from an already struggling under funded system. The only ones who would pay the price, would be the children and adults they served. Suing would only cause me to relive, be beat upon, and defend our family, Shay, and myself again. No one wins and everyone loses while the fight takes away precious time from the real task of serving children and families and adult clients.

Manfred had now become close to our family and knew of the other kid's issues. He understood that I was only one crisis away at times from disaster. Delonzo needs redirection and constant attention to stay out of trouble. Detamara melted down when she was tired or something went wrong. Becca requires great energy to keep up with her medical cares and pain. She needs redirection when she is obsessing. I was exhausted from Jim's five-year residency and managing the family alone. I was tired of fighting and working endlessly for the children, but I kept on keeping on.

My mental exhaustion was not from working with my children, but having to day in and day out navigate the tangled fragmented care system I needed to educate to help my children remain stable.

▼

We were told our children were not children who would victimize others and they would not be severely emotionally disturbed. I told the workers we would not put our other children at risk, especially Becca.

The children were told that we would be a forever family and it would be fun!

Jim and I knew the children would come with emotional baggage, but we had no idea how severe. We had no data on DeShawn's acting out behavior, except that he had cut a computer cord. Detamara and DeShawn's foster parents had requested an assessment for fetal alcohol and never received it, yet their preschool records noted they had asked for it.

After Becca's episode with DeShawn, he revealed he had been abused and child protection services came to interview him in our home. We worked with a Michigan child protection worker who told me I had more than I could handle. He told me my children would be impossible for anyone to handle. He warned me that I would be held accountable for anything that happened in my home and I could face charges of failing to protect. I had to understand that to make sure everyone was safe in my home. He walked away without telling me what to do. So for five years I had tried to be 'super mom' and always vigilant to protect my children, yet I didn't know what was wrong with them. We never saw the two - seventeen page psychologicals Shay had before we adopted her. The severity of her issues was hidden from us. We never saw the thirteen page data on DJ. Delonzo and Deangelo had never seen a therapist.

My vigilance carried us through fires, floods and victimizations. I would not reveal the severity of my children's needs to anyone for fear they would take them. Maybe we were lucky, but I like to believe we have been watched over. God gave me the intuition many times to prevent major disasters - the smoldering tissue box, the towel into the open door the gas hot water heater. My hand and eyes many times placed in just the right spot at just the right moment to stop a catastrophe. My intuition knowing the reality and my mouth sputtering out just the right thing to redirect a child. Becca's medical condition trained me to handle the stressors and develop coping mechanisms I would use with my adopted children.

Jim and I love all our children and all our children love us, but over time we came to realize that the way they show their love is different from our first set of six. Bridging the gap of broken attachments is difficult. Crossing over the chasm of generational poverty is complex. Not knowing the children you are raising are brain injured is unforgivable. Current brain research is showing us that trauma, abuse, neglect, malnutrition and chemical exposure changes children's brains.

Caregivers need knowledge of their children to care for them Professionals often mistake the stressed out parents and siblings standing behind a smiling child as not fit to care. They do not see the child who is hell bent on not letting anyone close or be told what to do. They do not see a parent doing their best to be vigilant around-the-clock to take care of the needs of the child, and while surrounded by the crisis needs of the child limit care for himself or herself. I feared that if child protection services swooped in to scoop up a melted down or misbehaving child, my biological and adoptive children would be taken too. And they would fail with Becca. Her medical needs were so great they would kill her.

▼

Manfred helped get the children assessed and their Medicaid cases opened by Mental Health. Detamara, Delonzo, DJ, all had fetal alcohol spectrum diagnoses. DJ and Delonzo had additional diagnosis of Bipolar Disorder. Delonzo also had ADHD.

Luckily for Deangelo we only see glimpses of the broken pieces since during his mother's pregnancy social services was working directly with her and it made a valuable difference for his future.

After that pregnancy she hid out from social services and ultimately it cost her the loss of all her children. For the three youngest kids, her road into deeper chemical dependency cost Delonzo, DeShawn and Detamara brain capacity and life skills.

My newest children were finally diagnosed and qualified for treatment. It had taken over five years! Slowly we found answers, and I got much needed respite for Becca, Delonzo and Detamara. We received in home help. I am incredibly grateful for the support that has allowed my children to thrive.

For the first time in years I took a hot bath without fear of disaster and I shut the door.

▼

Shay got help, and with Manfred's help, the others received the help they needed. In time Manfred and my acquaintances from the State helped other parents.

The small network of parents who I met through the Internet and my advocacy supported one another and learned to parent from afar or help each other fight for our children's rights to care and treatment, or to honorably let go. Every family has to do what is right for them. It is not our job to judge what is right for someone else. My friend whose testimony I carried to state Senate Hearings, name was cleared of neglect. Another parent's son was returned home with support services to help him thrive.

Not only did Shay make monumental progress, I did too. I was asked to help build a system of care for children in our community with the very people who wanted to betray our family. The new director of Mental Health launched an initiative to develop a Center of Excellence for Children with Neurobiological Disorders like my children. He appointed the new Deputy Director of Children's Mental Health and it was the same person who I felt had a vendetta against me because I did not listen to her clinical decisions since I could not bring Shay home. My intuition for my children spared us from disaster. If I had listened, I do not believe that we would have had the outcomes for our children. I doubted myself many times, but now I was validated when I called Manfred for a pep talk.

I was asked to sit next to her at meetings to develop a system of care in our community. I did not know what to think, so much was being asked of me. I was nervous and scared at the first meeting. I put aside my feelings and our history to work with her side-by-side. In time, she listened to my parent-expertise and she listened to other parents and acknowledged the barriers that frustrate families. Slowly, together we work together to better the system.

I have made great gains in speaking in front of others. I testified, spoke before the state mental health board and opened a conference with a Keynote address. I had to overcome my social phobia and fear of speaking.

Shay's highlight came when she graduated from high school a year after returning to our community. She smiled and handed me her diploma to lock in the safe for safekeeping. My daughter was not another statistic of those with disabilities without a high school diploma.

Looking back it is hard to believe that seven years have passed. Shay and I talk of our memories and discuss the future. Some say Shay is definitely my daughter and she mirrors my mission of offering others a hand up.

I am proud of my daughter, and I believe she is proud of me.

We both have come so far.

- 52 -
Forgiveness

When I talk to people about my children's past, they ask why I am not angry with their mother for causing all their problems. I feel sorry for their mother. She did not choose to be born with challenges like her children that made it virtually impossible for her to parent.

When we first got the kids, the stories made me angry. I listened to their cries and saw such pain on their faces. Yet even with the entire trauma they experienced, they still loved their mother. In time I learned I had to forgive her for not knowing what she did to them. As I came to understand my children and their needs, I realized that their vulnerable mother had no help, didn't understand cognitively or culturally what was being asked or her, or wouldn't accept help and fell through the cracks of an unknowing society. I realize today that her offspring left without the supports and the fight I was willing to give could easily suffer the same face.

I have found some of her history and I believe she is a product of intergenerational fetal alcohol syndrome. Their mother did not have insight into how to help her children. She buried her hidden disabilities and mental health problems in drugs and alcohol. She never made it past middle school, she could not read a phone book, and she lived a life of poverty and want.

Forgiveness for the kids' abusive father was not as easy. He beat their mother. He threw her down a flight of stairs in front of the children and when I went down the stairs, Shay was reliving the trauma of her past. Her posttraumatic stress disorder put her mind in another place and time. Perhaps she was throwing him down the stairs instead of me. The kids told me that when he was sober and not high, he was a caring dad who brought them toys and played with them. But the drugs, and alcohol, and withdrawal from self-medicating made him mean and nasty.

I had to learn to forgive him too. Without him, my children would not be here. He was their father and he had wounds that we may never understand, wounds that he maybe tried to bury in substance abuse. Perhaps, the only way he knew how to help himself was to self medicate.

Shay had brain damage caused by the drugs and alcohol before she was born. She had trauma responses from the abuse and neglect. She had attachment issues that kept her distant from the family. How can I blame her for her hurts?

Her wounds were compounded when the school failed to provide the support, structure and guidance for her to be successful. I had learned that she functioned at a higher and more stable level when things were calm and controlled and so I had worked diligently to maintain a very structured home for her and her siblings. I learned to protect my children I had to prepare for everything and with preparation we prevented many catastrophes. I could not help Shay's with her complex behavior from the medication prescribed and the doctor who failed to listen almost cost me my life and my daughter her family.

▼

Shay needed compassion. I had to forgive her for all the hurt she had caused the family, and the pain and lifelong challenges I will live with from my flight down the stairs. I cannot forget the moment because I will forever live with the pain, stiffness and spasms.

Fighting for Shay became the tool that helped me overcome my diagnosis of Post Traumatic Stress Disorder (PTSD). My flight down the stairs was not my first trauma; my first trauma was when Becca coded. I fought for my daughters, the first for her life, the second for her family. Shay has a right to a family, and the right to be all she can be, just like Becca.

I have taught my children that people can be forgiven, but to earn back trust behaviors have to change. The walk is greater than the talk. Shay is learning to live with her history and her fetal alcohol syndrome. Naming it, helps claim it. Just like with Becca, once we knew what we were dealing with, then we could find answers to help them cope.

My adopted children are survivors. They knew no stability; they had grown up in trauma, neglect and pain. They were brain damaged before they were born. Yet, in time, we have all moved forward together. It is that togetherness that has allowed us each to remain strong. Not all people are so lucky and as my children grow into adulthood they will struggle to integrate the pieces of their past into their future.

Perhaps I had to experience my own PTSD to understand how to help my children. My flight down the stairs was not my first trauma. I had to face the trauma of nearly losing Becca. I had to live it, to understand what my children could not tell me. Out of learning how to help myself, I came to understand how to help my children. Those traumatic times are forever etched in my memories, but I had to move past them. Just like my children have had to learn to let go of their traumatic pasts. My experience will forever be a piece of who and what I am, but I can choose to remain stuck or continue forward. I have learned to use the pain and struggles to empower me to continue on.

We all have choices of how we handle adversity. We can feel sorry for ourselves, or we can be survivors. Our scars become our stars if we let them. We all have the choice about how we see things, we can be bitter and angry over the circumstances of our lives, or we can find gratitude for each and every day that we are here. It is a choice. We all will have to face tragedy and loss, it is a part of our journeys. None of us will be spared.

We are all one moment away from losing our job or becoming homeless. We are all one moment away from facing serious illness of someone we love or ourselves. Most of us do not know it. We will all face losing someone. It is part of life.

DeShawn is lost from the family, but our prayers are with him. Our hope is that his new family will be able to reach him and teach him to love and care despite what the professionals have told us.

We have seen professionals proven wrong with kids who do not have a chance. We have seen miracles with Becca and Shay. So each day our prayers continue for DeShawn and the people who interact with him.

▼

My lips will never be the same, but my smile is bigger than ever. Until we have faced challenges, we can never find what we are truly capable of until we are required to. We do not know how blessed we are until we almost lose it.

Most of us walk around in denial that anything bad can happen to us. I did and my teens think they are immortal. It becomes a way of coping. For a long time, I could not think too far ahead and I was afraid of the future. I had to face the wound of the long ago loss of my devoted grandfather at the age of nine. I had to understand why I do not like flowers. I had to remember that flowers reminded me of the day we buried him so I could smell them again. I faced my fear of losing Becca and I went on with loving memories as others I lost who I cared for deeply. I lost friends and watched my friends bury their sick children. I was thankful that this time it was not I.

Each loss reminded me how precious and fragile life is.

Walking the walk of a parent with a child with a critical illness is not all sadness. We have a bit more idea that life is way too short. Families such as ours can choose to fight, be angry, be bitter; or become survivors. We can face each day striving for tomorrow, all the while enjoying the moment. No matter how strong the storm, we can look for and find rainbows. We know that eventually there is a sun shining on some tomorrow and so we hang on to hope.

We all have the courage in us; we just don't know it is there until we have to find it. Until we have faced adversity, we live our lives not taking risks. Some of us take the safe road. We take for granted today wishing for tomorrow.

I learned to live with the fact that every day I have Becca is a miracle. She can be challenging, and her obsessing can try my patience. I remind myself, she is still here to obsess. Life is too short to spend our time wishing for things to be different; we need to appreciate what we have.

Jim and I learned it is not about what we own, or how much money is in the bank. Those times looking back when we were strug gling, make us appreciate what we have today. Money does not buy happiness; and it will not buy us more time with Becca.

The Possibility Thinkers Creed

When faced with a mountain,

I will not quit!

I will keep on striving until I climb over,

Find a pass through, tunnel underneath, or simply stay..

And turn a mountain into a miracle with God's help.

Robert H. Schuller

As the wise old woman in our church foretold so many years ago, on Becca's dedication day, 'we were lucky.' We were blessed to have found out early on, what was truly important in life; we got to grow up sooner than later.

Out of that blessing, we would not waste our lives waiting for tomorrow. Good or bad, we will make it through.

We understood that everyday is a special present.

A gift of love, a gift of hope, and the joy of each moment.

▼

I have helped myself heal my wounds and our family's wounds by helping those on a similar journey. I can now help others and do the work that I promised myself so long ago I would do.

We use our hearts and talents to make a difference each and

everyday. I have had to teach my children how to love and give. They did not know the meaning of love and caring until someone was willing to teach them by setting an example. I have taught my children to do random acts of kindness whenever they can, whether it be opening the door for a stranger with a smile, or surprising an elderly person in the parking lot by offering to load their groceries or return their shopping cart to the cart corral.

We tell the kids we have shown them how to live and taught them lessons for where life will take them. We have given them the tools and now it is up to them to make their own way. Mom will be there to help them find supports they need to be successful, but they have will have to want to accept it and abide by the rules to keep it.

As our older biological children hit adulthood they finally understand the depths of the mental illness and trauma's impact on their adopted siblings. They have lived for years with the challenging behaviors, and now they understand why and how it impacts their siblings' futures. Each of my biological children struggles to forgive some of the past hurts. I tell them we have to leave the past in the past. We cannot go back and change it and our anger will cause us our own pain. They are beginning to understand what FASDs means.

They can forgive, but trust will have to be earned, as each of their siblings moves forward on the life path. Unlike, our oldest five children, the younger five may find the road they choose ultimately chosen for them. Because of their brain damage will those whose job it is to help and serve see my young adults as individuals who have hidden disabilities and provide abilities of protection, support and tools to achieve. Or they will choose to see them as "normal" and set them up in their vulnerabilities to fail.

All of my children have normal desires - to find love, to have money, to have food, to have a safe place to live, to have good health, to have fun and to 'be' normal. They need friends to help them move towards these life goals.

For DJ, Shay, Deangelo, Delonzo and Detamara we have given them a hand up. We have shown them another kind of life, far different than that of their parents. We ask them, what are they going to do with that gift? They can waste it and feel sorry for themselves or they can be thankful for the chance to see another way and reach for their dreams. Those dreams are not so different from any other kid. Sadly, the support systems for young adults with disabilities are few and far between to help them reach their dreams.

Each of my children with differences is only one step from the person who will set the compass on their lives. The road is not well traveled by those who are successful; the statistics after transition to adulthood are bleak for my children with disabilities.

Their hidden brain damage sets them up for failure and is com pounded by their struggle to appear and be normal. It is common for persons with FASDs to fail to be able to live on their own. Many require help or supervision consistently accomplish daily tasks and because of the nature of their disability some days they manage and other days they are incapable.

They may have the best of intentions and not be able to begin to figure out the first step. They may get the job of their dreams and not be able to keep it. Eighty percent of those with FASD lose their jobs. Relying on employment for complete income for many may be futile. If you lose your job you can't live on your own, because you will not be able to pay your bills. And the downward spiral of failure takes over.

▼

My job will not be over as the kids turn eighteen. It actually gets harder. No longer do I have any power to protect them from their impulsive choices. I realize these children will not be able to survive without society supports and for their own independent self-worth those supports include more than family care.

DJ fell, as so many kids from the system of child welfare do, to the street and homelessness, but DJ has returned home. He tried to walk the path of his mother. He called to tell us the day after Thanksgiving that he needed us. This family of ours is unique. We made phone calls across the country to fill in all our kids. We are in this together, but the Yurceks are a family. Has lost tons of trust because of his past choices, and some of the kids are bitter at DJ for his poor choices. Everyone voted to give him another chance to come home and the opportunity to earn his trust back.

DJ still struggles with accepting his cognitive differences. He defied working with mental health; and he 'hooked up' with a severely disturbed young lady and gave birth to twin baby girls. The babies were exposed to drugs and alcohol in utero just like DJ and he tried to help her and quit abusing chemicals. She told him she 'd quit when she was six months pregnant, but by then it was too late. The power of the drugs and alcohol began the cycle again. But as with much of our story, bad things happen and then good ultimately prevails. The birth of the twin baby girls brought DJ home.

Home to finally begin the road to mending his broken heart and understanding his broken brain. Our evenings are filled with helping him draft a course of success and a life plan. We talk to him. We show him. We help him process his mistakes.

Most days, DJ is no longer feeling sorry for himself. He is picking up the pieces of his life to move on. In our home he has stability to allow him to get back on track – he has clean clothes, food to eat, and people to help him with supports and rules.

I find myself sitting in courtrooms, meetings, and answering panicked cell phone calls. I help find and fill out paperwork to reinstate food stamps or reestablish identities due to lost state ID, social security card and birth certificate. Without an ID he could not get assistance, a job, enroll in community college, or establish paternity for the girls. Without ID, DJs life was on hold and it took me nearly a week to reestablish his identity. Since 9-ll getting a new birth certificate is nearly impossible and Minnesota never sent in the paperwork to change it so our names were on it.

DJ wavers with what to do.

Jim and I will join our son in court. We will sit beside him and walk him through the process of paternity or not. With his brain injury it would be unfair to make him do it alone.

I wonder if the mother of these little babies can get her life together, her older daughter already lives with her grandmother. I try not to think ahead.

I overhear Jim talking with DJ and DJ is saying that he thinks the babies are not his. Part is wishful thinking as an easy way out or perhaps they really aren't his.

Then I hear Jim tell him that maybe they need to be his babies. Jim went on further to explain that maybe they were destined to come into this family who understands and can help them get the help and services they will need to have a better life? Just like DJ did. DJ is very good with children and enjoys them. The county has filed a neglect charge against him for abandoning 'his' babies, babies he is not sure are his. I try to not think too far ahead on this one.

Colleen is telling me to say no, no, no! No babies! She threatens to put me in daily therapy if I take on this task. Friends say we don't need this. They are right, we did not need this to happen, but Jim and I do not trust the child welfare world with our grandchildren. We have found out how to help our children and we do not trust them with our children. We have seen the damage they knowingly and unknowingly caused by not understanding. We have learned way too much.

The cycle continues until we stop it. I cannot blame DJ's girlfriend, she came from a broken home. Her dad was in jail, and her mom died from alcoholism. She may be prenatally exposed like DJ, we do not know. She found refuge from her ghosts in self-medicating with chemicals.

The courts gave DJ kudos for being in court and taking responsibility. But in time the paternity tests revealed that DJ is not the babies' father. These little twin baby girls will not be forgotten – they were the catalyst that brought my wayward son home. Our hope and prayers go with these babies that they will get the help they need in their futures.

WHAT IS FAMILY?

By the Yurcek tribe

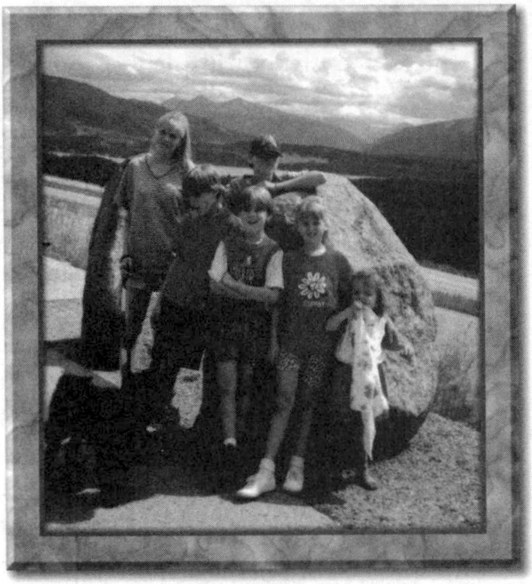

Families come in
all shapes and sizes.
People who love and
care for each other.
Everyone who lives in a house.
Some come together
through adoption.
Some through foster care.
Some live with their extended families.
Families don't always live together.
Some families are together for
only a little while.
But they are still part of a family.
Moms, Dad, Brothers, Sisters,
Grandparents, Foster Parents, Foster Siblings.
They always love and care for each other.

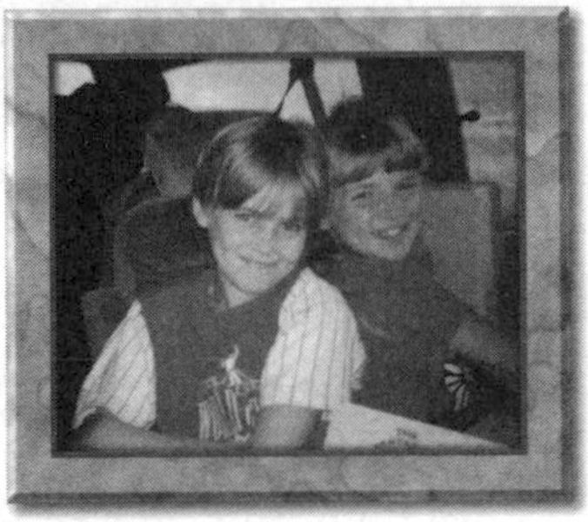

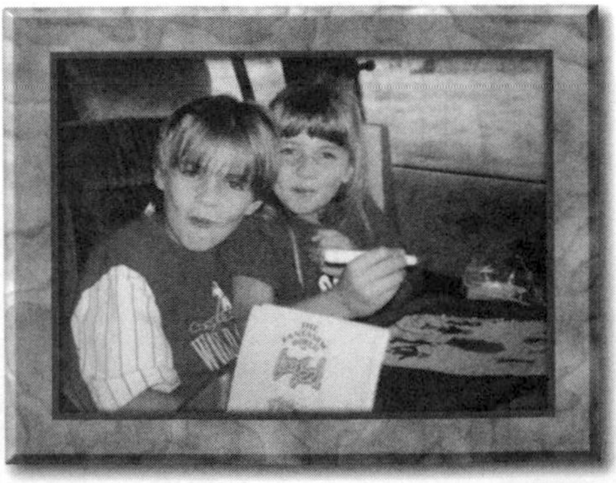

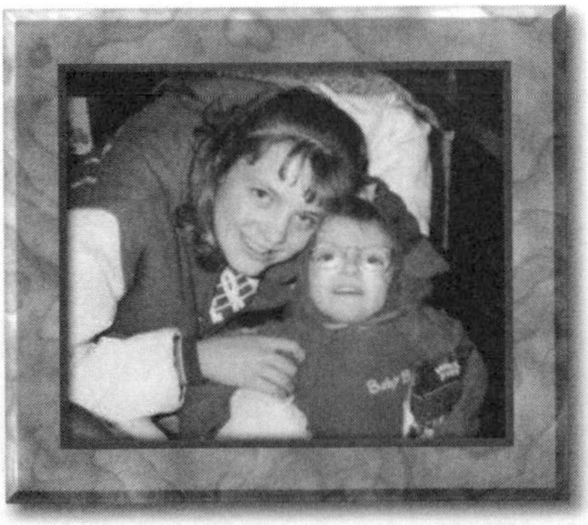

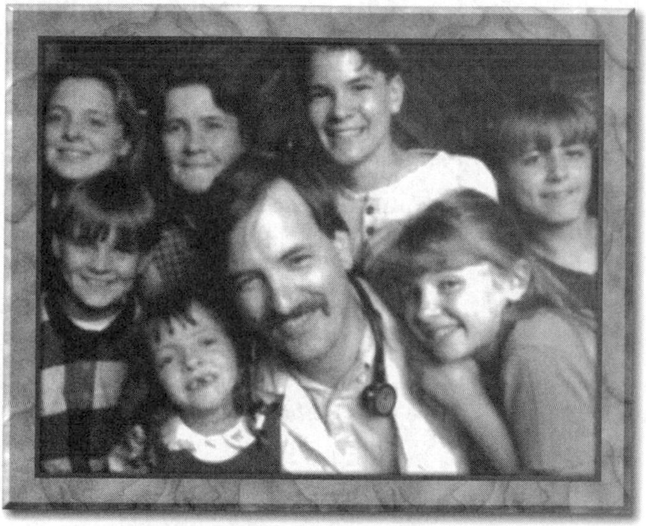

Special thanks to Kristy, Nathan, Ian, Marissa, Matt & Becca for sharing their family

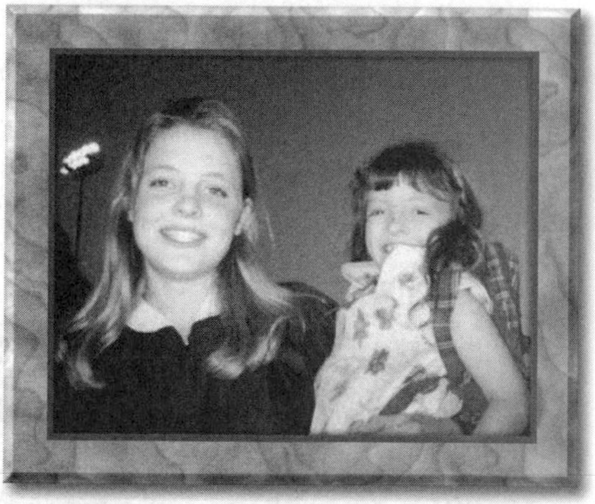

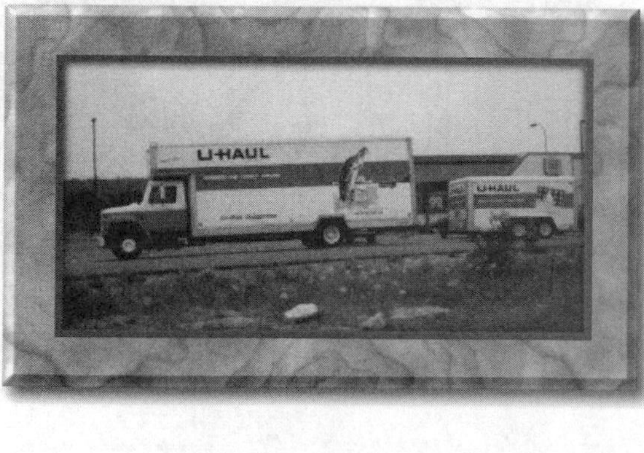

What is special about our family?

Birth and adopted kids, black, white and disabled,
It doesn't matter, we are expected to do our best.
A dog and a cat are family too.
We love them and they love us.
We love each other.
We were put together to become one big family.
We share our lives together.
We work, learn, and play together.
We all take care of each other and get along, most of the time.
We have others who share in our family.
Together we dream of a better future.

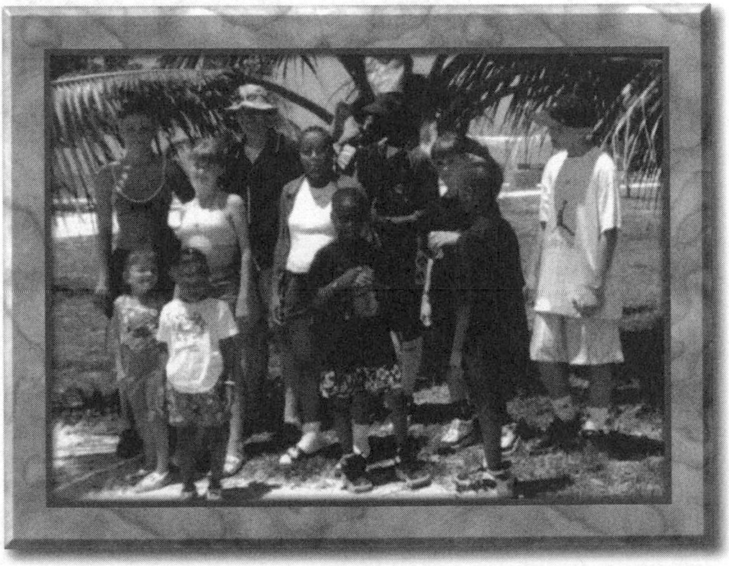

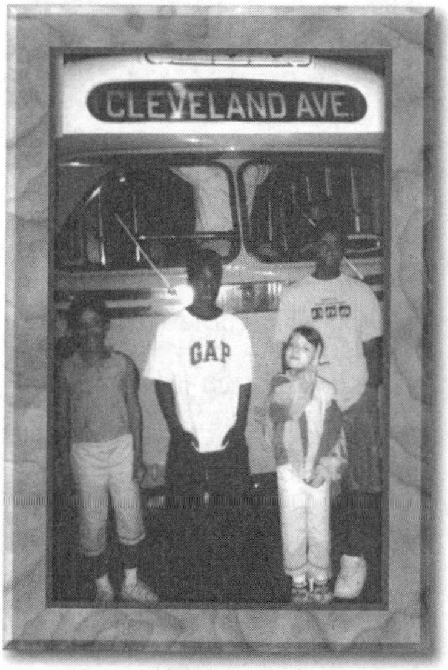

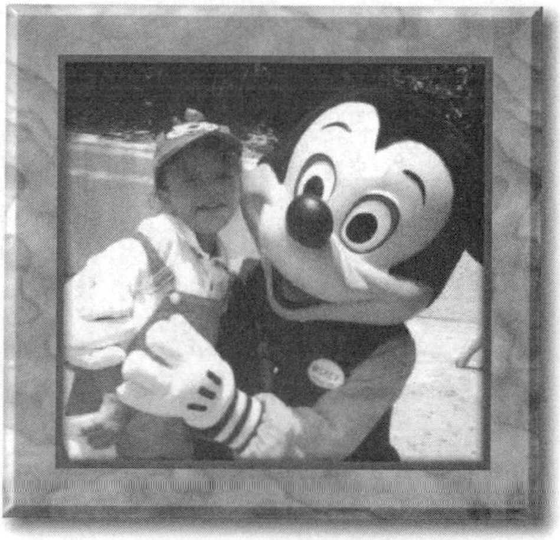

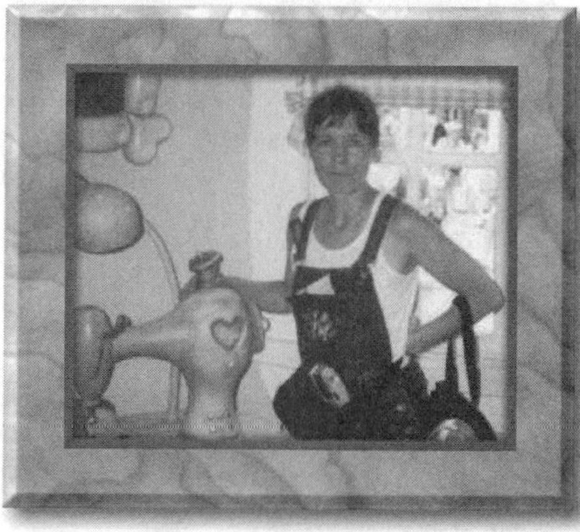

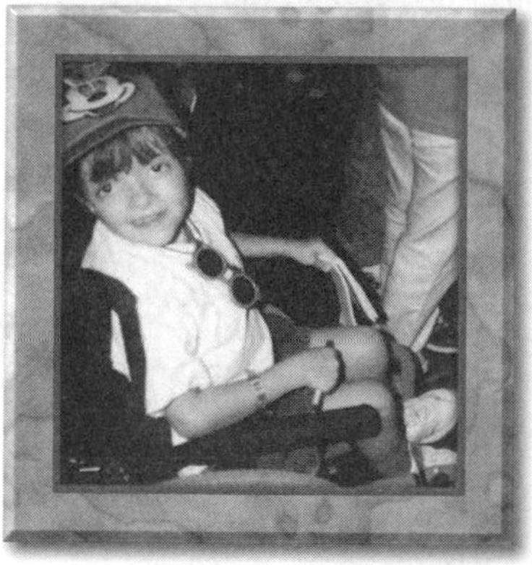

Special thanks to the Children's Wish Foundation, Atlanta, GA

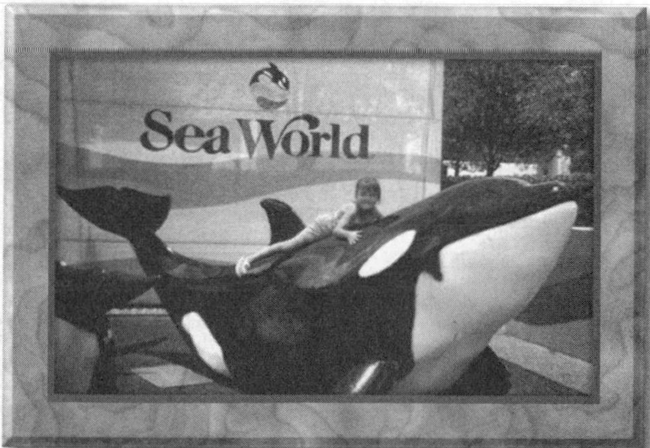

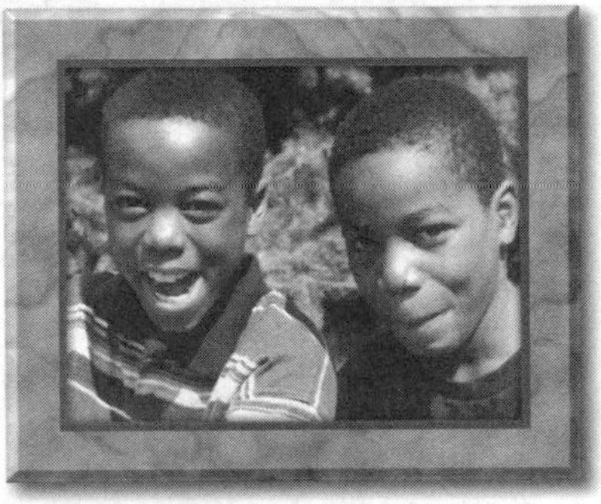

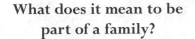

What does it mean to be part of a family?

Love each other.

Someone to hug and hold and love.

Helping each other out.

To care for each other.

Do your chores.

Not to fight and learn to get along together.

Listen to Mom and Dad they know best.

Follow the rules.

Sticking up for your brothers and sisters

when someone teases one.

Share with each other.

Someone will be there when you are

grown and need advice.

Someone who will always help you

when you need it.

A place to call home.

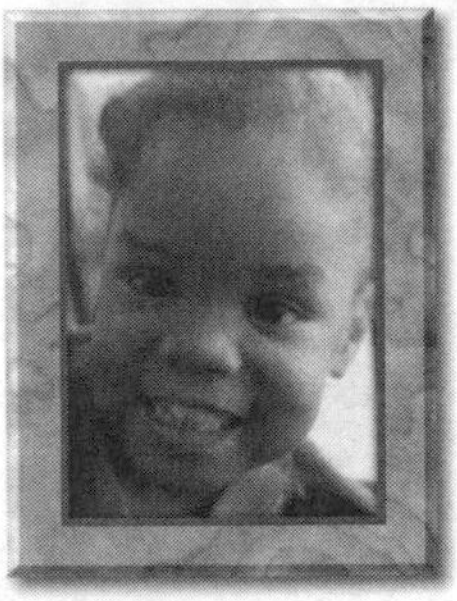

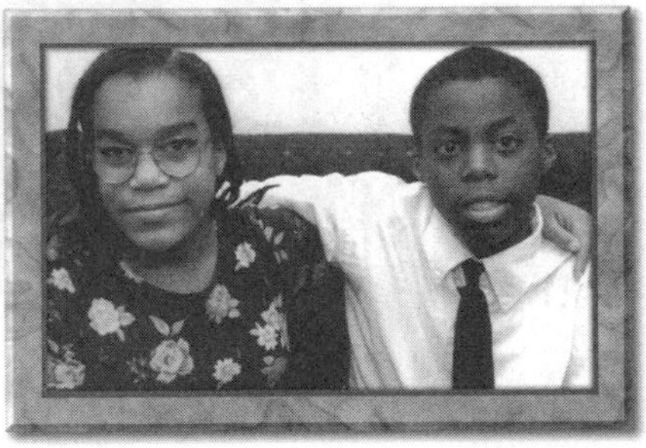

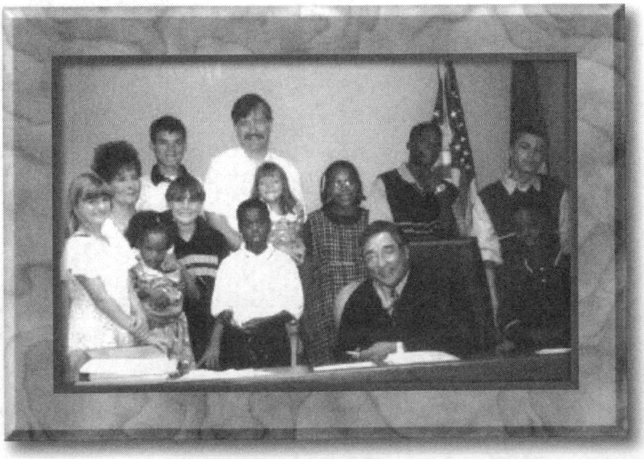

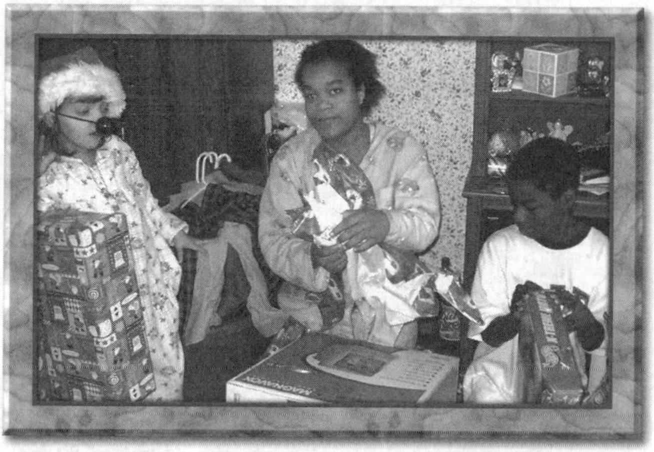

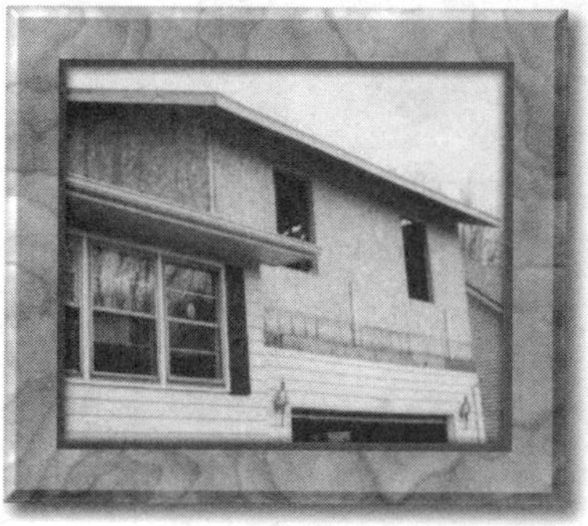

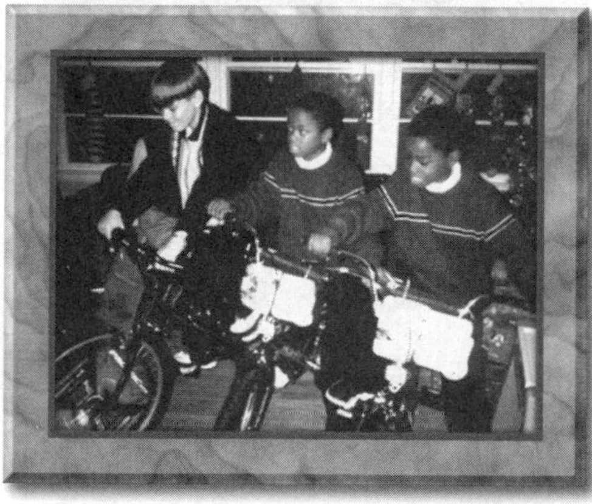

Special thanks to the Kalamazoo Community

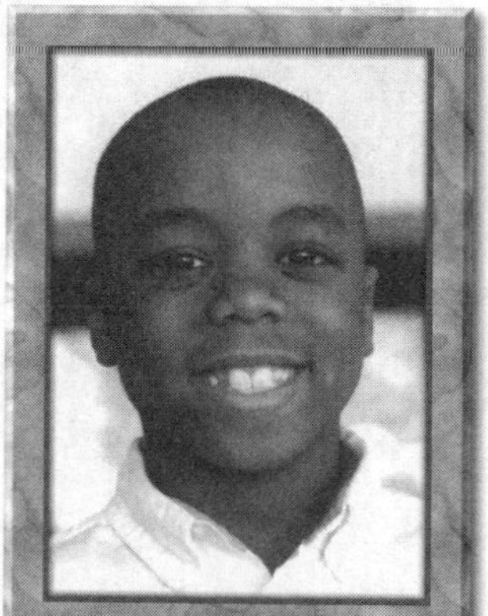

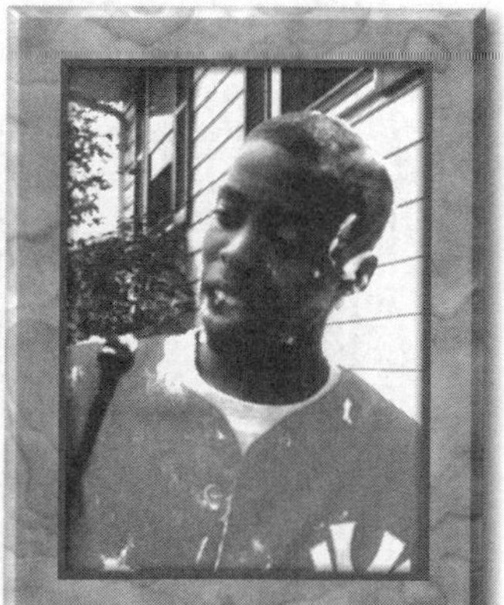

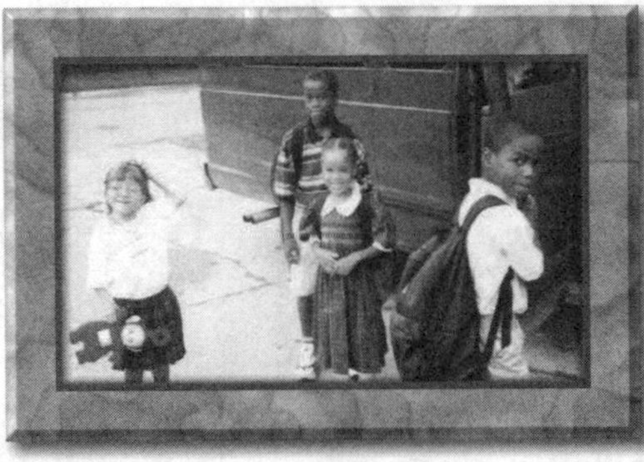
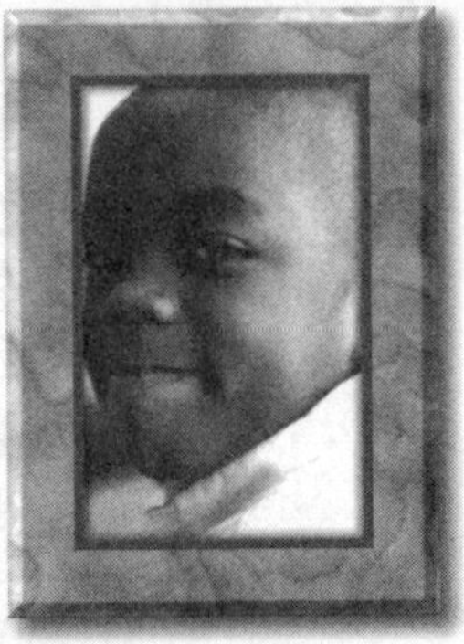
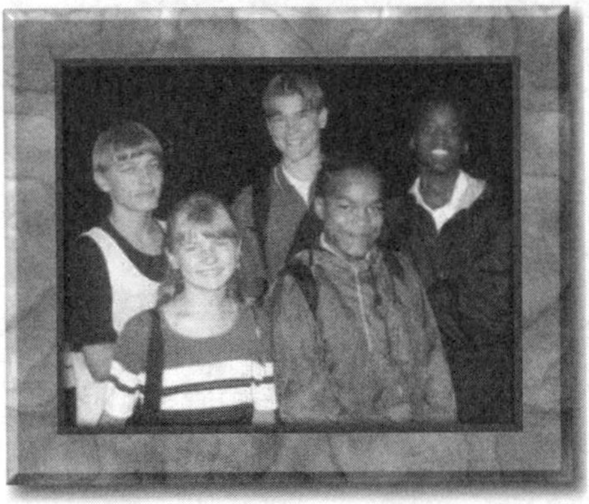
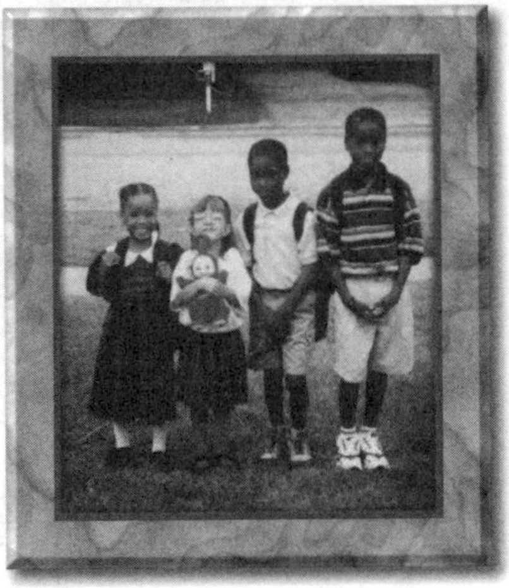
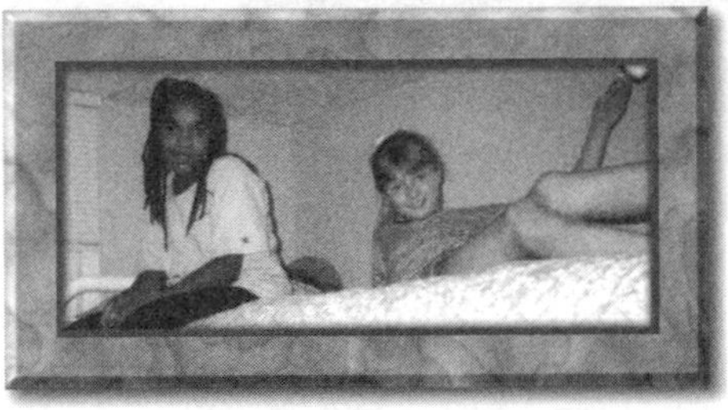
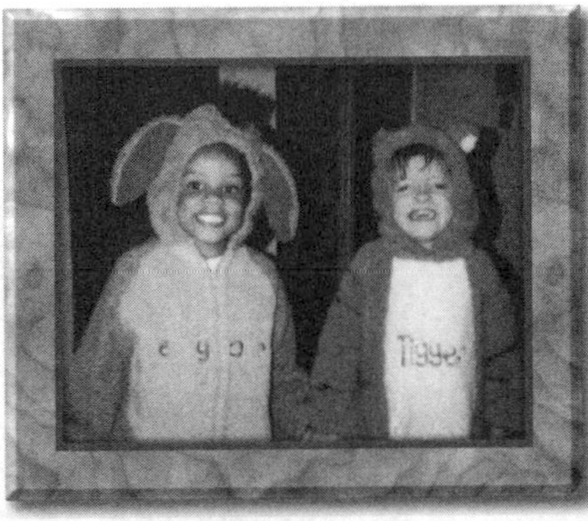
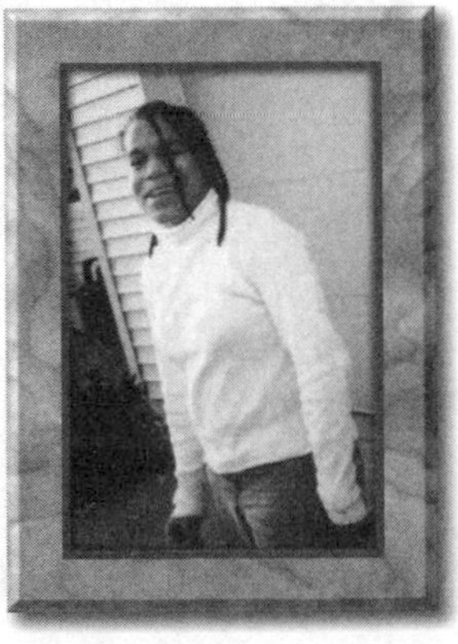

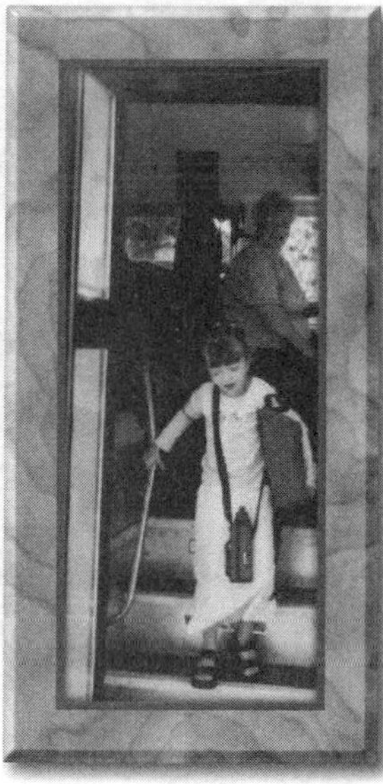

What is the part of having a family?

Hugs and kisses.

A safe place to call home.

Someone to tuck you in at night.

Someone to help you with your problems.

Sometime to cuddle.

Someone to take care of you.

It's MINE!

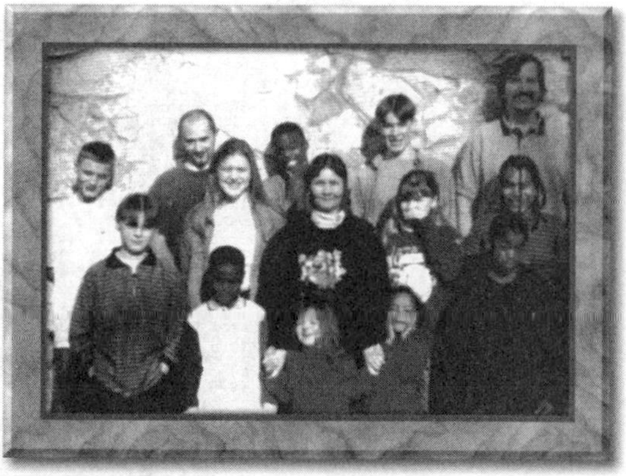

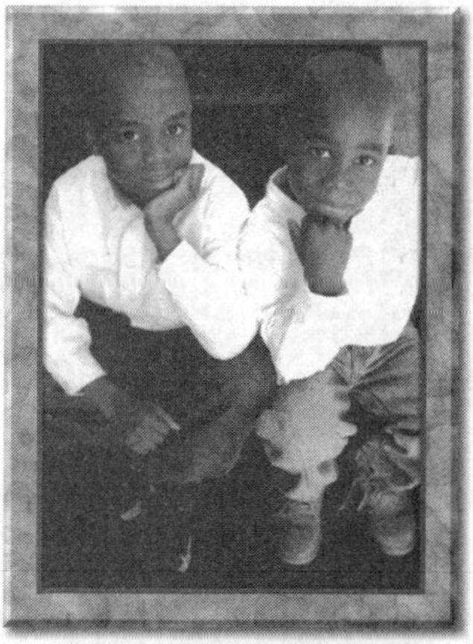

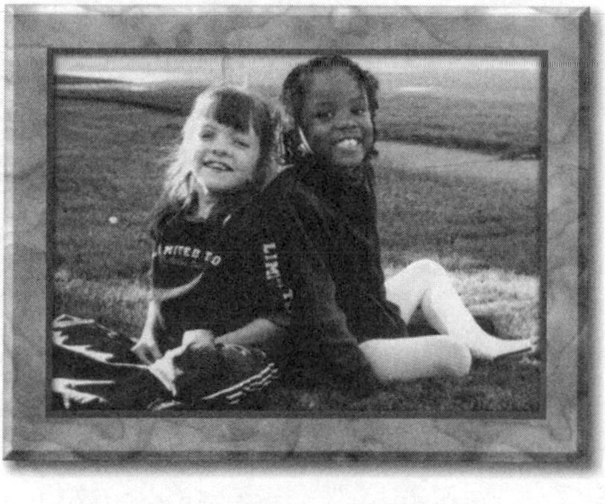

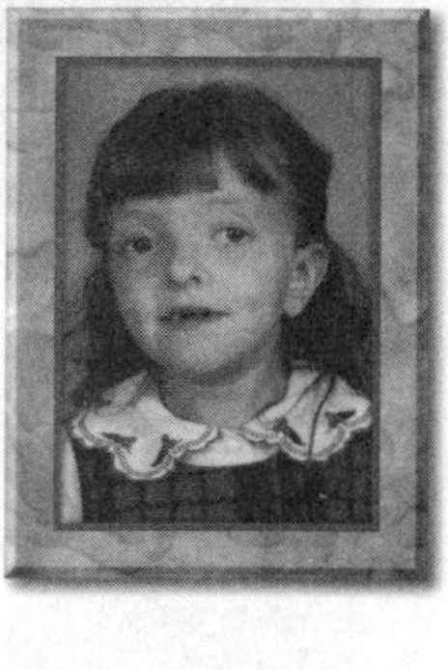

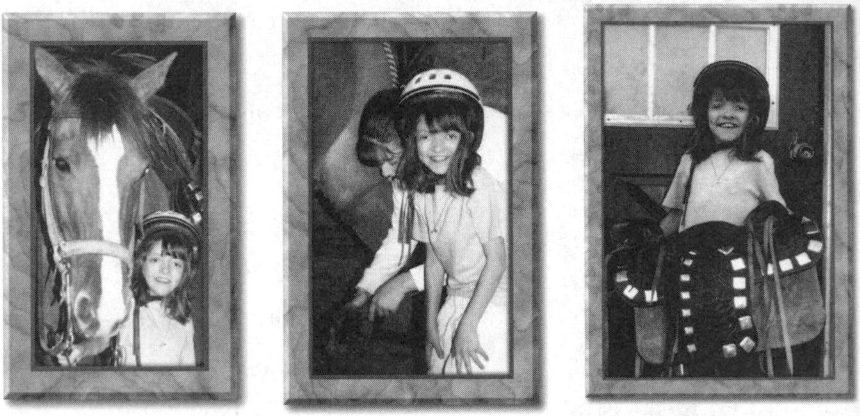

Special thank you to the Cheff Center

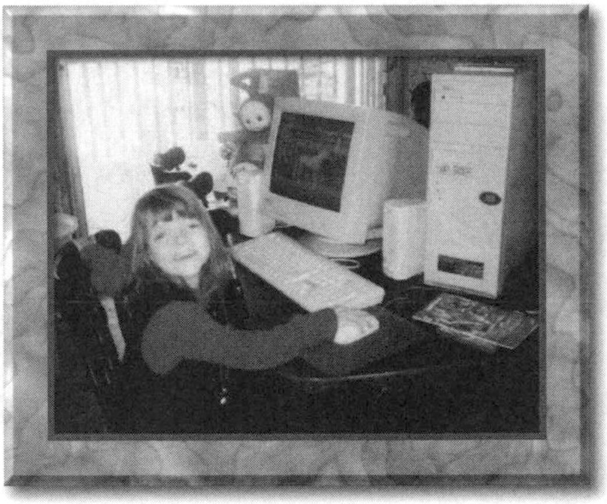

Special thanks to Crossroads Mall, Kalamazoo

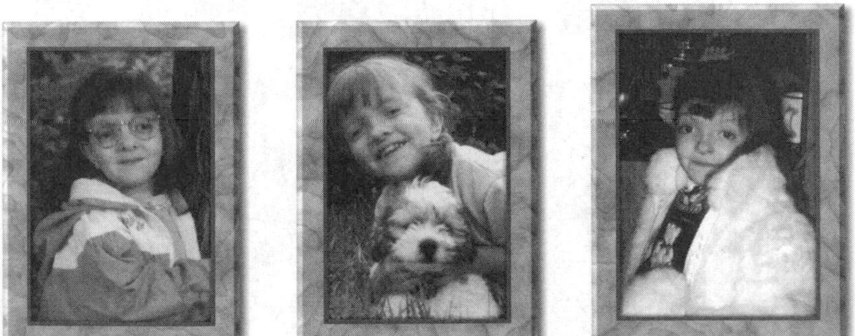

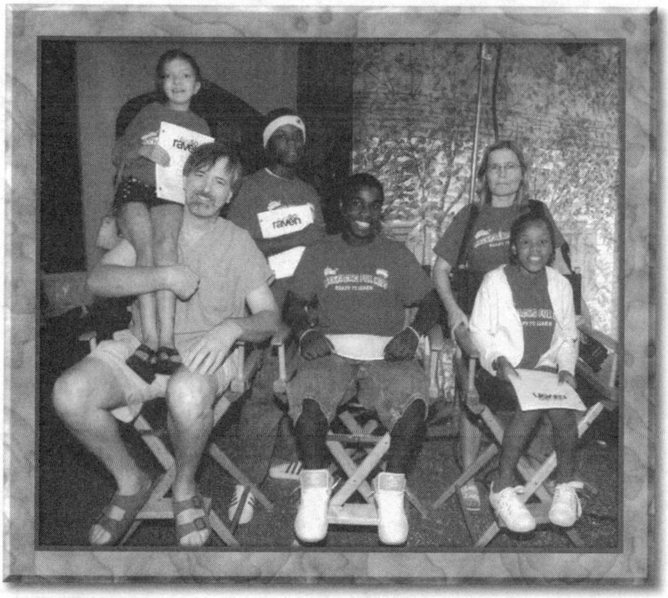

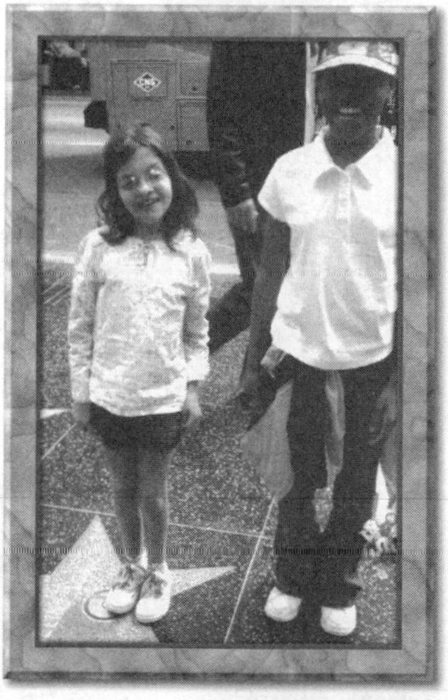

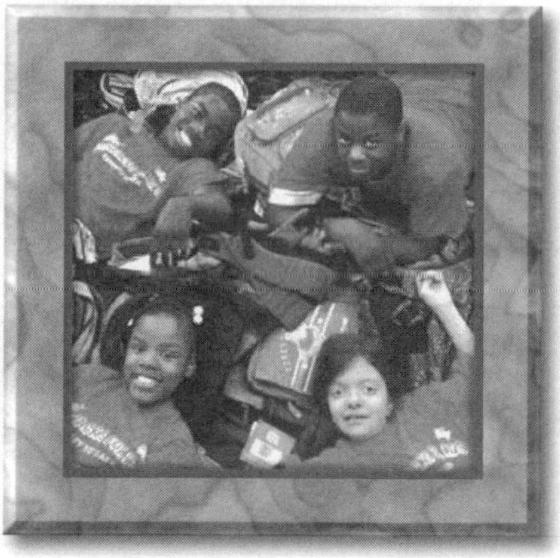

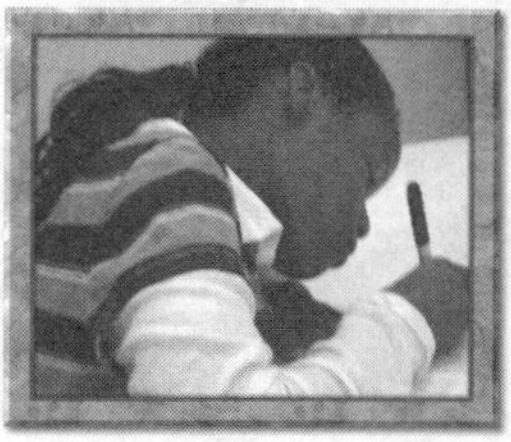

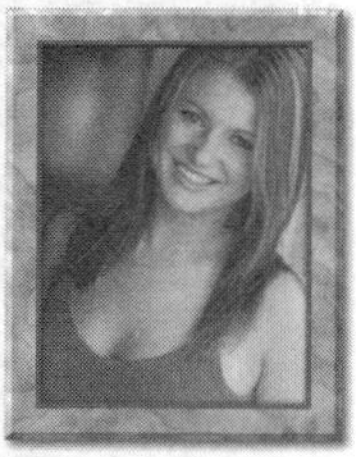

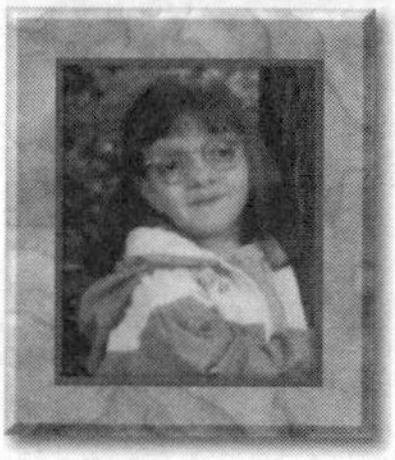

www.backpack-for-kids.org

Special thanks to Disney

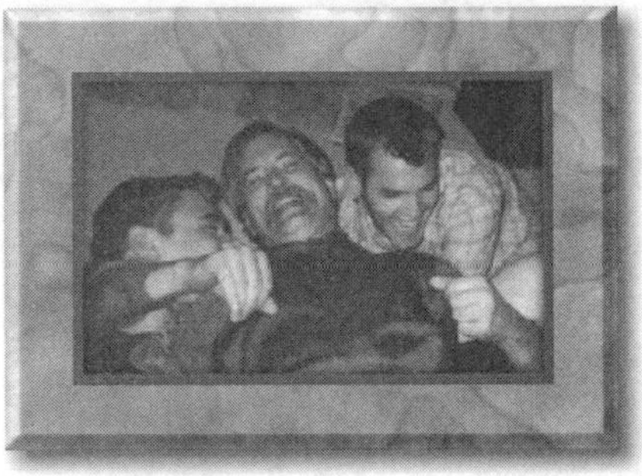

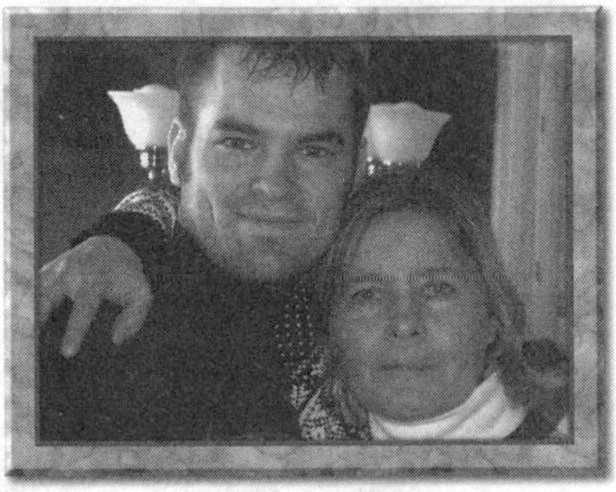

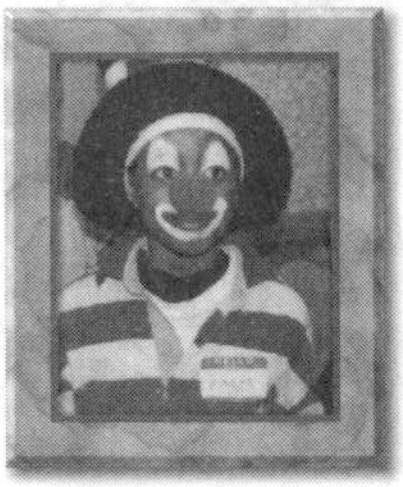

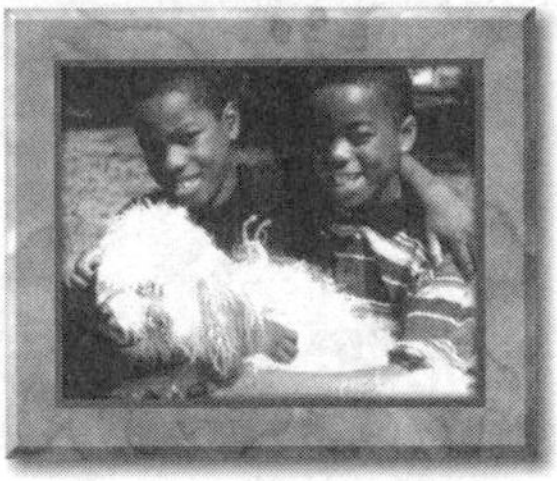

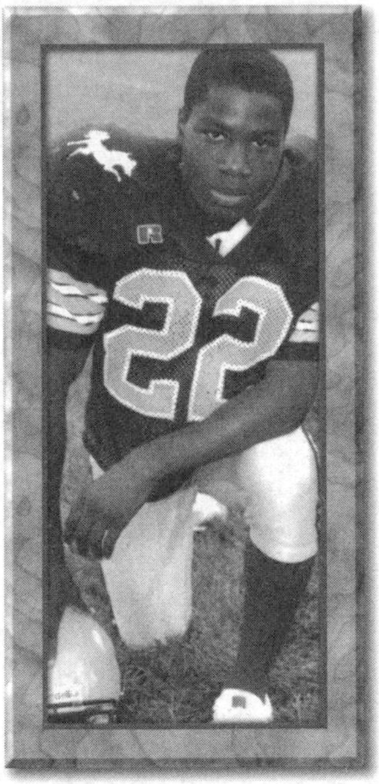
22

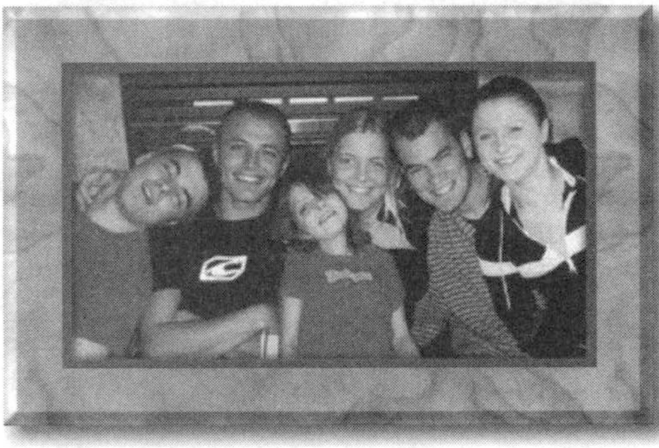

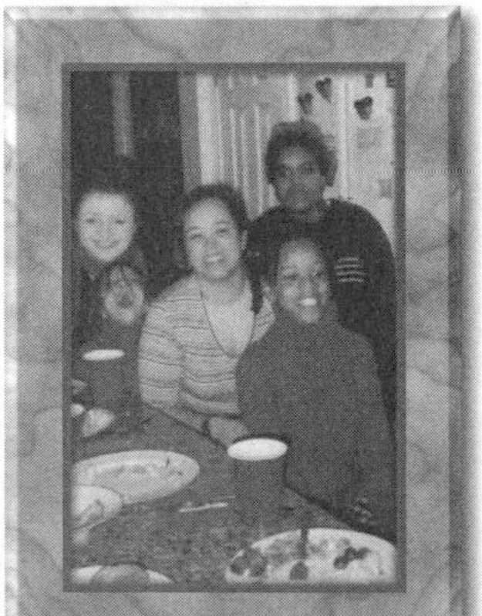

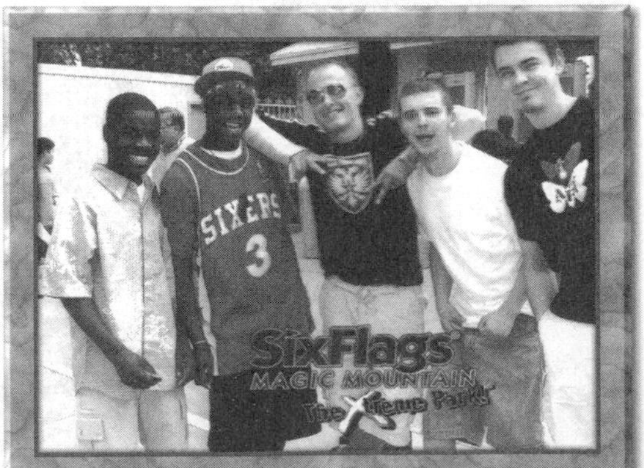
SIXERS
3
SixFlags
MAGIC MOUNTAIN

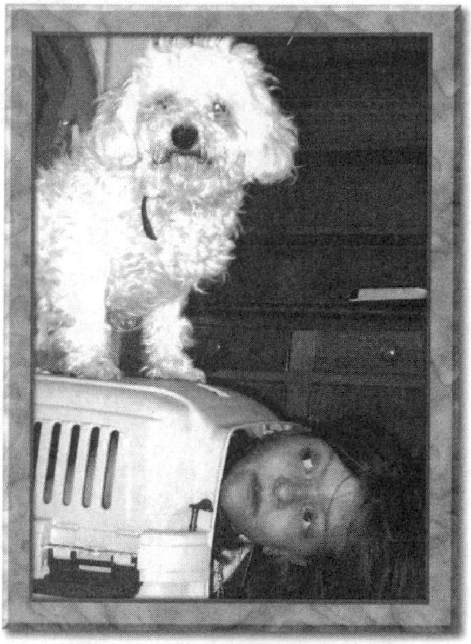

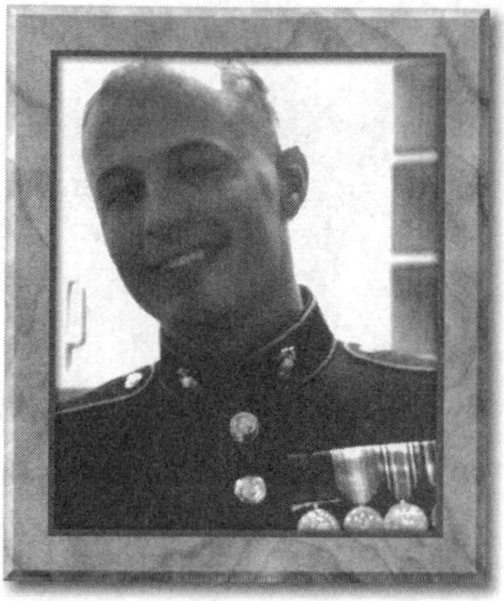

Special thank you to all the medical professionals and caregivers and Dr. Noonan.

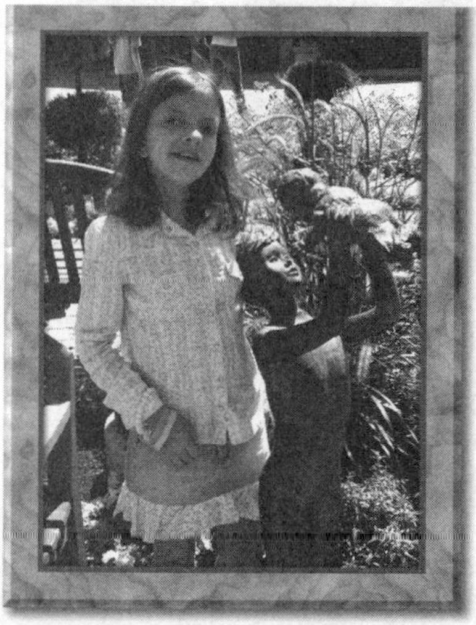

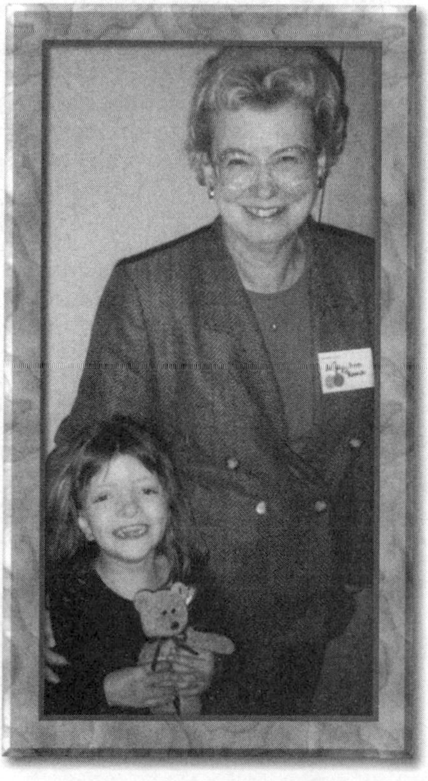

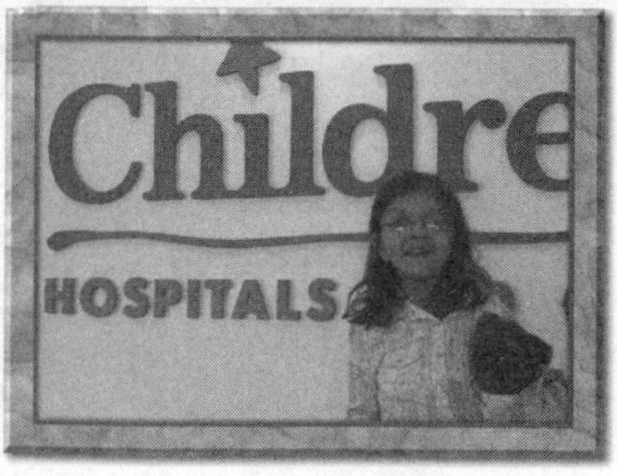

Thank God for the miracles

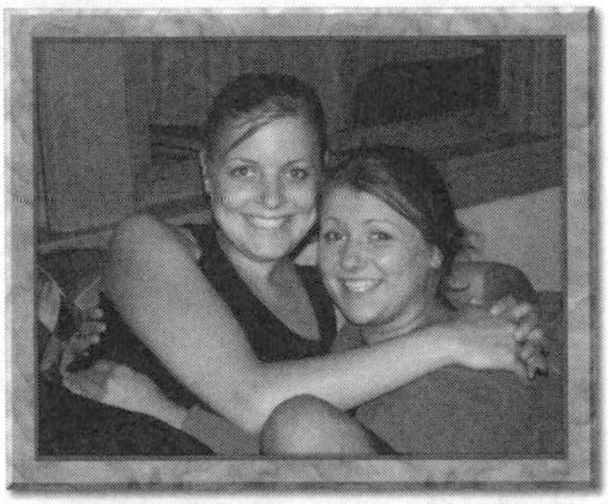

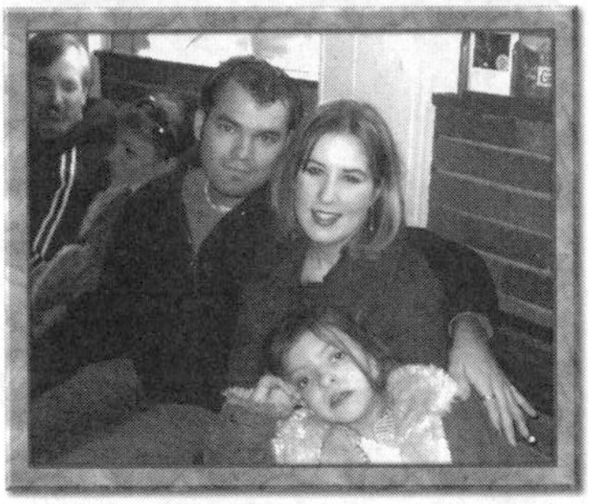

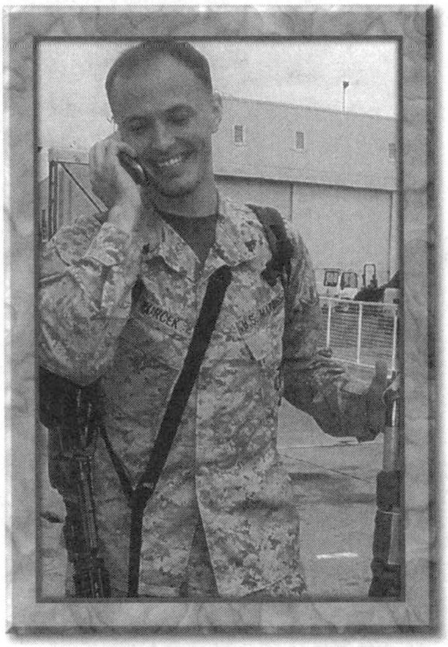

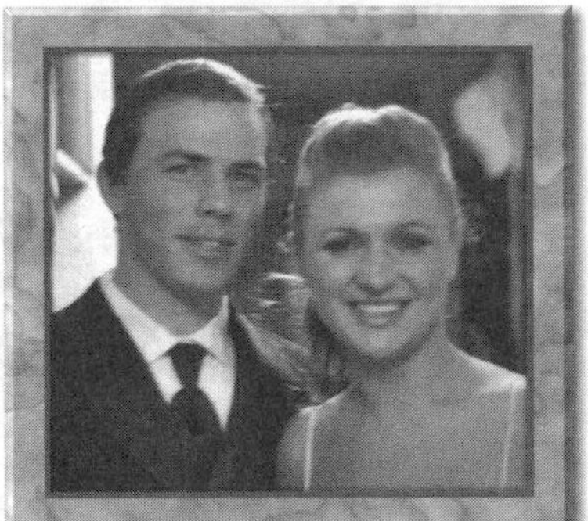

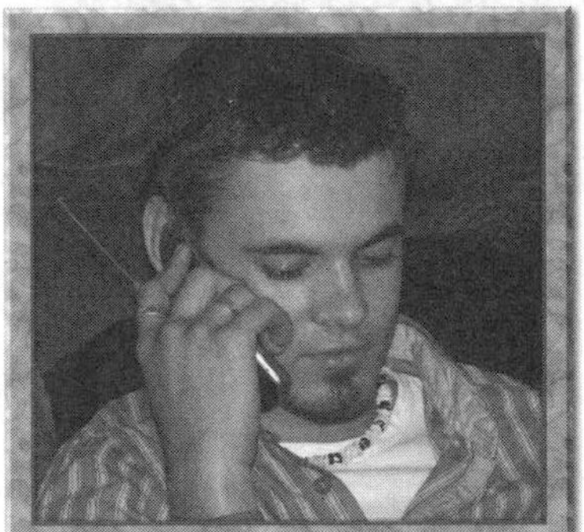

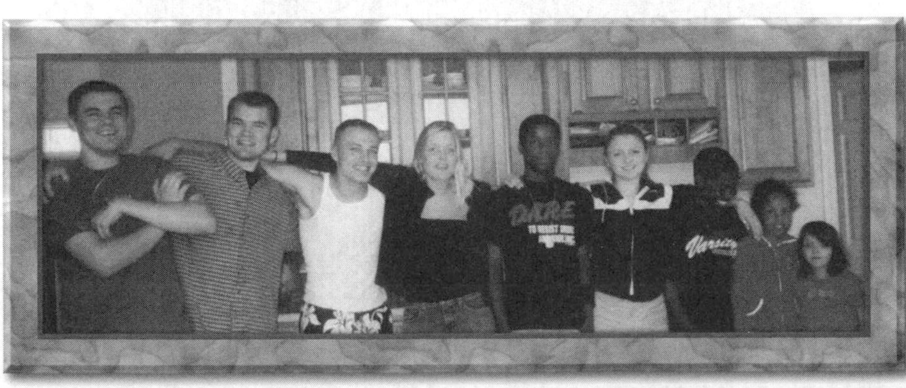

Part Three

The Journey Continues

Part Three - Miracles By the Dozen

- 53 -

All Grown Up

Time does not stand still. The kids have grown up while we journeyed ahead. Jim is now a surgeon, practicing medicine and still loving his work. It has been sixteen years since Becca's birth. Some parts of the journey are miles long, while others pass in the blink of an eye. When we first ventured into the world of special needs we had no idea of the journey that lay ahead. As I close our story I know that it is just the end of a chapter in our lives. The journey will continue on with our children's lives and the next generation.

Now that many of the kids are adults I can see the benefits of all the hard work. Time has helped heal many wounds. What many said was an impossible journey was not really so, we did it. Our kids are resilient and so is our family. Jim and I made it through together, stronger and united by our challenges. Today I see that same strength ingrained in each and every one of my children.

▼

Kristy graduated from the all women's college the year before Jim graduated residency. She spent her final year of college running the computer department, teaching a basic computer class, and going to school full time. She spent her winter vacation doing an internship at a Fortune 500 Company. On her second day of work, Kristy was offered a full time job in IT and department heads competed over who would prevail in getting her to agree to work for them. Kristy was up for a change, but was not about to leave the college in the lurch, she finished school while working at 3M, running the laptop leasing program and going to school.

After graduation she jumped into a Masters Program at St. Thomas the same college her grandfather Yurcek, uncle, aunt, and cousin had attended. In a little over two years she was done with school, which had been completely paid for her employer. Kristy advanced through the ranks and spent this last year flying back and forth between France, Spain, and the United States. She calls me from the Swiss Alps, from the Eiffel tower, and places I never dreamed my children would ever see. Kristy is moving up the corporate ladder fast and will no doubt continue into high management positions and found happiness with a new partner.

▼

Nathan will be married this spring, and Stacey his fiancée is Becca's hero and friend. She is excited to be able to be a bridesmaid in the wedding, and next weekend we will travel the six hundred miles to attend the bridal shower. Becca has been connected to her brother and almost sister-in-law via cell phone and they talk everyday. Nathan graduated from Augsburg two years ago and left the college computer job for a position keeping the computers, networks, and systems running for a banking regulations business. He has bought my parents home and is working on remodeling the basement. Stacey joins Nathan in his bargain hunting and they make my day when they call me to let me in on their finds.

▼

DJ has floundered these past few years, and it is good to have him back into the fold of the family. He has returned to the values of family he garnered from his three-year crash course in stability and caring. Presently, DJ is stuck in pieces of his past. He is stuck in being angry for all that he has been through. His rap writing is full of anger and bitterness. He has not yet come to terms with his history.

Yesterday, we bailed him out to pay for paternity testing for the twin baby girls before the hearing. The courts have given him thirty days after the summons, which he received last Wednesday and if we waited for county support, the testing and results would be too late. It they are his daughters, he would be found neglectful. As I close the book, DJ is now free to move with his life and is moving into his own one bedroom apartment and is off to community college.

▼

Ian is out of the Marines and I thank God safe and sound. My son is home. My heart goes out to all the mothers who are not so blessed. He and Matt and their friends will be renting the old house we never sold, now with completed above garage rooms. Soon he will be starting college and walk the long path to med school.

▼

Marissa graduated and reached for her dreams. She auditioned in Chicago along with the kids from prestigious acting schools. She did not settle for less. She sent in applications to the top colleges for performing arts across the country. She couldn't believe it when she was selected to audition for such places as Juilliard and The American Academy for the Dramatic Arts. She would get a chance to audition to the schools that train America's greatest actors and actresses. Marissa was surprised when she was accepted into her first choice. Their website lists some of the greatest actors and actresses of the past and our time. She was soon off to college at the American Academy of Dramatic Arts in Hollywood, California.

I worried how we would ever pay for it all and she had no financial aid. We managed to float her a loan by using our tax refund, and helped pay her rent and bills. The second year she took out loans and graduated at the top of her acting class.

Breaking into acting in Hollywood is expensive, and this past year she has worked to get enough money to pay her own way, including pay for the photography for her headshots. Marissa does not fit into Hollywood, but she is into serious acting. She felt lonely and out of place. Eventually, the loneliness was eased when she met her boyfriend Jordan. Marissa and Jordan flew home to meet this infamous family of ours. Jordan is an intern at a major television network for screenwriting out of thousands of applications. Marissa and Jordan are happy and working to realize their dreams together.

▼

Shay is thriving in the community, and learning to live her own life. Every Sunday she comes home for a family visit. She calls often and I help her whenever she needs me.

Shay is a helper. She continues to volunteer in group homes for adults with severe developmental delays served by community mental health. She helps our family on our volunteer projects and contributes her skills to Backpacks for Kids. Shay just started her first 'real' job; she did not want to be outdone by her younger brothers. She lives independently, calls our house home, is an active member of our family, and is definitely 'still' my daughter.

Manfred and I participate in the planning process to make sure that she can continue to grow and reach for her dreams. Shay has been lucky. My hope and prayer is that we begin to find out how to keep young adults like Shay stable through transition and build person-centered lifeplans.

▼

Not so little **Matt** has graduated from high school in June with never having any assistance with his learning disabilities. He has finally acknowledged he struggles with dyslexia, which I have known since second grade, but he had never failed enough to qualify for supports. Matt graduated early just to get away from high school.

Jim and Matt challenge each other over who is taller and Matt has now passed up both brothers. He has started community college, and works for the Pizzeria. He was pleased to show us his impressive 4.0 first semester grades in his English class this fall. He has a passion for working with cars and putting things together.

Matt had a close call with bullying in automotive class when another student lit him on fire behind his back and his shirt went up in flames. He wanted to learn instead of messing around and the unknown students actions were defended as 'just' a prank gone bad.

▼

Deangelo is now a junior in high school, on the varsity football and basketball teams, and runs track. He has his first job, and has grown into a very handsome, caring gentleman.

▼

Delonzo is a sophomore, and though there have been worries, with structure, love, support, medication, maturity and an outgoing personality we have hope for his future. He is the spokesman for the Backpack for Kids project, when Deangelo, Becca and Detamara are too shy to speak up. He carries the trophy for raising the most money for the Backpack for Kids project.

▼

Detamara is now thirteen, and at least for the moment, the baby of the family. She is a quiet caring sensitive young lady who is mom's girl. My helpful little lady has taken over for Marissa and is now my associate in cleaning our huge new home. Recently she has found a relationship with Jim and the two of them play around with corny jokes and sense of humor.

▼

Becca just celebrated her sixteenth and a half birthday with press releases sent out announcing *Tiny Titan* on Valentine's Day in honor of Congenital Heart Disease Awareness week. She is still very tiny. At sixteen, she is just over four feet and weighs in at an all time high of fifty-seven pounds. She finally wears a girl size 8 and whopping size one little girl shoes. Her slim jeans are getting 'too tight!'

Becca is my full time personal assistant. I don't need to have a planner; her amazing memory keeps me on track with all my appointments and schedule. Through the computer she just proved to the school district that the work they were giving her was too easy. In less than four hours, she mastered her newest adult level CSI computer game. The game reads for her, and her eye for detail and problem solving skills is amazing even to the professionals.

We have finally won a battle with the school district to offer her an education at home. The district is looking for assistive technology with voice recognition and read aloud programs. Technology for Becca is the key to unlock her abilities and keep up with her able bodied peers.

For five years I have taught her with little support and she has been left behind, I have battled through the special education system for help. We cannot fault the education for not knowing how to handle Becca. They have given it their best effort. Becca is one of a kind; she doesn't fit neatly in any box. My children tell me, I have to give up and 'just' do it myself. Becca and I will not settle for a life of nothingness like so many other children have had to because of lack of understanding and funding.

The doctors have returned to Becca's life with a vengeance. Her chronic pain is worsening, her joints falling apart. Finally the waiting lists for therapy opened up and we addressed her heel cord pain and her worsening elbow contractures that caused her arms to freeze. We also figured out the source of Becca's wheezing, her favorite fast food restaurant announced this week that the oil from their French fries contains both gluten and dairy products. The doctors had told me if she loved fries let her eat as many as she wanted to help her gain weight. Now the one safe place we thought she could eat was making her sick. That was why her mouth broke out in sores.

Becca is not happy, she believes the restaurant should change the recipe just for her. "Kids who eat gluten free deserve to have some place they can eat like other kids." Becca gave up her precious fries and already we are seeing changes in her behavior and pain levels. She is less obsessive which always escalates when she gets gluten.

As always every day is an up and down battle for our tiniest titan. She looks forward to Thursday night horseback riding. She volunteers with the younger kids and has found friends at the Cheff Center. Lauren is fourteen and Robin is almost eleven. Becca has now joined the ranks of having friends and teen girl sleepovers. She had her very first birthday party last year when Robin invited her to a clue party and Miss Becca attended as Miss Peacock all dressed up in a blue sequin dress and plumage.

After eight years in Michigan, we are again readjusting Becca's doctors. We took her back to the Noonan conference, this time at home in Minneapolis with both Dr. Pierpont and Dr. Noonan in attendance. The following week Becca was set up to be seen by Dr. Pierpont to help Becca's pediatrician lead her care.

As we walked into the Children's hospital through the glass

doors of the patio where I first saw myself with her in my arms, I teared up. I reminisced of the journey with Becca. Here she is alive sixteen years later, tiny and strong in her own way. This place saved my daughter's life, my intuition helped me help her not only survive but thrive. Within the last year or so one of the genes for Noonan syndrome had been discovered and Dr. Pierpont would at long last test Becca for the PTPN11 gene. Half of the persons with Noonan syndrome will test positive for this gene, the other half the gene has yet to be discovered. For the past sixteen years they felt the closest fit for Becca's severe condition was a variant of Noonan syndrome, and as the years had past, Becca exhibited virtually every finding.

October brought at long last our answer, Becca tested positive for the gene, a confirmed diagnosis from genetic testing; we had a final answer of Noonan syndrome. Dr. Pierpont made arrangements for Becca to be seen by some of the Minnesota doctors who had seen her when she was small and we came full circle.

Most of the babies who were as sick as our Becca did not see their first birthdays. Most children and adults affected with Noonan syndrome do not have the same severity as our tiny daughter. Dr. Pierpont, Jim and I talked about having her write Becca's case study to help those who will follow us. Within the list serve in the past few years, there have come to be other survivor kids, Autumn, and miracle four-year-old Evan. Evan's dad writes of their journey with beautiful portraits. Evan recently visited President Bush to let him know every person is important. He knows the beauty of living in today, as we have no guarantees of tomorrow.

How many of us are lucky enough to witness a miracle? In my journey with Becca I've seen plenty of miracles as I slowed down and paid attention to them. I am blessed to get the honor of hugging and caring for one each day of the past sixteen and a half years.

Pastor Rick foretold of Becca's mission, she is here to inspire, to teach and to love. She has inspired me to grow up as Alice foretold. I have become a better human being for all I have been through and now I honor the promise I made so long ago every day of my life, trying to make the journey lighter for another along the way.

- 53 -

THE DREAM

A miracle for many happened in Kalamazoo. Our community recently announced that anonymous donors had vowed to give a college education to every student who wanted to go to college. Out of generosity, the unknown benefactor will change the course of thousands of lives and families. Poverty will be lessened.

The requirements for the promise of free college are high. The kids must maintain a 2.0 GPA and take 12 credits per semester. The offer is good at any Michigan college and university. Whoever these funders are, they truly understand that education is what makes the American dream possible, but for many that possibility and dream is still too big.

The expectations to reach that vision needs to be set early to make a dream of college, and a career, and a better life. In our town, there is generational poverty that we've turned our backs on and we cannot close our eyes to the stark divide. Even with funding and grades, it remains impossible to attend college for some children. It will take the community to band together with tutoring, mentoring and basic necessities to support these children so they can realize their dreams.

For kids with disabilities the dream of college remains far from their grasp. Our college and universities will accommodate a small handful, but in general these children are not prepared to make that reality come true.

▼

It was an exception Jim and I remained a team as we worked, learned and struggled. Many of my friends were not so lucky.

I called a couple of the parents who I work with before bedtime telling them their wishes had come true and they could send their children to college. One mom who said she had never gotten a break just got a gift beyond her wildest dream. This mom was in tears with the possibility that her talented son could now go to college. Her son proudly carries an impressive 3.7 GPA while struggling to live with a sister who can be out of control. Her daughter is affected by Bi-Polar disorder and her mood swings affect her entire family. Sadly, this daughter's needs often override the unseen needs and dreams of her son.

The long-term price of living with children who are severely disturbed or have special needs without adequate supports take an emotional and physical toll. The bureaucracy of red tape for assistance programs, insurance nightmares, lack of resources and time drive these families to the bottom – out of money, out of energy, out of hope. The stress of living with and parenting a child with special needs, the financial struggles, and the lack of support cause these families to split and the families who stay together are few and far between.

Many of these parents struggle with raising children with neurobiological problems in poverty without a spouse. The men and women doing this job singley are especially vulnerable. They juggle too much. They answer too many phone calls to pick up a sick or 'misbehaving' child, and take too much time off work for the countless medical and therapy appointments. They are parenting against the odds, trying to hold down a job.

I remembered the words of Becca's pediatrician when he gave me the statistics for our family to be intact at the end of our journey.

Jim and I worked hard to make sure we did not give up on each other, our kids, or our family and education was our way out.

Families do not get shift changes. They parent day in and day out with breaks few and far between. Families are raising children even RTC's or intermediate care facilities cannot manage and they are bound by family law that they cannot use techniques allowed by the professionals who work an eight to ten hour shift and go home.

That toll affects the caregivers. They are exhausted and burned out. I have noticed many of my friend's who are raising these children, now face debilitating illnesses such as cancer, multiple sclerosis, fibro myalgia, arthritis, autoimmune disorders, severe asthma, and other immune compromises. The adoption of the children and five years of isolated caregiving played a huge toll on my physical health. My asthma flared, my fiber myalgia worsened and compromised my ability to care for my children. I needed to be rested and recharged but had no supports to allow me that freedom. There was no place I knew I could ask for help to care for myself.

If we are going to expect to maintain children in our homes and communities we need to remember to take care of the caregiver first or he or she cannot take care of the children. We must not simply pay lip service to this need. When a caregiver calls social services for help, they have most likely exhausted themselves and all the options they can think of. There are not enough hours in the day to fight for service and supports and navigate the maze and complexities of a broken and fragmented support system. It is too much to expect for each individual caregiver to become the casemanager, therapist, nurse, pharmacist, occupational therapist, physical therapist, tutor, transport, supports coordinator, insurance clerk, and advocate besides being a mom or dad.

For parents with kids who have complex behaviors they face misunderstanding and judgment, by the community, their place the worship and schools. Their extended families and old friends may abandon them, afraid to reach in or out, and not understand the reality of parenting complex young people. They lack respite and supports. If they are lucky, they find some shelter in other families with children with special needs where they are understood. Like Becca at her Noonan's conference, when families are among peers they have liberty to share their true feelings. They can dialogue, share, laugh, and discover new ways of coping.

I can do my job to help my children success when I am rested. When I do better my children also do better. When my perspective gets clouded my friends or Colleen remind me that I am doing too much. So I remember myself to cope again. Since Manfred got our family regularly scheduled in home help, I can get away, I can clear my head and I can take care of me. My health has recovered. I learned I must take care of myself or I cannot take care of others. I found appropriate medications for my children that work to stabilize the chemical imbalances in their brains.

My children do not want to use their disabilities as excuses, but rather their knowledge of their disabilities as guides to empower them to overcome their individual challenges. It is vital that they know and understand themselves to help them soar and fully participate in the community as adults.

People without disabilities commonly make decisions for us not with us. 'With' Manfred and the director of community mental health I accessed services to help me do the work to help stabilize their lives. Development of system change needs to be designed with us not for us. We cannot afford to waste funding. As administration discusses protocol, policy and strategies another child loses a longed-for family due to adoption disruption, divorce, and the child becomes another statistic. The dream for permanency and education becomes another loss.

▼

I think of Becca. During these past four years of schooling Becca myself, I understand her challenges. When Becca graduated from the early intervention program the wise occupational therapist told me that Becca was born in the right age. Computers would be her key to the world and she would need one to achieve. But the move to Michigan cost us that. The teachers told us that she needed to write and she needed to learn to read phonics. But what if one's body and brain cannot learn that way? We have lost four years of schooling from the educational system's lack of understanding that she needs 'abilities' from technology to achieve like her peers. In struggling to learn in a method too difficult, we may end up holding back the child and wasting precious time. The lost educational years for Becca cannot be made up easily. The frustrations of kids with disabilities and school failure can doom them to a life of poverty, isolation, and depression as they struggle through employment, housing and public services.

Since third grade, I fought for Becca to do schoolwork on a computer. Six years ago, Santa took care of her and her brothers took care of keeping the computer up and running for the next few years. Jim bought Becca her next computer before he got his SUV when he finished residency. Technology keeps changing and once again we need to update her electronic supports to help her achieve.

Becca is glad she is not in school anymore. She does not have to listen to being called a shrimp, shorty, or the countless other sayings her peers are so good at. She does not have to watch as others ignore her. She is no longer forced to sit at the SPED table because that is where the paraprofessionals can keep an eye on her. She doesn't always have to explain that she isn't a first grader and that she really is sixteen!

She no longer has to come out of the bathroom with her pants unbuttoned and ask for help, since her hands at times cannot even snap or button buttons.

At home her handwriting no longer makes her stand out, she is learning to use voice recognition software. Becca can write with a pencil for only a few seconds because her hands fatigue from holding the pencil while her brain struggles to understand how to move it to make each letter. 'In the process' of trying to write she loses 'what she was' trying to write. No amount of teaching will overcome her physical barriers. The computer helps her, but the keyboard is too big for her tiny fingers and she struggles to peck and reach for every letter, once again in the process of trying to achieve she loses what she wants to say. Her hand freezes around a large mouse with the hours she spends navigating the world on her computer. We searched for small mice and smaller keyboards to fix that barrier.

Although written into her IEP, claims were made that the technology was too new and expensive. It was argued as not fair that Becca could use it and not others. Once out of school, we wait while the district begins to learn how to make assistive technology a reality for Becca and others.

Becca is up to academic challenges using her strengths, while schoolteachers struggle to teach to her weaknesses. She uses a near perfect memory to build her reading vocabulary by sight-reading. She scoffs at reading third grade 'baby stories' as she discusses literature she's listened to on tapes with her family. She remembers the minute details I struggle to catch. Her eye for detail and problem solving are age appropriate if not advanced. She happily solved the new adult CSI forensics game in three and a half hours.

I will not allow Becca or my children to have their hopes and dreams squelched by having to settle for a life of nothingness. I don't think nothingness is a word, but for me it accurately describes the life that I have watched DJ and Shay try to live in. No one will hire them, because employers do not understand their hidden disabilities. They are grown adults and should be able to care for themselves. I don't want them to remain a part of the seventy-five percent of persons with disabilities who are unemployed. Work gives purpose to living and builds self-confidence.

As our culture moves from manufacturing to information, our children with excellent repetitive skills are lost as jobs are lost to other countries. On the other hand, for people like Becca doors are opened. Becca will probably never be able to work a full-time job because her body will fatigue, but that doesn't mean she cannot use her brilliant little mind to serve society and be fairly compensated for her skills. Persons with disabilities deserve an adult life of self-worth and the needs and dreams of my children are the same as the needs of others without disabilities.

Some of my children need prompts and reminders daily about what to do when. The medications that helps them stay stable, sticks them with living on social security checks to get Medicaid or Medicare. With future government cutting backs, who will care about them? Will they be shepherded off into group homes, day activity centers and menial jobs no one else wants to do? Will they be lost to the street using shelters for temporary housing because they 'appear' normal? Will structured living become the justice system for those with hidden disabilities, when much cheaper supports are viable?

We promised our children a new life, but our promises remain hard to keep. I wonder what the future holds for my children still at home. I have a lot of learning to do, and much advocating for system change so they can have a chance of a life of self worth. If they have access to technology or we utilize their areas of strengths all children can achieve, but they achieve differently from others.

If we had chosen not to adopt our children and they had remained in foster children they were eligible for free college and supported independence. But our family took away the promise of college and transition services by adopting them and we live in the wrong city to get the promised scholarship. The college dream is far out of these children's reach. Who pays for the technology for students with disabilities in college? Who pays for the paraprofessionals for them to be successful? There are no IEP's in college, just the Americans with Disabilities Act, and how do you modify tests and essays for a young adult who cannot write or remember the answers without assistance?

The adoptive families who adopt these kids are not rich, and many have other children. To get help from our child welfare system you have to utilize your resources first. Our children with disabilities often end up with emotional problems as they hit middle school. Families go broke trying to help their children survive and have a better future. As the rules tighten families exhaust their 401K retirement incomes to pay for out-of-home placements, or buy into the fragmented mental health system. Despite the education of inclusion, many pick on our kids. They struggle to keep up. Some give up and settle for being unable to learn. Some shut down from taunting and teasing of being a SPED kid. Kids can be cruel.

Graduation standards are changing and our kids with learning differences struggle to meet the standard, and without meeting the standard, even the technical colleges may remain out of reach. On the flip side, a student who focuses solely on passing the standards may find because of that 'hard-won' accomplishment, they are questioned when applying for support services they truly need as adult. Who will be there to go to college with Becca? Which program will pay for the technology for Becca to handle college?

Not all families can make it without help, the Yurceks worked out of poverty, but we didn't do it alone. Many people helped us along the way. Jim and I dreamed of the day that we would not have to rely on systems for Becca's care, but no one can survive catastrophic care without help, even a surgeon.

The nearly four thousand dollars for Becca's formula and feeding package are excluded from our health insurance. The insurance companies claim it is nutrition and insurance companies do not pay for food or vitamins. Without food Becca does not survive. She does not stay healthy. Her tiny impaired GI tract cannot break down all the nutrients needed to keep her sustained.

The insurance company does not pay for wheelchairs. They do not pay for her foot braces or her hand splints. They sometimes pay for physical therapy and rarely occupational therapy. The insurance excludes therapists for chronic conditions. Last month Becca's therapy cost over three thousand dollars and became covered after she 'fell apart' and was in enough pain to get help for her joint contractures and muscle pain. She spent weeks with casts on her feet and elbows. If we had gotten braces sooner, Becca would have been spared the pain and the insurance company spared the later costs.

I will never figure out their reasoning. Once you get something covered, there is no guarantee it remains covered. Jim's insurance covered Becca's growth hormone when he first went into practice, but then when they switched plans within the same company they claimed it was experimental. Becca needs to grow. You get different answers, even from the same company or government program. It is a full time job to help her get what she needs, let alone covered, submitted and followed up on where I discovered our doctors were writing off the co-pay I thought Medicaid picked up. But, our family is blessed by the taxpayers of the United States with Medicaid for our children. They already have Becca on their rolls for her formula and feeding package, braces, therapy, wheelchairs, and the rest of the things our insurance company refuses to pay for.

The medical system is manageable for a veteran to navigate if you have countless hours and patience. But the mental health care world I entered with my adopted children is another story. Since the fight for Shay beginning in 2000, much has been written about our broken mental health system, its fragmentation, its failures to adults and children with serious emotional disturbances and the failure to integrate medicine and the mind.

How can we separate the body from the mind?

Insurance companies do, they are not forced to have the same benefits for mental health problems as medical. We have exhausted what little we had to help our children come through their traumatic histories. We have paid for therapy, hospitalizations, psychological assessments and whatever they needed.

You have probably figured it out by now. I don't give up.

I am no longer 'just' a mom; I have become the MOM expert on getting kids through medical and mental health's door. I teach parents how to navigate the system, one family at a time.

My sister asked me whether I would return to school after the kids are grown? I don't need to. I have a full time job managing my children's healthcare and needs, along with the full time job of helping families get the help and support that they deserve. These past couple of years since my experience with Shay I have helped several dozen families from across the country not give up their seriously mentally ill children to the system. We have supported each other. We brainstorm together as we try to navigate the maze of broken systems. Some have prevailed; they found hope for their children.

There have been others who have been lucky like Shay, but they are few and far between. In the real world, American families 'are' forced to abandon their children in hospitals, or disrupt (unadopt) their adopted children. Both biological parents and adoptive parents have lost the battle because of inadequate support. They gave up because they loved their children enough to get them help, breaking their hearts in the process.

What does this fix?

The kid may not survive. If they do, they are destined to a life of failure, homelessness, and despair. They no longer have anyone to call family. There is no family home to call when you need support or you want to share your success. There are no birthday or holiday gifts from those you call family. No one monitors how you are 'really' doing or speaks on your behalf. The children float through child welfare into the rough sea of transition and many get lost in systems of social welfare, mental health and criminal justice. That is why I did not give up on Shay. If she lost the rest of her family, she would have no hope. But doing the right thing costs us a huge price. We cannot be forced to keep families in chaos because we do not have the supports available to help them help our children.

Fifteen to twenty-eight percent of older adoptions do not work and there is a small percent of children who are too complex to remain safely in homes and communities. Some of the kids of the system cannot be salvaged and even the professionals do not know how to help them with our current research. It is too late to make them whole again. To leave them in families where they cannot function destroys the family. We need a continuum of care. Families who are raising children with special needs need to be supported. Prenatal exposures mixed with child abuse, neglect and trauma in their biological homes complicates the process of integration into adoptive and foster families. At this moment, there is no process to put back what alcohol and trauma have removed. We can teach them to learn to cope and support them to grow and move forward, but we need to have the supports and a system of care to be able to 'earn' that trust.

No one can do it all.

Budget cuts, and fragmented systems have a price...broken

families, needy families, and despair.

I have known for a long time that I had to write this book. Maybe the reason I felt I needed to write was to explain how difficult it is for all families raising children with special needs. I hope my writing this chapter gets in the hands of higher powers, the government legislators, officials, the insurance company executives, the teachers, the professionals, the corporations, the non-profits. They have the power to make a difference for many. May they begin to understand the stresses and the hopes in our lives. Most families I know do not want to live on the system. They want out of it. It is too complicated and stifling. If educated parents cannot make it through, what hope does a single parent with a limited education, juggling the stress of a minimum wage job, trying to parent children with special needs, and living in poverty have?

The systems that make promises to support children from the child welfare system and place them with families should honor their promises. Children need to be helped early and not shuffled back and forth like airport baggage. What's wrong with a society where we talk about helping people with disabilities but fail to provide them with the tools or methods to get their even most basic needs met? How can it be, that even a doctor does not have access to the resources his child needs to thrive without assistance!

I have seen things begin to change in our community. Our community received a huge system of care grant from the federal government to help us break down the barriers and simplify the fragmentation for families with children who have complex mental health needs. Parents, youth and professionals are working together to develop programs for youth and families to drive their own care.

I want all my children to reach the American Dream, regardless of able-bodies and able minds. My job will not be done as they reach adulthood. In many ways it is just beginning. I will be there to help them figure out the maze of insurance if they are lucky enough to get it on their own. I will walk with them through the governmental bureaucracy of Social Security and Medicaid. I will sit with them as they speak with Mental Health or Rehab Service professionals. I will make sure their cases are kept open after caseworkers close them because of misplaced paperwork or computer glitches. Those systems are crucial to the support of persons with disabilities. The patchwork system is more problem than help.

My job will never be boring. My children with special needs will need assistance for life in some way or another. I will always have a challenge ahead of me. They need case workers and support workers and hopefully in time they will need these less and less. I am not their case manager; I have to let them go. I cannot manage their lives, nor should I. Their independence at whatever level is important to their self worth. I don't want my children dependent on me. There is a balance between sheltering them and helping them. I will give them a hand up when they fall down. I will dust off their backside and help wash up parts of the mess. I will encourage them to get to the places they need to be and I will monitor their services. They will need to make their own mistakes, but without the ability of cause and effect this mistakes may have huge repercussions. I cannot do it all, because now that they are adults I need to become 'just a mom' because that is what they need me to be.

In the last twenty years, medical science has helped children survive. Are we ready to support them to be all that they can be in adulthood and the transition to get there?

We have to expect that the government, society, and communities value each individual to make the American Dream a reality for those who are challenged. For my adopted children, research in the areas of prenatal exposure and early life trauma is opening understanding of the changes to the structure of the brain. By understanding the brain differences, we may gain pathways to help. Parents who are living with these brain differences become experts in strategies to help them learn and achieve and are sharing their resources and ideas. The new trend of family centered practice and family empowerment is a step in the right direction. Parents and professionals working side-by-side is part of the solution.

A miracle happened in Kalamazoo, 'College Hope' for so many.

May God bless the mysterious benefactors for their gift of Hope. We in our community are now beginning the work to change the way we support families with children with neurobiological differences. We have the task to carefully use the six million dollars to make life easier for families to navigate systems I was blessed to find. I pray other benefactors across the country will do the same for children with disabilities, seeing them not for their weaknesses, but for their strength, determination and different abilities.

Someday Becca may want to take a couple college classes. Perhaps I was wrong when my sister asked if I was going back to college. Perhaps, I will go back to school, not by myself, but with my daughter at my side. Someone needs to step up to the plate and leave no child or family behind. I made a promise to my children. I will do everything in my power to make a difference. I spend each and everyday honoring my promise.

These children are societies children; they belong to all of us. When the systems take these children away from their abusive neglectful families it should only be on last resort.

When we remove them we make promises to those children to give them better futures.

Those promises need to be kept, and the foster, adoptive and kinship care families have the resources and training to be able to help those children succeed.

How can we do this as a great community? We need to care about these children.

Just like the families who take these kids in. Our media needs to not only tell the horror stories of the broken families who fall to the stress and lack of support or whatever happened. But we need more stories of the heroics of these children who are achieving and the families that support them. We need to honor these children and families hard work by giving them the PROMISE of a college or vocational training. These children can get a free college education if they make it that far if they age out of the foster care system, these children who are receiving federally or state funded adoption subsidies lose that benefit. We need to help those who helped get these children through school rewarding them for all their hard work with scholarships for our former foster children, they had done their jobs well and changed the course of a child's life. These adoptive families have many times exhausted their savings with tutoring, meeting these complex children's needs or have simply given up money for retirement by doing the work called to us to help a child have a better futures.

Each and every one of us can help in some way or another. Be a voice and demand our legislators and policymakers to make children matter. They are our future; we have the power to better the outcomes for children from the child welfare system and children with disabilities. We can be mentors, donate to non-profit organizations so they can do the work of serving children and families. One voice can turn the tide by creating a ripple than can turn into a wave that has the power to change the course of better endings and new beginnings for OUR children.

Our tiniest titan has shown me to believe in miracles, I knew I had to write this book for a reason. Little is ever gained out of the easy times; only the hard truths make real change. The hard truth is we as a society are not giving our children with extraordinary gifts and challenges the supports to be successful, we are holding them back from better endings and new beginnings by the barriers of policies and lack of money and caring.

We need to help ALL children succeed, and understand that some of these children will need lifelong support by a caring society.

My Tiny Titan showed me how to believe, and may her story change our hearts to reach out one person at a time, creating a wave to listen to the voices of our children and the needs of families. I close this chapter with HOPE that those who read this book will turn the tide of compassion for those who need a hand up in life.

- 54 -
FULL CIRCLE

The people in the government and child's social services had the right idea. Families need to be kept together when possible. However, in their wisdom these broken and hurt children have been planted in unsuspecting homes where adoption disruption, divorce and the trauma of the new children's lives have been transplanted. No one can understand their pain and chaos unless you become one with them.

We cannot expect social service professionals to understand and personally I am not surprised at the number of allegations made against these hardworking and struggling adoptive and foster families. From the children's mouths come accusations of historic pain against safe new caregivers. From their imprinted histories come challenges to the new families to repeat the abuse and neglect. From the beginning they recreate the trauma they know because that feels comfortable. In this *Alice in Wonderland* kind of existence, looking glass families are set up from the beginning to fail.

When we move these children to foster and adoptive families we make promises to help them. But when the families cannot access help, they are forced to become another rung on a ladder of broken promises in these children's lives. Unknowingly these systems set up the family to fail when they needed to trust that the family's request for help was probably their last resort. In most cases the call for 'help' comes after they have already exhausted their inner support systems. Reaching out for help, especially to child welfare, is daunting and families struggle exposing the realities of their children.

It is a fail first mentality. To get help for our children in the educational, child welfare or mental health system our families must first fall apart. Our children must be far enough behind in school to finally get help. Only the severest children get services and we wait until they become more severe to qualify. Sadly as a last resort, the juvenile justice and adult penal system provides the next level of structure and supportive care. One could hardly call that a family, ashes of broken promises and heartfelt tears are lost on the trail.

We need prevention.

A tiny titan changed me by showing me the strength I never knew I had when I was 'just' a mom. We are never free of the shadows of the past. They are always behind us, ready to haunt us. Without the shadows we wouldn't be as strong. We need to be thankful for the shadows, without my experiences I would not have been given the seeds of beauty, character and strength to blaze the path for those who follow. I keep moving forward remembering my history is only shadows and I continue to walk in the light. Hope.

Jim and I are more committed to each other while others think we need to be committed. But God didn't plan the Yurcek path for them. Over the years many told us God wouldn't give us anything more than we can handle. Now I simply answer, some of us don't fall down very easily. God doesn't promise a life without storms. He is there with us through the turmoil of the storms and shadows in the darkness. He is there through the calm. He reminds us when he allows us to see the miracles, when he paints the sky with a rainbow and lets his Son shine.

Our journey took us from the crisis of Becca's birth, and lean times through Medical School on faith and hard work. With a leap of faith, we left our home of twenty years on to a new life, added a family nobody wanted, learned to help my new children and Jim adjusted to a new career. Our family was here for a reason. All of our work here was to leave a lasting legacy, a seed planted for others to move forward. We were just a small change agent.

▼

As I finish this book, our lives have taken a turn. We don't know where will be going and we don't know when we will get there. Only God has our day planner. I know the chapters of our lives will continue, each of the kid's moving forward on their own journeys. Some will beat the odds, others may not. I will continue to allow them to move forward, guide them, encourage them, whether it be a phone call of a job promotion or sitting in the court room watching and encouraging them as they face sentencing.

Becca's sixteen years of medical history can be written as the case study, making a difference for all those who follow behind her. She survived for a reason. The tiny titan has not just changed our lives, but the lives of those who read her story. Becca in her critically ill, traumatized and fragile beginning came as a teacher bearing a rare disorder no one suspected. And because of our love and commitment to fight with our tiny titan for her life, we learned to hang in there for the long haul. Through thick and thin, good times and bad times, richer and poorer times, in sickness and in health, Jim and I, and our family are a united front.

When we merged our two families into one, we were once again catapulted into critically ill children. This time the disabilities were hidden in their life experiences and brains, they were psychologically, not medically fragile. Somehow on this part of our journey we had come full circle.

My children are extraordinary. Becca and her generation are the first such critically ill children who are living to adulthood. DJ, Shay, Deangelo, Delonzo and Detamara are only the second generation of children diagnosed with Fetal Alcohol Spectrum Disorders. We are in our infancy of knowledge to build adult support strategies.

People judge others by what they see - and with their snapshot vision they often judge Becca as incapable and treat her like a little girl. Becca is a young woman with untapped abilities. On the other hand some of my handsome sons with hidden brain damage remain little boys in man-size bodies, needing legitimate support and care.

Their path is uncharted. Tomorrow is a new day and we believe in better endings and new beginnings. Our children with physical and mental complexities need to have services and support to thrive and become the best they can be. There is much to learn from these tiny teachers, they are more determined than any of us would ever dare be. For all my children, I continue to step back as they step up to adulthood. We have come full circle. I enjoy being 'just' a mom.

Once again, the Yurceks, stand at a place where we know life will be changing, Jim, I, Kristy, Nathan, DJ, Ian, Marissa, Shay, Matt, Deangelo, Becca, Delonzo and Detamara, wait at the starting gate for the next chapter.

And we thank
God for Becca,
our Tiny Titan
who taught us to stand
on the hopes
and dreams
of impossibility.

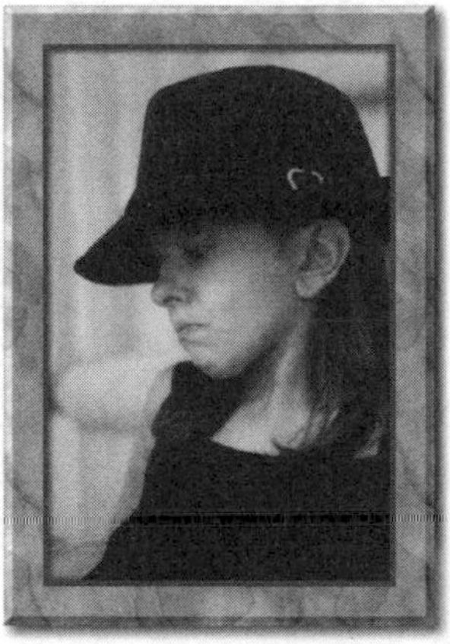

WHO CARES ABOUT ME

written by Ann Yurcek on behalf of her daughter Rebecca

I am but a little girl
Who's life has taken a different twirl
I am disabled, that's what I'm labeled
I'm trying so hard to be able.
I am fed different than my friends each day,
for me it is the only way.
Mom worries for that day,
that nobody will want or care to pay.
WHO WILL FEED ME?

They say dollars have all but dried.
They say everything needs to be cut.
The programs that help me have to be shut.
WHO WILL PAY FOR ME?

The doctors and home healthcare help me out.
My therapies and medicines I cannot be without.
My braces and wheelchair help me about.
My glasses, I cannot see without.
WHO WILL CARE FOR ME?

School budgets are already stressed.
My needs are trying to be met.
It costs a lot to educate me.
How will anything be left for me.
HOW WILL I LEARN?

I am a little girl who fights to be alive.
But without healthcare, I won't survive.
With all the wonderful care
I have thrived.
My family and I have always strived.
WHO CARES ABOUT ME?

Without help we won't be able to cope.
We cannot give up hope.
There is a choice.
Just listen to one little voice.
WHO WILL HELP ME?
I am just a little girl who wants to be,
as happy, healthy, the best little girl I can be.

RESOURCES

Special thank you to all the charities who made a difference in the success of our Tiny Titan and our family. For those readers who give generously we ask that you support those organizations who made a difference in our lives, so that they can continue to reach out to others.

CHARITABLE SUPPORT

Becca's Hope Foundation providing hope to extraodinary children and families. *www.tinytitan.org*

Noonan Syndrome Support Group consider makig a donation in honor of our tiny titan. Checks to TNSSG-Becca's Hope. *www.noonansyndrome.org*

Backpack For Kids is a program designed with Kids, FOR other Kids by kids. *www.backpack-for-kids.org*

Cheff Center therapeutic horseback riding. *www.cheffcenter.com*

Children's Wish Foundation International grants wishes to children with medical conditions. *www.childrenswish.org*

Habitat for Humanity International A nonprofit, Christian housing organization building simple, decent, affordable housing in partnership with people in need. *www.habitat.org*

Hour of Power walking the road of possibility. *www.hourofpower.org*

Lions Club International answers the needs that challenge communities of the world. *www.lionsclubs.org*

Make-A-Wish grants wishes to children with life threatening medical conditions. *www.wish.org*

Toys for Tots is the US Marine Corps community action program *www.toysfortots.org*

US Citizens — A special thank you to the taxpayers and citizens of the USA for helping us support our extraordimary children

Your local place of faith

WEB RESOURCES:

Autism Society of America
www.autism-society.org

Child and Adolescent BiPolar Organization www.bpkids.org

Child Trauma Academy
www.childtrauma.org

Congenital Heart Information Network www.tchin.org

Hays Kids
www.hayskids.org

National Organization on Fetal Alcohol Syndrome
www.nofas.org

National Hemophilia Organization
www.hemophilia.org

Noonan's Syndrome
www.noonansyndrome.org

North American Countil on Adoptable Children
www.nacac.org

RAD - Reactive Attachment Disorder www.radkid.org

Sensory Integration International
www.sensoryint.com

For more resourcss & support ***www.tinytitan.org***

BETTER ENDINGS NEW BEGINNINGS

Giving ordinary people, extraordinary voices to show that better endings are possible and new beginnings can be achieved with powerful stories to inspire, build hope and provide wisdom to change the world one person at a time.
www.betterendings.org

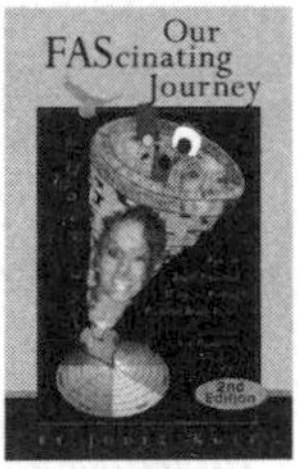

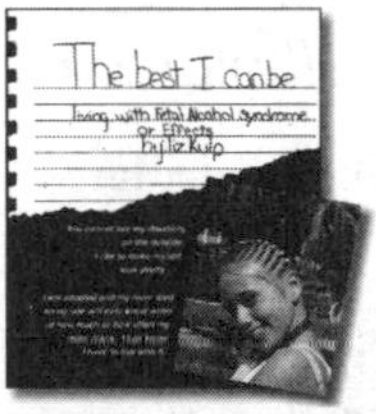

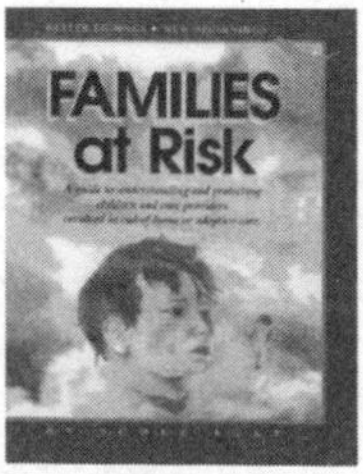

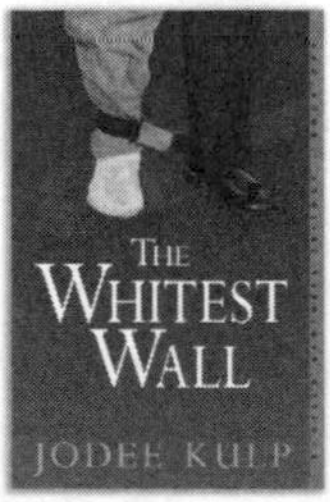

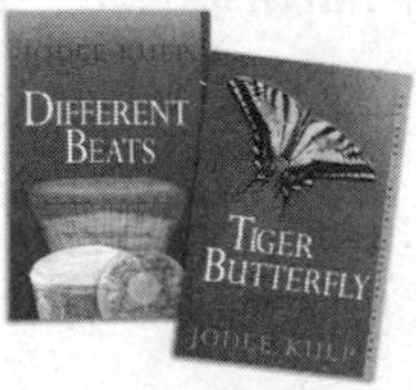